WE LOVE YOUR BODY

Lani Miller and Diane Rodgers

Illustrated by
Joanie Oliver

MORSE PRESS, INC.

PUBLISHED BY MORSE PRESS, INC.
417 E. Pine
Seattle, Washington 98122

•

Library of Congress Catalog Card
No. 80-81842

ISBN 0-933350-32-5

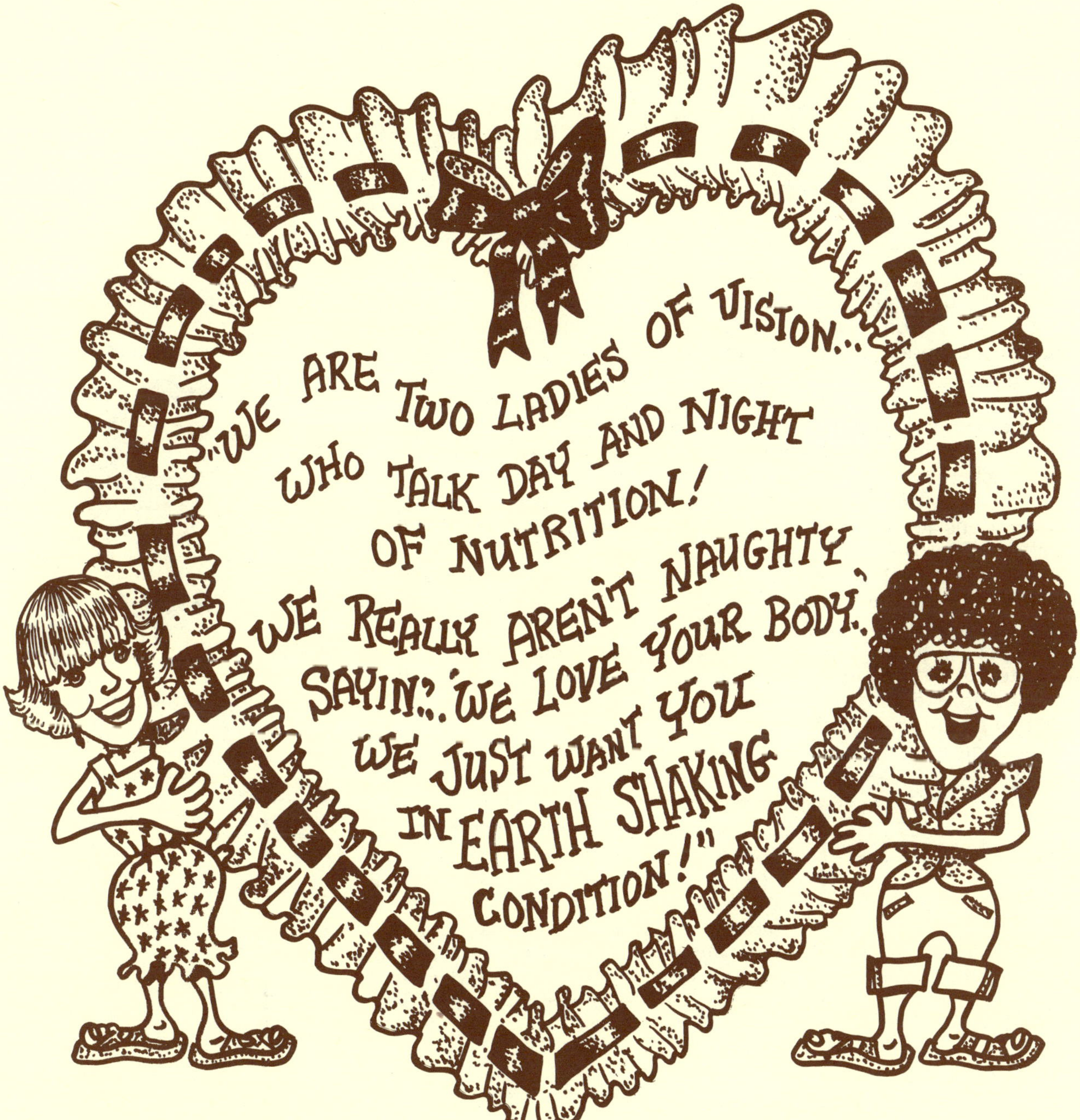
"WE ARE TWO LADIES OF VISION...
WHO TALK DAY AND NIGHT
OF NUTRITION!
WE REALLY AREN'T NAUGHTY,
SAYIN'... 'WE LOVE YOUR BODY.'
WE JUST WANT YOU
IN EARTH SHAKING
CONDITION!"

A Note to Our Readers

"We Love Your Body" is a natural foods cookbook with sound information for helping families make the transition from processed junk food to nutritious, wholesome, yet thoroughly enjoyable eating. From personal experience, we found that we could better handle daily stress and become more in tune with our purpose in life once we discovered the keys to vibrant living.

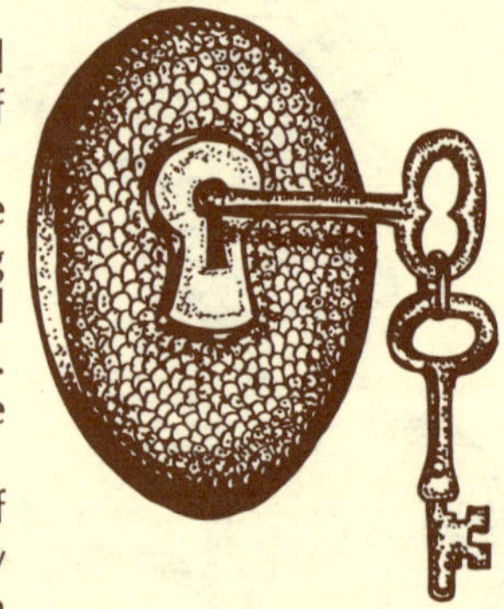

Since diet is only ONE of the keys necessary for improved health, we've tried to open other doors by also sharing our philosophy and practical applications of exercise routines, relaxation techniques and concern for our environment.

Tucked lovingly within the pages of this guidebook, you will find the highlights of fourteen cumulative years of trial and error experiences, including suggestions for positive alternatives, attainable goals, time-saving hints and delicious, proven-on-husbands-kids-friends-relatives-and-customers recipes. Rather than dwell on what should be "given up," emphasis is placed on the beneficial results achieved through pursuing a more natural lifestyle.

Like weaving an original tapestry, we strive to create a different kind of cookbook: one that speaks to the palate about taste, to the heart about vitality and to the head about common sense. A handbook, if you will, that awakens a truth — inherent in the heart and soul of each individual but often, in the name of convenience, denied — *that a genuinely healthy body provides the foundation for improved physical, mental and spiritual communication with our families, our friends and our God.*

It is not our desire to identify or prescribe treatment for specific diseases. We strive only to introduce each individual to inherent powers of self-development through sensible eating, moderate exercise and positive thinking. If you have a physical limitation which may require medical supervision, you should consult your physician before beginning any new health program.

Sincerely,
The Authors

Do you not know that your body is a temple of the Holy Spirit within you, which you have from God? . . . So glorify God in your body. — *1 Corinthians 6:19,20*

What's Happening?

Dear Friends . . .

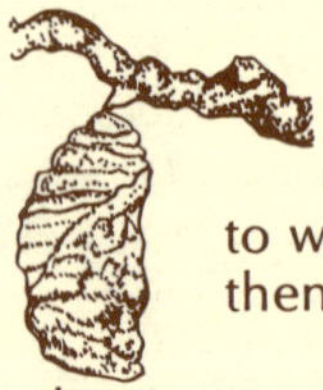

Darkness

Changing long established eating patterns from the "typical" processed American diet to wholesome, natural foods was to us like being a caterpillar, confined to a dark chrysalis, then emerging as a beautiful butterfly, free to explore and determine the directions of life.

In innocence and ignorance we were blind to the nutritive needs of the human body and content to leave the responsibility for nourishment to the advanced technological innovations of the food industry.

Due to the traumatic shock of crippling diseases and death early in the lives of our loved ones, we were suddenly forced to become more aware of the relationship of diet to over-all health.

Metamorphosis

We discovered that changing our families' diets for disease prevention resulted in such unsolicited benefits as decreased food expenses, calmer kids, fewer colds, increased stamina, endless energy, and an insatiable desire to read and learn more. Not just our diets, but our lifestyles were becoming more naturally oriented. In short, we took the responsibility for individual and family health into our own hands.

The results of our changes were so profound that we couldn't contain ourselves any longer. We had to share them with you. If you find yourself stifled by your own cocoon, we hope this book will free you, so that you too, will emerge inspired, enlightened and hungry for change.

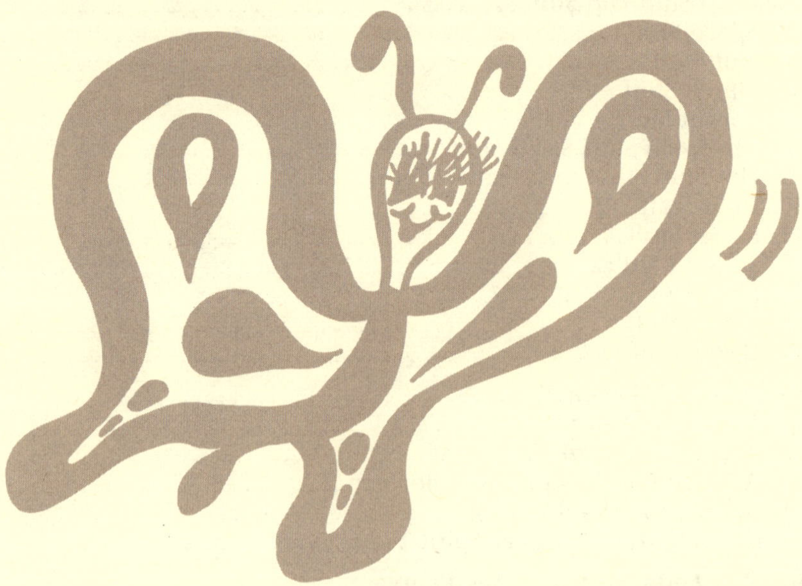

The mark of your ignorance is the depth of your belief in injustice and tragedy. What the caterpillar calls the end of the world, the master calls a butterfly. — *Richard Bach, Illusions* (Dell Publishing Co.)

Dedication

To The Seven Super-Duper Kids who were the incentive for our adventure into good nutrition, our experiments in whole foods cooking and our restaurant.

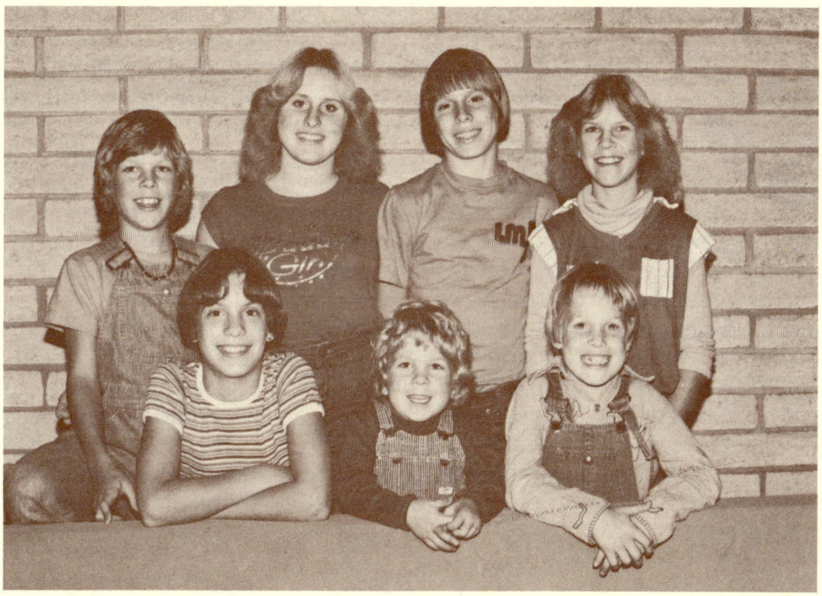

Matt Heidi Dan Mona
Wendy Randy Chris

A Word from Dr. Lendon H. Smith, M.D.

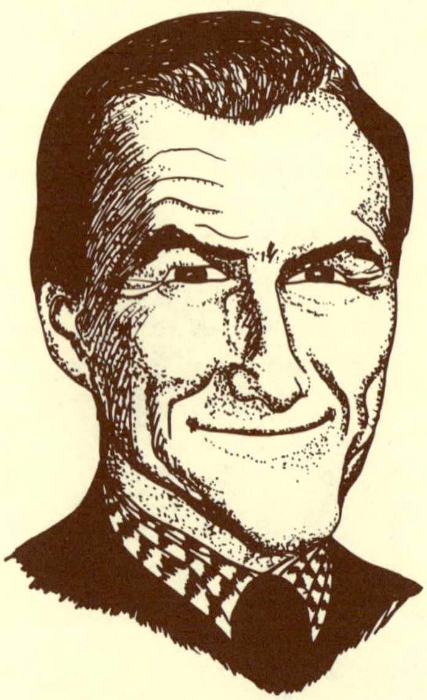

I have been giving advice about diet, vitamins and nutrition for the past five years and have finally figured out that I really don't know what I am saying when I tell someone to eat better, or tell a mother that she has to feed her child better. She thought she was or she would have changed the eating habits of the family long before she came to see me.

I tell them to nibble on raw vegetables, nuts, seeds, fruits, cooked eggs, legumes, fish and sprinkle brewer's yeast and wheat germ on everything they serve. That's my lesson in nutrition. And I expect them to extrapolate from those remarks a whole new life style in the kitchen. I'm telling them to serve more nourishing food. I'm telling them to do it naturally, like my wife does it. She makes it look so easy that I thought everyone could do it with equal facility. (Watch an expert violinist; he makes it look easy. He will tell you, also, that it is easy.)

The present generation of parents was reared by parents who, in general, had many convenience foods. They have no practical experience in making things from scratch. They didn't do it, so they don't know how to do it. We have to teach the feeders and providers of the next generation what our ancestors knew automatically 10,000 years ago. We have a stone age body and we have to eat stone age food. Actually, that means as little preparation as you can get by with and still call it cooking.

You will notice that Lani and Diane don't mention red animal meats (fish is used); the reader may certainly have that option. They show, however, that people can eat well, feel better, and get by more inexpensively, by using vegetables, eggs, dairy foods and fruit. All the statistics indicate that sugar, salt, beef and processed foods are anti-nutrients; the body has to *work* to metabolize them.

This book is for anyone who can eat and taste and swallow. It is especially aimed at the parents of children who seem to need sweet and exotic looking snacks (a la Saturday morning television). The recipes are easy and your children might just think they are eating forbidden junk because they taste so good.

Now I have a book that I can recommend to parents and patients who want to feel better easily. I won't have to worry that they will go home and say to each other, "What did he say?" Or "I can't do that; I don't know where to start."

Thanks, ladies.

Lendon H. Smith

A nationally known author of several books, the most recent, *Improving Your Child's Behavior Chemistry* (1976) and *Feed Your Kids Right* (1979), Dr. Lendon H. Smith has made his own special niche in the field of good nutrition. Strong in his belief that many so-called behavior problems and irritating childhood habits are the result of physiological and chemical imbalances rather than parental or psychological pressures, this pediatrician offers practical, down-to-earth, nutritional and vitamin treatment, thus helping to eliminate parents' feelings of frustration, guilt and anxiety.

His quick wit and spontaneous humor entice people to sit up and listen. You may have seen him most recently as a guest and repeat guest on "The Phil Donahue Show." Whether as a Doctor, Parent, Teacher, Lecturer, Author, or Person, thousands have enjoyed Dr. Lendon Smith . . . "The Children's Doctor."

Thank You . . .

The preparation of this book was very much like having a baby; thoughts and ideas conceived in a loving and generous spirit were carried in our notebooks, next to our hearts, literally everywhere we went for nine months. We nurtured our embryo and saw growth take place daily, before our very eyes. Admittedly, there were minor aches and pains, along with some strange cravings, but our zeal never diminished, from the planting of the seed to the final contraction.

The natural delivery of our finished copy, though two weeks overdue, was an emotional, somewhat painful experience. We hope that you will adopt our "baby" warmly into your hearts and homes.

Without the constant encouragement from our mid-wife/artist, Joanie; our Pediatrician, Dr. Lendon Smith; our supportive friends, and our ever-so-patient families, this initiative may have never reached fruition. Therefore, we must give thanks:

Thanks to all of our customers who encouraged us to temporarily exchange batter and bowl for pen and paper.

Thanks to our students-in-waiting who expressed continual interest and eager anticipation of our due date.

Thanks to Jean, Suzanne and Chris for their sisterly advice, constructive criticism and editing of the manuscript.

Thanks to all our friends who shared recipes and ideas as well as some old wives tales.

Thanks to Todd, our typographer, and Chris, our cameraman for their sense of humor, expertise and patience.

Thanks to our obstetrician/publisher, David Island and Morse Press, who saw us through delivery and believed in our abilities as parents and human beings.

Thanks and love to our moms who were enthusiastic and offered positive thoughts and grandmotherly words of encouragement.

Special thanks to all our children, who provided us with the opportunity to be mothers; who permitted us the freedom to experiment with their tastebuds and who furnished ample suggestions from the kid's point of view. (Please forgive us if we missed a super play at a baseball game because we were jotting down an idea or a recipe.) Thanks also for preparing and cleaning up after all those meals, folding all those clothes, and sprucing up the house when you saw the need. You have been champs throughout all the phases of this book and we couldn't have done it without you.

We thank one another for the way we work together in harmony — complementing and balancing each other's style and methods of research; compensating for each other's strengths and weaknesses; acting as restrainer, critic, inspirator, devil's advocate and *terra firma,* each guiding the other when necessary, with a brightly lit candle through a corridor of uncertainty and mixed emotions.

Last, but not least, we thank our husbands, Stan and Dennis — patient husbands who tolerated rooms piled with books, papers and research materials; kind husbands who endured lentil loaf served five different ways five nights in a row; compassionate husbands who took over the child-rearing and home-making throughout the entire "pregnancy"; nervous husbands who walked the waiting room floor many nights while we stayed up until wee hours typing away; loving husbands who stood by our sides and coached us through our labor pains, and who sincerely hope that this will be our last baby!

Lani & Diane

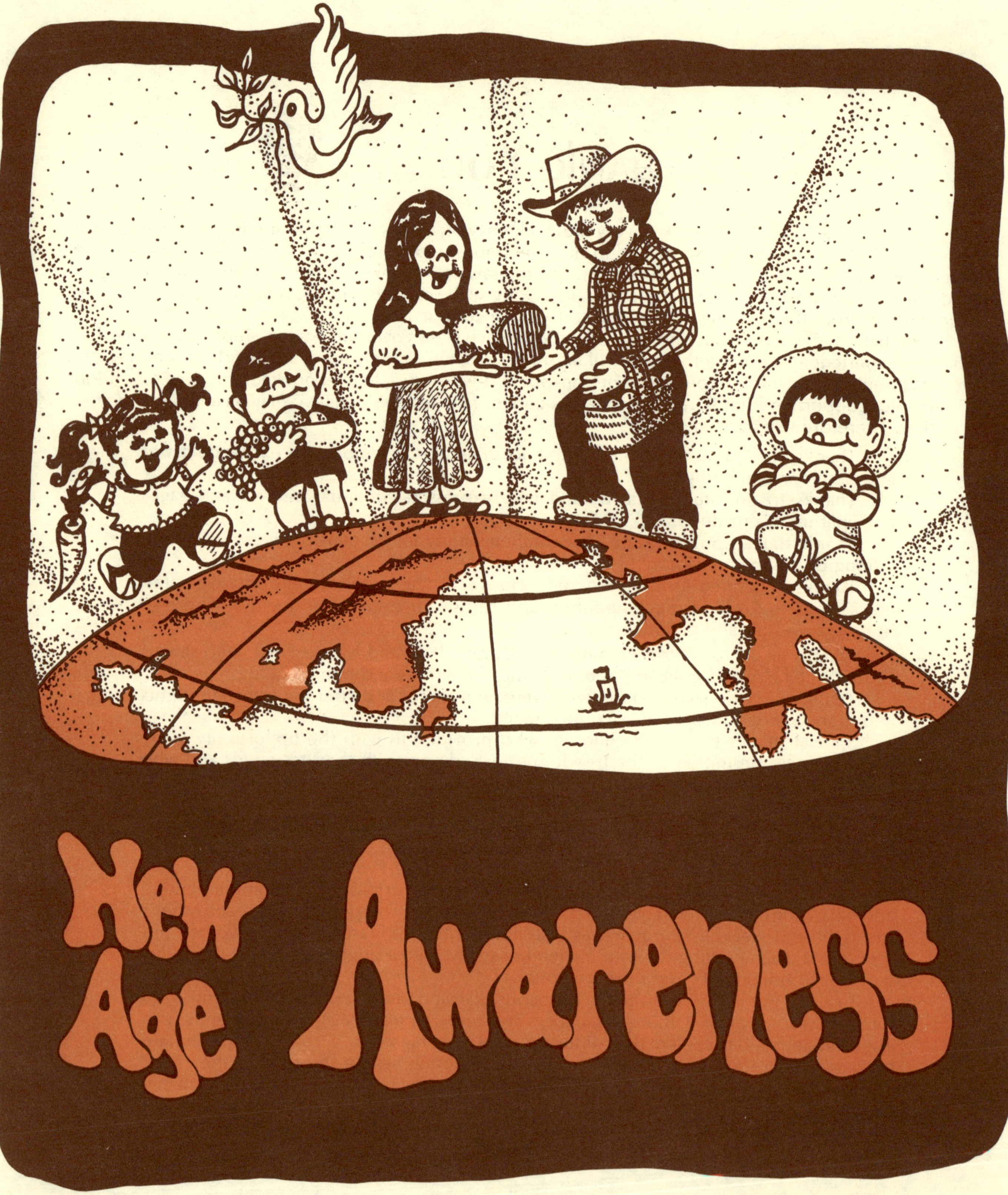

New Age Awareness

New Age Awareness

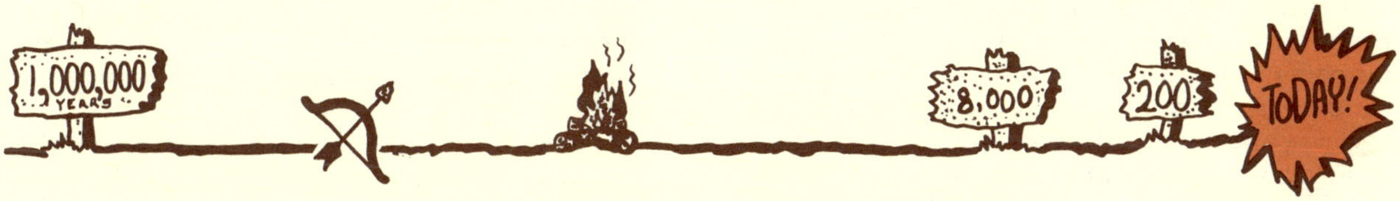

Food for Survival

Imagine a time line of one million years. We can be fairly certain that mankind has been around this long. For many thousands of years, he traveled in small groups in search of food; a nomad who couldn't settle down because survival depended upon his ability to find nourishment. Food was fresh and uncooked and had to be sought out daily. A typical meal might have been composed of nuts, seeds, berries, various roots and leaves, and small insects.

Somewhere along the line, tools were developed and the fight for survival became a more aggressive one. Depending upon environment and climate, various animals were hunted and killed for food. These were also eaten raw, the skins and fur used for clothing; hooves, antlers, horns or tusks for fashioning new tools. At some point in time fire was discovered and utilized, but the diet was still primarily raw.

It wasn't until about 8,000 years ago that animals were domesticated and crops were grown. Later, communities were formed where cows and goats were raised for milk, butter and cheese; chickens, for eggs and meat; and cattle, for meat and its by-products.

While man progressed rapidly in all aspects of life during the next few thousand years, his food was still basically one of grains, nuts, seeds, meat, dairy products, and fruits and vegetables, all of which were whole and natural. Only in about the last 200 years, merely a hair's breadth from the present on the time line, has man begun to adulterate his food.

In the Name of Progress?

During the Industrial Revolution the steel roller mills were invented to separate the bran and germ from the rest of the grain, creating a pale, white, nutrient-depleted flour. Sugar refineries were built to refine sugar from its natural state of beet, cane or corn, to white granules, devoid of minerals and vitamins. Soil was saturated with chemicals. Pesticides and other sprays bombarded our plants as well as the atmosphere. Factories began producing colorful boxes, wrappers, packages, bottles and cans, which were then filled with instant, dehydrated, frozen, heated, dyed, flavored, chemical-laden non-foods which would later be found to be of so little nutritional value that they would have to be fortified with vitamins and iron.

Is it any wonder that such a finely adapted

body, nearly free of degenerative diseases for thousands of years, is now suddenly "out of tune?" Can we be expected to absorb the onslaught of chemicals, pesticides, pollutants, synthetic colors, flavors and preservatives without any ill effects? What a shock to the human system! After hundreds of thousands of years of a natural diet, the human body cannot adjust to this whirlwind of changes overnight. Compare it to an auto that has run smoothly for many years, is suddenly filled with alcohol, sugar, lard, chemicals and other junk, then expected to run as efficiently as with regular fuel.

Consider the way technology has handled the feeding of today's adolescents. Their steady diet is one of soda pop, salty potato chips and french fries, white bread with nitrite-laden lunchmeat sandwiches, and sugary cookies and candy bars. Can this diet be expected to meet the teenagers' increased nutritional requirements brought on by high emotional and physical activity and growth?

Livestock and dairy cows are not fed instant T.V. dinners. Every farmer knows that the healthiest stock or crops are a result of knowledge and application of sound nutritional principles. When was the last time you saw an ear of corn with a hearing aid? A spud with spectacles? A pig with pimples? A cow with cavities? Or a hypoglycemic hen? Millions of dollars are spent each year in research for the development of animal feed that supplies all nutrients — protein, fats, carbohydrates, vitamins, minerals and fiber, in the exact proportions required by each group of animals, so that each succeeding generation will be healthier, sturdier and more productive than the last. What a contrast to the food conglomerates' research into faster preparation — tastier — more colorful — cheaper — non-food products for human consumption!

Can anyone predict the health of the next generation of humans? Is the teens' peer group entirely to blame for their poor nutritional habits? Certainly not! Examine their parents' diets and how their eating habits developed. Unfortunately each generation tends to be victims or imitators of the preceding generation. Somewhere along the line, in the name of progress and labor-saving products, we were captivated by and enslaved to the conveniences of modern living.

Making Changes

Now, with our very planet in danger of succumbing to the polluted by-products of progress, we must again take a look at our lifestyle and think about simplicity and quality of life. What is really necessary? What is beneficial to our planet? How might we feed more people, live healthier lives, and suppress our materialistic greed? The Western World has an obsession with possessions, but we can change.

We feel very strongly that no one has the right to adulterate our planet, the very source of life, for the sake of profit or any other reason. In order to maintain a freedom of choice, we encourage each individual to take his or her share of the responsibility for increasing the harmony of life on Mother Earth.

New Age people are doing something positive about their present state of living. And we are all New Age people if we are sensitive to the heartbeat of our planet, concerned for the quality of our future, and aware that each person can play a major role in preserving the air, land and water for future generations of people and all living things.

Getting rid of the plastic clutter in their lives, New Age people are living on less — less food, less fuel and less factory-produced items. They are people of the earth who are reaching out for roots; who garden, farm, cook, sew and create with their hands, regardless of the increase in time and labor. Their lives take on a meaningful purpose when they take a part in the handiwork of their own existence.

James Thurber once said, "Let us not look back in anger, nor forward in fear, but around in awareness." Start today; set the example; soon others will respond. Now, more than ever before, New Age Awareness is a necessity for survival into the Twenty-First Century.

Back to the Beginning

The nourishment of the spirit and the propagation of the human race, basically depends upon love and food. In order to be fully loving and radiantly healthy, we must return to the original food supply. Was not Adam's fruit in the Garden of Eden pure? Yet today's chemical concoctions that look like, feel like and, in some instances even taste like the real thing, can never equal the quality of Nature's own craftsmanship. Of course the chemist's lab can reduce an apple to known nutrients. But since man cannot create from synthetics a whole apple, complete with seeds that will sprout a new plant and continue the life cycle, then we must place our trust in the time-tested foods of our ancestors.

How can you as an individual get back to Mother Earth and lead a productive, satisfying life? You can begin by examining your own lifestyle and noting the changes you might make to conserve and preserve the earth's resources. You might consider incorporating some of the following suggestions that we feel emphasize quality of life rather than quantity.

By applying some of these ideas to your own life, people — friendships and gatherings — will become the center of re-creation rather than night clubs, movies and television. Money will take a back seat in the trip through life. Individuals, making small but effective changes, will herald a New Age of brotherhood and mutual concern for the planet Earth.

We are all one, a part of the Universal Creative Force, and if we use our energies for the highest good, our vibrations will become contagious; then more and more people will tune in to this great force — this energy and great Spirit.

WHAT YOU CAN DO

1. **Conserve gasoline and oil by car-pooling when possible to work, school or when taking a group of children to athletic events or other activities. Plan your errands for one day of the week and map out the route using the least mileage. Better yet, ride a bike or walk.**
2. **Burn cheap brush and dead wood for home heating, remodel or build energy-efficient homes and utilize solar energy. Using storm windows, weather-stripping or caulking cracks in doors, and re-insulating walls and attic of your home can save dollars as well as fuel. Be on the alert for energy-efficient ideas and implement them whenever possible.**
3. **Read the facts about chemical pesticides and fertilizers. Help distribute pamphlets concerning the potential dangers to humans, animals, plant life and the water supply in areas where toxic sprays are used.**
4. **Raise your consciousness and level of awareness to the world hunger problem, affecting millions of people and for which we all are responsible. Increased land usage for grain crops can decrease mass starvation. In *Diet for a Small Planet,* Frances Moore Lappe' states that an acre of grains can produce five times more protein than an acre devoted to meat production; an acre of legumes can produce ten times more protein. Yet the majority of grains and legumes that the U.S. grows — corn, wheat, soybeans, barley and oats is fed to animals rather than people. Ms. Lappe' further points out that an average steer produces only one pound of beef for the family dinner table for every sixteen pounds of grain and soybeans it is fed. This fifteen pounds of wasted protein per one pound of edible meat is equal to ninety per cent of the world's yearly protein deficit. According to "A Shift in the Wind" newsletter from The Hunger Project, over a billion people are hungry or mal-nourished in this world today. Thousands of people — most of them children — are dying each day from hunger or malnutrition. By eating the grains firsthand, there would be less waste of land and food, with enough protein to feed everybody.**
5. **Use bio-degradable products (soaps and paper, etc.) whenever possible.**
6. **Conserve precious resources that go into the plastics and synthetics of modern-day artifacts by recycling bottles, cans and plastics or reducing use of products packaged this way. According to the U.S. Department of Commerce over 600 pounds of packaging materials go into the products used by each American every year. Packaging alone, consumes about 80% of all paperboard produced, 65% of all glass, 25% of all plastic, 22% of all paper, 15% of all wood and 7% of all steel. Half of all packaging is used to decorate and promote food, so consider this the next time you go to purchase that fancy little package. You have a choice!**

7. **Raise your own bees for honey and hens for eggs. Grow your own fruits and vegetables. Experiment in hydroponic gardening. Even city dwellers can grow indoor gardens! Everyone can grow year-round pesticide-free salad ingredients in glass jars: alfalfa sprouts, mixed sprouts, and buckwheat lettuce.**
8. **When you can, by-pass big business in favor of local merchants. The chains and conglomerates will survive without your dollars, but the small business person depends on your support.**
9. **Learn to barter or trade your skills and services for your neighbor's fresh milk, eggs or bountiful garden harvest. Trade the products of your sewing talent for your friend's repair skills, etc.**

A LETTER FROM CHIEF SEALTH

One hundred and twenty five years ago, Chief Sealth of the Duwamish Tribe, in what is now the state of Washington, wrote very prophetically to President Franklin Pierce, protesting the government's proposal to purchase tribal lands. Though his letter spoke of the white man's devastating and destructive ways of the 1850's in his quest for land, gold and new settlements, regardless of the cost to the dignity and rights of the Indians, he speaks to each and every one of us *today.*

How can you buy or sell the sky — the warmth of the land? The idea is strange to us. We do not own the freshness of the air or the sparkle of the water. How can you buy them from us?

We know that the white man does not understand our ways. One portion of the land is the same to him as the next for he is a stranger who comes in the night and takes from the land whatever he needs. The earth is not his brother, but his enemy, and when he has conquered it, he moves on. He leaves his father's graves, and his children's birthright is forgotten.

The air is precious to the red man. For all things share the same breath — the beasts, the trees, the man. The white man does not seem to notice the air he breathes. Like a man dying for many days, he is numb to the stench . . .

The white man must treat the beasts of this land as his brother. I am a savage and I do not understand the other way. I have seen a thousand rotting buffaloes on the prairies left by the white man who shot them from a passing train . . . What is man without the beasts? If all the beasts were gone, men would die from great loneliness of spirit, for whatever happens to the beast also happens to man. All things are connected. Whatever befalls the earth befalls the sons of the earth.

One thing we know which the white man will one day discover. Our God is the same God. You may think now that you own him as you wish to own our land. But you cannot. He is the Body of man. And his compassion is equal for the red man and the white man. This earth is precious to him. And to harm the earth is to heap contempt on its creator . . . Continue to contaminate your bed and you will one night suffocate in your own waste.

We might understand if we knew what it was that the white man dreams, what hopes he describes to his children on long winter nights, what visions he burns into their minds . . .

Our warriors have felt shame. And after defeat, they turn their days in idleness and contaminate their bodies with sweet food and strong drink.

East West Journal, Boston
letter from Dale Jones of
Seattle

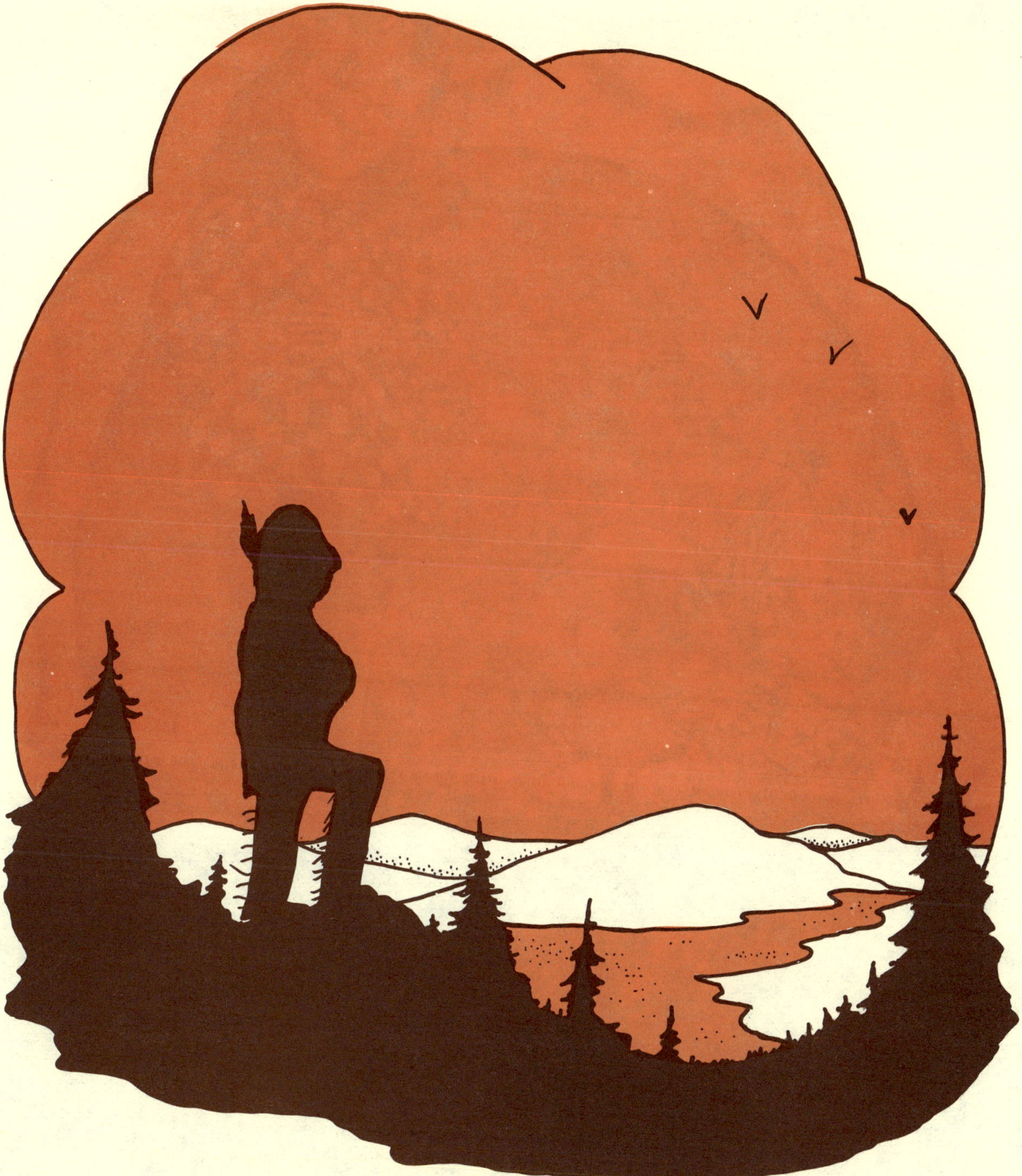

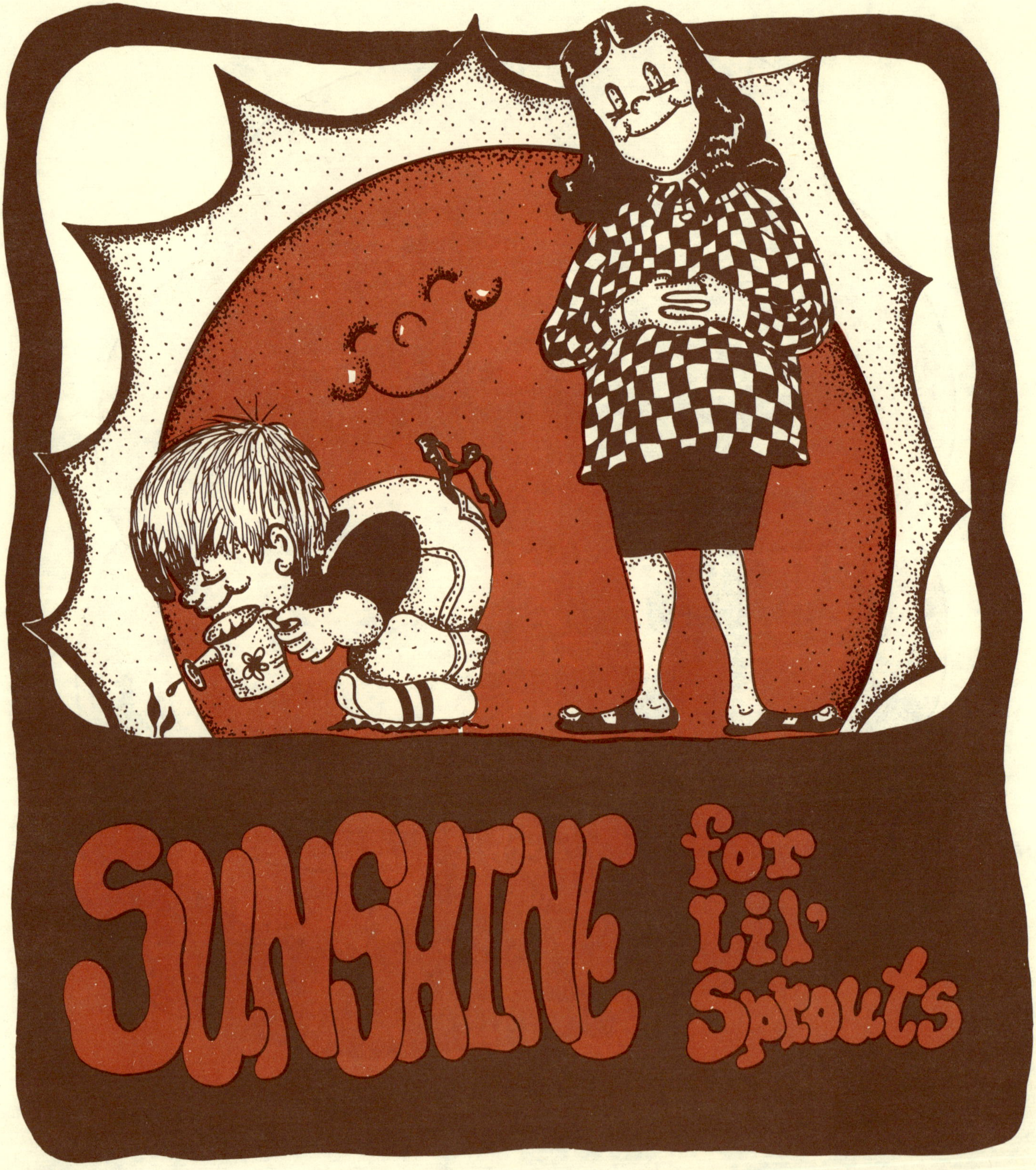
SUNSHINE
for
Lil'
Sprouts

Sunshine For Lil' Sprouts

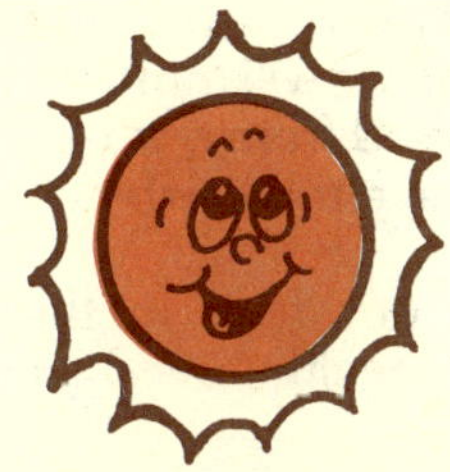

As We Sow, Shall We Reap

It is, perhaps, from plant life that we attained the maxim, "survival of the fittest." Look around the base of trees in the forest — there are literally hundreds of little seedlings, standing brave in the battle for life. By their very constitution, the strongest plants thrive. Some seedlings have fallen, or been carried by the wind, far enough from mature plants to get extra sunlight — just the boost needed to be counted among the strong. Still others grow slowly, slight of stature and easily attacked by natural foes, surviving, but forsaken to a life of mere existence. We can't help but think that, given a choice, the struggling plants would prefer to thrive.

Within every seed lies the very source of hope for the future generations of that species; every resource necessary to carry on their race and produce plants true to their heritage. Given suitable conditions, the embryo will awaken from its sleeping state — live temporarily on stored nourishment — until suddenly, bursting with energy, it sends forth an incredible system of self-preservation called roots.

While man and animals can travel in search of a food supply, plants must be satisfied with the food they can reach by means of their roots. To compensate for this apparent limitation, some plants send out highly complex root systems. Even when growing in soil depleted of nutrients, many plants have a remarkable ability to send a tap-root twenty or thirty feet deep in search of sustenance. (We see these independent plants in a dry, barren field and unable, or unwilling to recognize the courage and sheer determination of their fight for survival, we refer to them as weeds.)

An intricate network of rootlets provides a solid foundation, holding the plant firmly in the ground and enabling it to spring back even after an onslaught of human-induced adversities. The roots make a lifetime commitment with the stem to complement one another's purposes and goals, to "hang in there" and to channel food, as well as guidance, to the rest of the plant.

The humble stem is the catalyst that performs the most noble task of all. The stem raises the leaves up above the surrounding growth, to be blessed by the sun's golden rays. Some plants unashamedly transmit food from the air and energy from the sun through the stem, back into the soil, thus leaving the earth richer than before. It is this sense of unity, this synergistic force, that gives food, beauty, fresh air and life to us all.

Caught up in the breathtaking brilliance of flowers, we sometimes forget that it is in the flower that fertilization takes place and seeds are formed — those same seeds that will carry on their ancestry and produce the next generation, the seeds from which new little seedlings will someday sprout.

Seedling Survival

For a more complete understanding of how we feel that children grow, go back and reread "As We Sow, Shall We Reap," substituting the words, "child/ren" in place of "plant/s," trying to perceive the entire story as it relates to the growth and development of children.

We would like to dedicate this chapter to all of the children of the world — the Lil' Sprouts — our hope for the future. We started this book in 1979, *The International Year of the Child,* but shouldn't EVERY year be the year of the child? It is our prayer that we will transmit the knowledge and energy gained from our new awareness, so that we may leave this earth richer than before we came.

We place our faith in the growth of a generation of healthy seeds, complete with every resource necessary to carry on their race and produce seedlings true to their heritage. Please join us in our effort to provide every child with wholesome food, sunshine, tender kindness, respect for Nature and bountiful love so that they may grow strong of body, mind and spirit, as God intended us all to be.

> *Divine Love is the seed, devotion is the sapling, faith is the fertilizer, good company is the rain. Unconditional dedication to the Supreme is the flower and God-Realization is the fruit.*
>
> *Sai Baba*

Sunshine For Lil' Sprouts

Ten, count 'em, ten fingers, ten toes,
Pink cheeks, blue eyes, and Daddy's nose.
Go ahead and take credit,
With God's help you did it!
Now here's how your Lil' Sprout grows:

From Birth to Seven Years

The nutrients in Mother's milk
Keep baby's skin as smooth as silk.
Antibodies work night and day
To keep all kinds of illness away.

When solid foods are on your mind
Remember variety, some of each kind.
Keep portions small, don't satiate.
Force feeding contributes to overweight.

You set the example as you set the table.
And when children see that you're strong and able
They will follow your pattern right from the start,
As long as the message comes from your heart.

Even a toddler can understand.
He wants to grow up and become a strong man.
"Put good food in your mouth, then relax and chew,
Soon you'll grow an inch or two!"

Naming foods with texture and tastes that vary
Will help to build vocabulary.
Games of association help a child to relate:
Milk/teeth, eggs/muscles, exercise/heart rate.

You're in control at home, it's true,
But you have your work cut out for you,
The moment a child enters first grade,
Your hassles and headaches are ready-made.

Schools have holiday parties and candy sales;
Colored frostings and drinks; it's a sorry tale.
Birthday treats unwisely "chose"
Are waved before your child's unsuspecting nose.

Breads and rolls made of pure white fluff
Are just part of the high starch cafeteria stuff.
Vegetables cooked to a mush and salted,
Into the garbage cans get vaulted.

"Support our athletic department at half-time!"
"Buy candy bars and colas for only a dime!"
"Do a good job, get a sweet reward."
How much of this can their teeth afford?

From Seven to Twelve

No one else will look after your child's health;
The sugar industry is more concerned about wealth.
Sweet commercials are designed to keep kids mesmerized,
But children have the right to know they're being victimized.

With some "private eye" help from parents; they'll see,
The phoniness and the fallacy.
The ads that were once the most effective,
Will be blatantly mocked by your little detective!

Children lend themselves well to physical fitness,
Observe any playground and you will witness:
Running back and forth doesn't seem like repetition
When healthy children are involved in healthy competition.

Now, don't panic if your child misjudges a food.
An unknowing adult may say, "Eat it, it's good!
Sure, it's full of sugar, but that's OK,
You need sugar for energy, every day!"

At first your child may hesitate,
To tell the adult, "No, thanks, I'll wait."
But after children learn what's BEST to eat,
They'll opt for fresh fruit and ignore the sugary treat.

Let's don't train our youth to link feelings with food.
Whether lonely, or ill, smart, pretty or good,
Junk food just serves to plug up their ignition;
There are much better ways to give recognition.

Try a pat on the back, a handshake or another action
That permits the child some self-satisfaction.
A "Thank You!", says "You're #1,"
Honest appreciation for a job well done.

Young people co-operate when they have a voice.
Offer different fruits, nuts and cheeses, then give them a choice.
Their sack lunch will taste even better, we guarantee,
When the note inside says, "You're SPECIAL to me!"

From Twelve to Fourteen

Good public relations skills will be needed
To assure that, by junior high, your wise counsel is heeded.
Neither coax, nag, bribe, nor concede your ideal,
Sooner or later they'll know you're for real.

The world's starving children are no laughing matter
For thoughtless remarks or idle chatter.
Adolescents need to know, in this democratic society,
About unjust food practices and conglomerate piety.

Needless processing, less nutrition, higher cost,
Young people can understand how humanity is lost,
When agri-business cares more about high-dollar gains,
And ignores Third World people with severe hunger pains.

Humans the world over need the same nutrient accounts,
Albeit in wide and varied amounts.
Some cups runneth over while some go dry,
Depending on distribution of the world's food supply.

In this country we're constantly hearing it said
That American people are the best fed.
Unfortunately we've confused "best" with "most."
Check our dis-ease statistics, we really shouldn't boast.

School health books say acne's not caused by what you eat,
But by hormonal changes. Now, isn't that neat?
So "pig-out" on junk food, cram everything in,
Even the "experts" claim no effects on your skin!

But, what do they think regulates hormone change?
Street Lights? My word they must be deranged!
Hormones are secreted by a gland system: endocrine,
That must all be kept healthy if we're to have clear skin.

We simply can't separate one body part from another;
The bond is as strong as a babe to its mother.
We're only as good as the sum of our parts.
To build a strong world, we must start with strong hearts.

From Fourteen to Sixteen

Never give up your role as advisor and coach,
Remember that teenagers require a more delicate approach.
They're not lost in Burger City, as was previously suspected,
Just sorting out their values, some confusion is expected.

Your world and theirs may seem miles apart,
But someday they'll understand the love in your heart.
They'll miss your good vibes when you're not always around,
And think "My parents got me this far, healthy and sound."

"I appreciate the guidance they gave to me,
Now it's my own responsibility
To feed myself, keep fit and strong,
With the good habits they taught me all along."

Yes, youth have the right to make their own decisions,
But the media boggles their minds with value revisions.
We believe in "rights": the rights to sturdy muscles, bones and teeth.
These are the legacy, we as parents bequeath.

We're such gullible adults and vulnerable kids,
When the soft drink and cigarette companies make their bids.
Those ads with sexy girls and macho guys,
First attract attention, then with false hopes, hypnotize.

They know from statistics, teens have money to burn;
And that once addicted, a customer will return.
That's why they seduce kids in the formative years; if they wait
Their victims get wiser, the pitch comes too late.

Hey kids, "You've come a long way baby!", so keep it that way.
Good health and vitality every way and every day.
You don't need a crutch or a pacifier,
You're strong and you can set your goals much higher

Than being just another "one of the guys"
With pimples and greasy hair and glassy eyes.
Your health is all-important; ignore peer pressure and the current fad,
Dare to be different, one day you'll be glad!

Read, research, learn from the people you admire
Who run, bike, love Nature and never seem to tire.
You don't need a smoke, swig or other body pollution.
Why be part of the problem when you can be part of the solution?!

From Sixteen to Forever

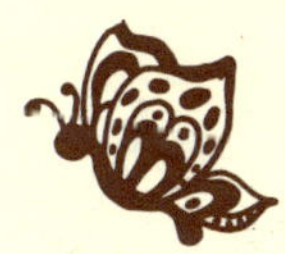

In a remote village on the other side of the world,
A fine young man and a sturdy young girl
Work extra hard, eat special foods and pray in preparation
For the day that they will marry and birth the next generation.

In America we give our teens cars, ersatz food and television,
Then gripe about crime, disrespect, greed and no ambition.
Our young adults are our future, not just temporary vegetation,
It's time families get involved in whole person wellness education.

Your young athlete is most open and will surely devour,
Food that's prepared to build muscle-power.
When he starts dating girls, you'll know there is hope,
He's gone from mud puddles to knee patches to car grease to soap!

When he has a wife and a daughter or a son,
He'll communicate with them, each one on one.
He'll teach them to look at both the pros and the cons,
So their minds won't be garbled with hard-sell put-ons.

Your ever-dieting slim, skinny teenage girl,
Runs possibly the greatest risk in all the world.
For she is the flower, wherein lies the seed
That will carry on the heritage, true to her breed.

Being fashion conscious is certainly OK,
But some girls go about dieting in the very worst way.
Encourage her to read, urge her to think
About inherent dangers in that no-calorie soft drink.

At a time in her life when iron needs skyrocket
Have her keep raisins and sunflower seeds in her pocket.
If she refuses to eat the balanced dinner you bring;
Feed it to her boyfriend — he'll eat ANY thing!

Yes, someday when they have children of their own
They'll appreciate your dedication and caring tone.
They'll thank you for helping them get on the right track.
Self-satisfaction's enough; now pat your own back.

You've given wholesome food, understanding and love
With God's bountiful guidance, on the wings of a dove.
In your children are your roots, the foundation for all their days,
Cradled by moonbeams and kissed by sunrays.

You respected each child and their individual needs;
You tilled, sowed, composted and kept out the weeds.
You've done your best; set your mind at ease
Those healthy Lil' Sprouts are now Strong, Sturdy Trees!

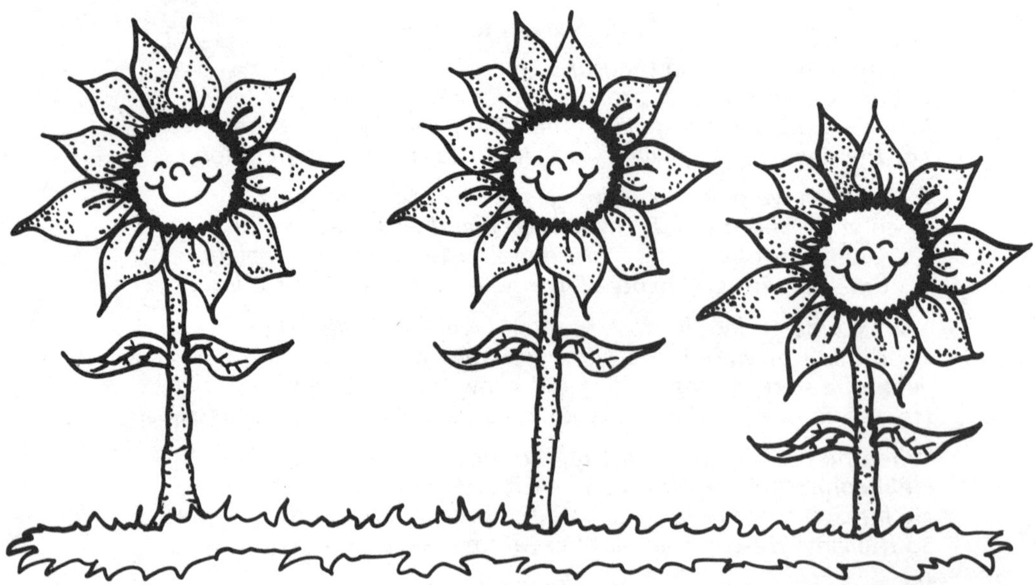

WHAT YOU CAN DO WITH YOUNG CHILDREN

1. An intellectually and physically stimulating environment in the first four years of a child's life is of utmost importance in increasing natural abilities and developing body and mind in preparation for later, more formal education. Take children shopping and let them compare labels and products. Let them help bag, weigh and mark groceries. Use every opportunity to teach practical skills: size, shape, weight, color, smell, texture, origin, price and taste.
2. Give young children a bigger responsibility in preparing food, from scrubbing and washing vegetables, shelling nuts or peas, peeling bananas or carrots, to actually putting together a recipe. Activities like chopping, whipping, shredding, slicing, squeezing, kneading, freezing, drying and so on, help develop coordination, design, color arrangement, vocabulary and an understanding of acceptable forms of food processing.
3. An old proverb states, "I hear and I forget, I see and I remember, I do and I understand." Children need to see food from the beginning stages of growth until it is put on the table. In the summer plant, weed, water, harvest and prepare fresh vegetables. In winter, help them grow sprouts. They will love having their own jar and rinsing daily to see the sprouts and leaves emerge from the seed; then placing in the light, to observe the chlorophyll develop in the leaves, and finally eating them in their salads and sandwiches.
4. The importance of keeping records can be established early by giving children their own recipe file complete with cards. Each time they prepare or help prepare food, acknowledge that help; give them a pat on the back and tell them how much you appreciate working together. Have them write down their favorite recipes. Over the years they will accumulate a complete recipe file and the skills needed to feed themselves when they are on their own.
5. Commercials attract attention by splashes of bright colors and catchy slogans and jingles. Let children put their own artwork on their recipe cards and give their own funny names to the foods they prepare. Many of the names of foods in *KIDSTUFF* originated just this way.
6. Help make children aware that the junk foods advertised don't meet the body's nutritional requirements and physical needs. Explain to them the nutritional superiority of food made from scratch over canned or packaged foods. Encourage them to trust their own judgment.
7. When it's their turn to take treats to Sunday School, scouts or school, help children make the snacks the night before. Include the recipe for their leader or teacher. The next time a parent asks for some good snack ideas, s/he can pass yours along.
8. Hold a jingle or slogan contest. The kids can make up catchy tunes and colorful posters to promote their own favorite foods. For the funniest, the most informational, the cutest tune, etc., award home-made certificates good for a free afternoon, having an overnight guest, or a book of their choice. See that everyone earns an award.
9. Arrange field trips to a farm, a creamery, a cannery, or whatever places there are in your community that deal with the many levels of food growth, preparation and distribution. Point out the detrimental as well as the beneficial practices that you see, and don't be afraid to ask questions of the management.
10. Read *Feed Your Kids Right* by Dr. Lendon Smith (See booklist, *Inspiration for Independence)* and become familiar with the right foods as well as the right reasons for making dietary changes.
11. As a community service project for your scout or 4-H group, visit a convalescent home or home for the retired. Prepare samples for the people to enjoy the good tastes of yogurt, kefir, tahini and other nut butters, carob, whole wheat crackers and undyed cheese, and smoothies and shakes. Encourage kids to "adopt a grandparent."
12. Give children old magazines full of colorful pictures of foods. Let them cut out pictures of nutritious foods and junk foods. They can make and display a collage with the good foods and throw the junk foods into the wastebasket.
13. If a child's only exercise comes during school physical education classes, s/he is likely to be a spectator, rather than a participant, of physical fitness activities as an adult. Organize your own

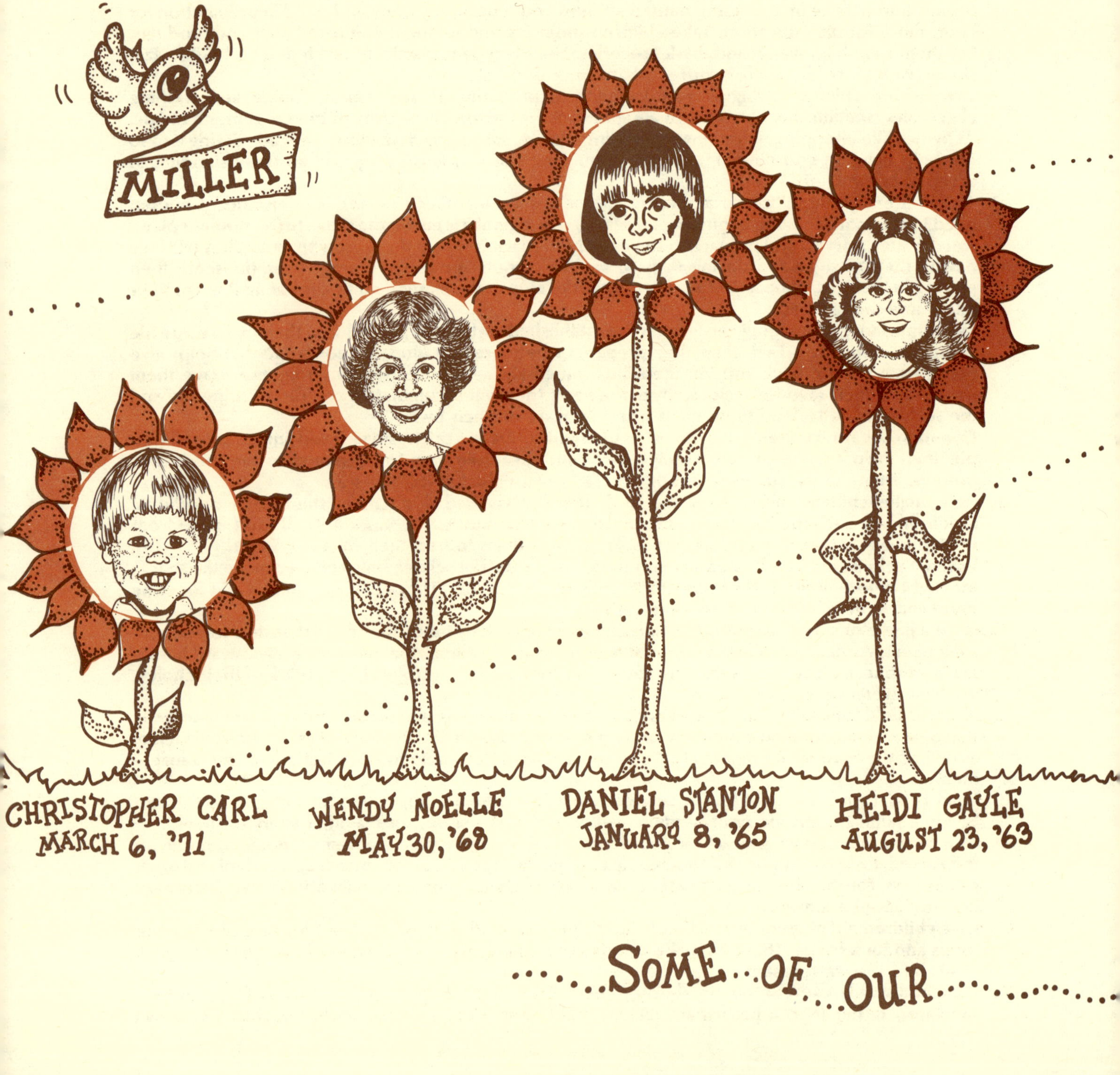
MILLER
CHRISTOPHER CARL
MARCH 6, '71
WENDY NOELLE
MAY 30, '68
DANIEL STANTON
JANUARY 8, '65
HEIDI GAYLE
AUGUST 23, '63
SOME OF OUR

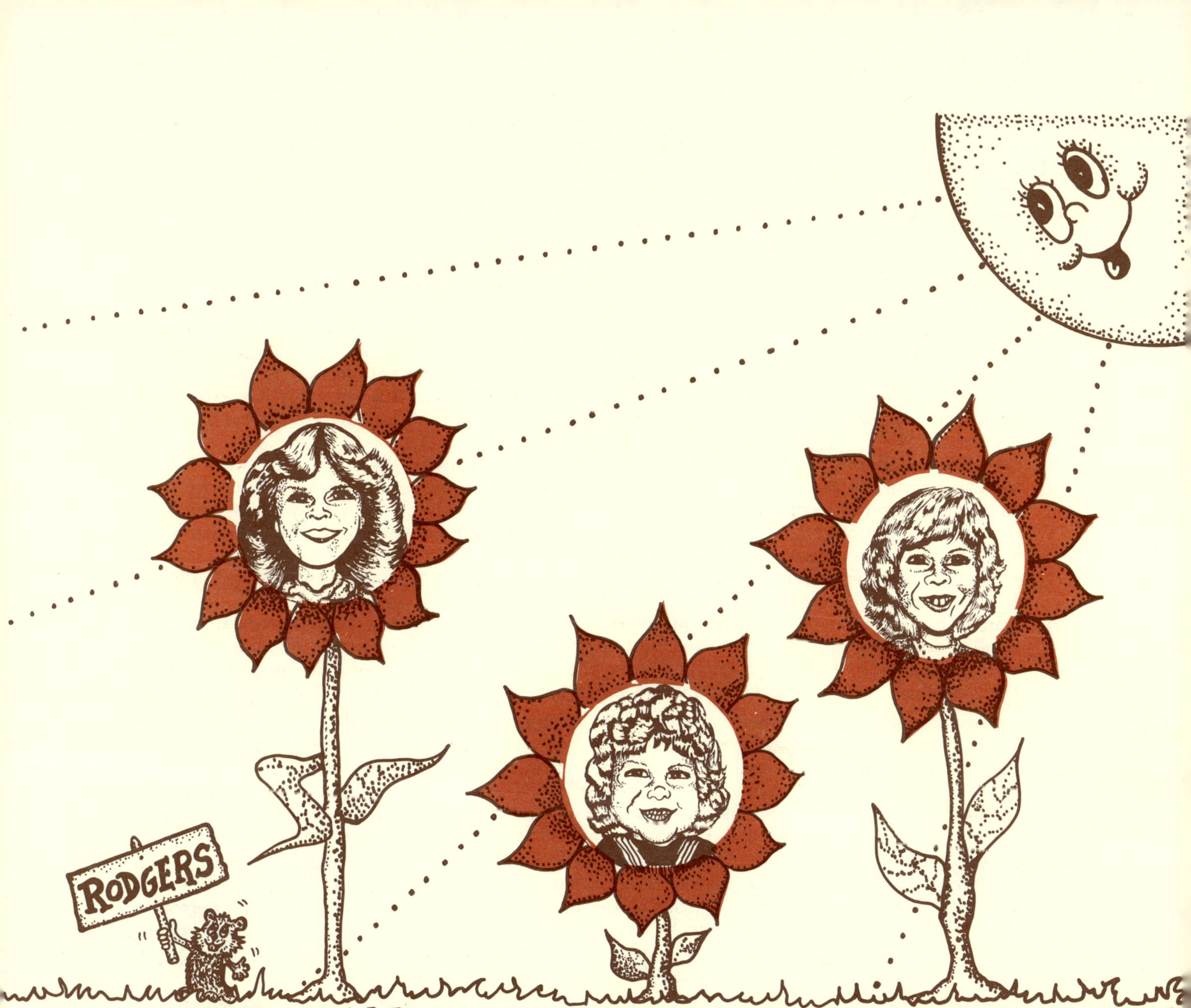

RAMONA LEANNE
MARCH 13, '67

RANDY ALLEN
JULY 4, '74

MATTHEW ALLEN
AUGUST 12, '68

......FAVORITE.....LIL'......SPROUTS...

sports: bike-a-thons, jog-a-thons, backyard decathlons, obstacle courses and your own summer and winter olympics. Make exercise a part of every day.

14. Give young children opportunities to make choices and participate in decisions regarding family problems early in life. By exercising their own skills in problem-solving, they will learn to become confident about their choices and less likely to let other people persuade them into doing things they might be uncomfortable with when they become older.
15. Food has long been associated with love, but it is an injustice to manipulate feelings and attitudes by means of food (especially sweets) as a reward or punishment. Food is a source of nourishment, a form of creativity and pleasure, and a means for gathering to break bread with loved ones. But it is not, and should not be used as, a medium of exchange for behavior modification. Reward jobs well done, good grades and chores with words of praise or a hug and kiss. This will encourage children to become motivated for the intrinsic rewards — feelings of self-worth, self-accomplishment and self-satisfaction. Awards are fun but should come as a surprise rather than an every day expectancy. For special occasions make prizes non-food items or tickets for skating rinks, a concert or a sports event, etc.
16. We all know there's an over-supply of violence on television and the crime rate in our country increases annually. We feel diet, family relationships, television, peer pressure, and environment all play a part in this complicated drama. Monitor your children's television viewing. Be firm. Don't let the kids control you. Together you can select some of the excellent programs available that educate as well as entertain, and that deal with human values and feelings, and are designed to open doors of communication between parent and child. Television is *not* an outside influence. It's right in your home and there's a plug you can pull.
17. Schedule a family U.S.S.R. (Uninterrupted Sustained Silent Reading) hour twice a week, or alternate reading nights with a game, poetry, or music night. In U.S.S.R. a certain time is set aside for silence; no T.V., no stereo, no sibling rivalry, no noise of any kind. Just peace and quiet for one solid hour. Have children write about personal life experiences or keep a diary during this quiet time.
18. Go to your city or school library and obtain a reading list of favorite children's books. Then select books with your child — some at their reading level and others that you can read to them. Books open doors to imagination and fantasy with which television can't begin to compete.
19. Using *Creative Food Experiences for Children* or *We Love Your Body,* offer to teach a class in grade school on "How to Prepare" yogurt, kefir, frozen fruit shakes or smoothies. Better yet, donate the book to your school PTA so they can use the lesson plans or recipes for future activities.
20. Interest your children's school cafeteria staff in reading and using, *From Classroom to Cafeteria,* by Sara Sloan, Director of Food and Nutrition Programs, Fulton County School, Atlanta, Ga. This book is a curriculum resource guide to be used by teachers, students, parents and food service personnel. *Nutra Lunches & Natural Foods,* also by Ms. Sloan is a guide designed for use by homes, schools, camps and institutions interested in converting from a diet rich in refined products to a diet featuring whole foods such as grains, seeds, nuts, honey, fresh fruits and vegetables.
21. If you are concerned about use of too much sugar and starch in cafeteria lunches or sales of junk foods in schools, write letters to your local school board and send copies to the State School Supt., Letters to the Editor of your local newspaper, the FDA, and Carol Tucker Foreman, Department of Agriculture, Food and Consumer Service, 14th Street and Independence Avenue S.W., Washington, D.C. 20250.
22. To increase awareness of the world hunger problem in a positive way, discuss it with your children. By serving rice in a bowl with chopsticks for one evening meal a month, the family can relate in a very personal way to this food problem. Many affirmative steps can be taken — donating to world hunger programs; helping out in local food programs, etc.
23. There is almost no basic skill that cannot be learned using food relationships:

    A. SPELLING. From simple food words for early grades (fig, corn, milk, nut) to more challenging

words for older kids (persimmon, pomegranate, distribution, inequity); the list is endless. Follow up each lesson with discussions about the words.

B. TEXTURE. Feel the smooth apple, rough coconut, fuzzy kiwi berry, crunchy cracker, crisp carrot, soft banana. Don't panic if a child breaks crisp food, mashes soft food or mixes food into a mountain of "glop." Different foods have fascinating textures and it is the natural curiosity of the child to experiment with food. (Of course, if the child is sixteen and still mashing bananas between his/her fingers, it may be time to encourage a new source of entertainment!)

C. COLOR. Make a game out of color identification. For small children: "I'm thinking of the color red; can you name a food that is red?" For older children: (close eyes) "In my mind's eye, I see a vegetable that grows on a bush, starts out green, then turns red when it's ripe. We grow them in wire frames to support the heavy branches."

D. VOCABULARY. Teach action words and their meanings: dice, chop — slice, pop; grate, shred — dip, spread; peel, core— stir, pour; grind, baste — toss, taste! Give older children a topic and ask them to write a poem: "The Life and Adventures of Englebert Eggplant!" or a report: "How Pineapple is Planted, Harvested, Processed and Shipped."

E. MATH. Count foods, estimate sizes (small, medium, large), compare raw weight with cooked; divide one food two, three or four ways; note cooking time, how long for personal labor and how long in oven. Older kids can prepare cost accounts for meals, breaking it down per serving, wages, etc.

F. AWARENESS. Teach about growing food by having your own garden; marketing, by selling some of your produce; distribution, by sharing or trading your abundance; finances, by leaving a bill at each person's plate showing how much their meal cost to prepare. Have a hunger awareness meal in which each person eats only a bowl of rice or a potato with their fingers instead of silverware, and a glass of water dipped from a jar with everyone sharing the same cup.

24. **Take the Organoleptic Test — touch, see, taste, smell and listen every time you introduce a new food.**
25. **Add to this list your own solutions and methods for dealing with outside influences. Let us know the ones that work for you and your children.**

Full Circle

O' beautiful child, my precious child,
What mysteries have I learned from you?
I, as your student, and you as my guide
Taught me all about life — and we grew.

You were a helpless mass of movement and noise
Whose mind struggled to know and be free.
Yet, through your inquisitive, sunny bright eyes
It was I who learned how to see.

You showed me how to look at a single leaf,
To see each exquisite green vein;
To marvel at the tree's enchanting ballet
As it quivered in a gentle rain.

My hopes and fears, my dreams and schemes
Soon revealed their realities,
And you were the center from which all truths evolved,
My little miracle in faded blue jeans.

You taught me to make the most of each God-given day;
This moment is all we possess.
Then my worries and fears about future and past
Disappeared in Love's present caress.

You nudged me through the difficult days
By giving me a confident shove,
So that the past, the present and future
Merged into eternal love.

O' delightful child, my closest friend,
The time has come for you to leave.
But, because our visions were clear and defined
Sweet memories won't allow me to grieve.

So blessed child, when you have one of your own,
Here's some wisdom that ever holds true:
To have an exciting, fulfilling and joyful life,
Be the student, and let your child be — the guru.

WHAT YOU CAN DO WITH TEEN-AGERS

1. **The automatic dishwasher has replaced old-fashioned mother-child conversations over a sink full of dishes, but sharing time together in food preparation can re-open the lines of communication, closeness and camaraderie. Take teens shopping; plan menus and enlist them in school lunch preparation.**
2. **We are indeed a nation of gullible adults and vulnerable youth. Suggest that your teen-agers watch T.V. commentaries dealing with consumer rip-offs.**
3. **Let your kids trade pertinent newspaper or magazine articles they read for a special family night, an article of clothing or special privilege. Six chapters read from a book about the hazards of refined sugar, for example, might become the ticket for a night at the skating rink, a new pair of socks, or unlimited time for one night on the telephone. An article from a health oriented magazine might be an incentive for them to read and you to rake the leaves — good exercise for you and a learning experience for them!**
4. **Having their own Diet Diary notebook will encourage teens to keep track of the foods they eat outside of the home. They will soon learn to correlate food with over-all ill health, skin outbreaks, tension, and energy output as well as the more positive signs of improved health when they stick to a sensible plan.**
5. **Invite them to attend lectures and workshops in your community with guest speakers who, through a fresh point of view, may have a greater influence than mom and dad. They are exposed daily to convenience food promotion; they need to hear both sides of the story in order to make a critical evaluation.**
6. **Hold an Ethnic Awareness Day. Have teens represent a different country and prepare native foods, using the same method of preparation if possible, the same spices and seasonings, similar containers to serve their provisions and traditional table decorations as the country they have chosen to study. Reports on history, native customs, and the making of costumes can be fun and interesting. Everyone can try their hand at the languages; at least learn the names of the dishes plus "please" and "thank you."**
7. **The appeal of take-out fast food is: quick service, familiar tastes and low prices. Keep plenty of homemade fast food in your refrigerator that can be "taken-out" and enjoyed en route to practice, the game, or wherever they go. Homemade pizza (frozen), fruit and cheese, trail mix, or pocketbread ready to fill with a variety of mixtures are fast and tasty. Don't forget the shakes and smoothies.**

8. **Strike a "cook's night out" bargain with your teen-agers for special celebrations. Instead of going to a restaurant for dinner, let them plan, prepare, serve and clean up after, a dinner menu of their choice, served to you and your spouse on the best linen, with candlelight and live music. You would pay $25 to dine in a restaurant of equal caliber, so pay your kids instead. And don't forget to leave a tip!**
9. **Discuss peer pressure with your teens. Let them know that you, too, deal with this universal problem, and share ways that you handle various situations. Once you know where pressure is most demanding, you will be able to plan family activities accordingly. For instance, if everyone is smoking and drinking at parties — host your own parties! Birthdays, seasons, sports events can all be great themes around which you can plan festivities. A progressive dinner party is great fun and teaches that parents and kids can cooperate in planning and preparing for good times without drugs to spoil the fun.**
10. **Many schools are beginning to offer more classes that deal with emotional growth but the major responsibility for educating teens and pre-teens about sex, tobacco, alcohol and drugs, should come from home. This may mean some research on your part. There are excellent materials available in the library, through law enforcement offices, and churches and civic groups often sponsor parent-teen workshops that deal honestly and effectively with these subjects. Counseling sessions are available in almost every community (through the County Health Department) where parents and teens gather on equal ground to discuss controversial issues.**
11. **Organize a "Depression Week." Plan a shortage of gasoline, water, electricity, money and food. Teach thrift and resourcefulness using** *only* **food from the pantry; do no laundry or wash** *only* **by hand and line dry; walk or ride bikes everywhere; recycle whatever possible; read by daylight or candle light; wear layers of clothes to keep warm and pray together for people who are worse off than yourselves.**
12. **Spend some time with your teens concocting and using facial creams, lotions or shampoos made from ingredients found in your refrigerator. A yogurt-cucumber or mayonnaise face mask, an almond or oatmeal cleanser, and a honey-egg shampoo with lemon juice rinse and an herbal bath with luffa sponge can all contribute to that "picture of health" look and "peaches 'n cream" complexion they strive for. Acne is best treated by a good diet, some vitamin and mineral supplements, plenty of exercise, fresh air and rest, along with an even state of emotions. (See** *Nothing New; Tried and True* **— Natural Cosmetics.)**
13. **Athletes will usually listen to their coaches. Gain the confidence of your school coaches by sharing your reading materials relating strength and stamina to diet. Try to get the film** *Better Food for Students* **where the late Gena Larson was in charge of an all natural foods cafeteria, during which time Helix High School excelled in athletic events.**
14. **Start a Brown Bag Conspiracy in your junior high or high school. Meet with groups of interested students once a month at school, everyone bringing sack lunches. The kids ask questions or bring up issues dealing with diet, exercise and health. You provide answers or sources for information. These same teens can then volunteer to work with children in the elementary schools to teach them good nutrition habits. Using puppets or mime, students can act out a junk food junkie vs. health food enthusiast scene. Puppets can be made to look like ice cream sodas, bottles of pop, carrots, apples, pizza, etc.**
15. **Add to this list your own solutions and methods for dealing with outside influences. Enlist the help of your teens, ask what kind of activities** *they* **would like to do to increase their awareness of better health. Let us know the ones that are the most successful!**

And now here is my secret, a very simple secret;
It is only with the heart that one can see rightly;
What is essential is invisible to the eye.

The Little Prince

BROWN BAG CONSPIRACY CREDO

I have the right to be me. I have the right to be healthy enough to live to my maximum ability; not just free from disease, but bursting with energy, stamina and creativity.

I have the right to strong bones, teeth and muscles, clear skin, shining hair, sparkling eyes, endless energy, an even blood sugar level and the opportunity to smile and be happy each and every day.

I have the right to a clear mind that will enable me to learn anything that I choose. I have the right to read and explore the works of the great naturalists of all time in order that I too, may become more in tune with my own body, mind and spirit through a closer bond with Mother Earth.

I have the right to choose whole, natural foods whenever possible and to say "No, thank you" when the only foods being served are junk.

I have the right and responsibility to develop myself to my own fullest potential.

I AM ______________________________

Some Human Rights Issues

We recognize the individual's inalienable right
To smoke, drink or take RX, but we also hear the plight,
Of children who must suffer the side effects of these actions,
For which medical evidence clearly exists, showing adverse reactions.

Smoking

Observe children closed in a vehicle or a room with no ventilation,
Absorbing toxic lead right through their skin, as well as with each inhalation.
Side stream smoke has been documented as being more dangerous than
The main stream smoke that blackens the lungs of the smoking woman or man.

So, while the parents have rights that they want respected,
CHILDREN'S rights must not be totally neglected.
The gift that would make any family relationship stronger
Is the one that says "I quit smoking — so we can ALL live longer."

Drinking

Physical or emotional abuse by an alcoholic parent
May never be reported but is often sadly apparent
In the children's personalities and attitudes of apathy and despair.
They love their parents, so they stay and pray that someday, someone will care.

Even those kids whose folks only drink on infrequent occasion,
Receive the message loud and clear that drinking is a social obligation.
Everywhere they go, booze is being served, even in the name of charity,
And the price one pays for not going along? Criticism and unpopularity.

Alcoholism is this country's #1 addiction and drug misuse.
How many parents sanction social drinking, yet shudder at hard drug use?
This way of thinking surely reflects our gross lack of education,
It's time we took a second look at this appalling situation!

Drugs

Medicine cabinets all over the country are bursting at the seams,
Drugstore aisles with their colorful vials, fulfill the pill-poppers' dreams.
Have a sniffle, sore throat, headache, droopy eyes, heartburn or constipation?
Don't worry, some pharmaceutical company has prepared just the right medication.

But try to understand that each and every symptom is your body's way
Of telling you that, somewhere along the way, you've gone astray.
Please listen to your body, for it is like an open book;
When it gives you the warning signals, STOP and take a closer look

At the reasons you're experiencing those "minor" aches and pains,
They're the sign of deeper trouble, listen now, pull in the reins
On a lifestyle that has made you dependent on prescriptions,
When all you really need are some new-life directions.

Over-the-counter drug poisoning is a sorrowful killer of kids.
Granted, some help came about from the new child-proof lids,
But they are no deterrent for curious adolescents and teens.
Surely you know what the wrong combination of supposedly safe drugs means!

Quality of Life

The current methadone program has about a 1% success rate,
Substituting legal drugs for illegal ones and causing quite a debate.
But it has often been said and found to endure:
"An ounce of prevention is worth a pound of cure."

We must alert our young people to become totally aware
Of the influence of ALL drugs on future generations they'll bear.
Thus PREVENT the addictions before they ever take place,
And improve the quality of life for the whole human race.

If Your Lil' Sprout Has A Problem

Healthy Children are active, noisy, even rambunctious, but they can sit still when they need to. They tire after a busy day and sleep well, preparing their bodies for another day of activity. Healthy children may have off days, but for the most part can adjust to changes in schedule, authority figures and surroundings. They are usually cooperative, eager to learn and respond favorably to encouragement and affection. Eyes are bright, bodies are agile and minds are inquisitive.

Hypo-active Children show little motivation toward work or play. Appetites are often poor and the television receives preference over stories or games. Erratic blood sugar levels may cause the otherwise lethargic child to become violently upset at changes in routine. They may be "clinging vines" and unable to adjust to day care, pre-school or even an occasional babysitter. Signs of excess weight may begin early due to lack of exercise. They may sleep nine to eleven hours a night and still appear run down throughout the day. Lapse in memory may make school work a monumental task.

Hyper-active Children may be impulsive, aggressive, fidgety and/or easily frustrated. Boys are involved 7:1 and may have a high I.Q. but do poorly in school. Some type of sleep problems are usually apparent; light, restless, late-to-bed-early-to-rise sleep may be accompanied by bed-wetting, head-rocking or mobility during dreams. Personality characteristics may change unexpectedly from receptive and sweet-tempered to stubborn and destructive.

Learning Disabled Children find it difficult to learn in the normal classroom environment. They usually need a one-to-one instructional approach and a firmly-outlined activity plan, requiring complete cooperation between school and home, teacher and parent. Academic and/or physical limitations may be increased by short attention span, low self-esteem and various forms of frustration. Tremendous patience is required on the part of all who come in contact with learning disabled children.

Influences

The foods that nourish life from birth to toddler to teen, directly influence resistance to childhood diseases, allergies, moods and temperament, ability to read and write, social development, physical development, (bone structure, teeth and dental caries, hair, complexion, strength) mental alertness and stability, and various patterns of behavior. We feel that all of these conditions and many others too numerous to detail here, are as much related to diet as to environment or heredity.

When foods were whole and processing was minimal and without profuse chemical additives, parents were able to cope with naturally rambunctious children. They called them the "terrible twos" (no matter how long they lasted!) and both parent and child weathered the storm. Children were able to play hard and fast, to the point of exhaustion, yet calm down when asked to do so. Discipline could be administered and understood and students could sit still in school long enough to learn.

Except Tom Sawyer, of course. Now there's your classic hyperactive boy. Just think of the adventures we would have missed had Aunt Polly administered Ritalin to ole' Tom!

A Sad Situation

Perhaps future studies concerning the diets of both abusive parents and battered children will confirm our suspicion: the combination of low-blood sugar in the parent and a refined sugar or chemical additive-induced period of hyperactivity in a child is sheer dynamite. The child is totally unaware of the cause of sudden bursts of energy, possibly alternating with episodes of anger, stubbornness or depression. The effect proves to be too much for a parent who may be experiencing a hypoglycemic (low-blood sugar — short-fused) reaction.

The same meal may have caused problems in the parent and the child that are opposing, but equally disturbing. This contrast of physical reactions is more than either parent or child can handle and the resultant response is unhealthy, traumatic, conflict, leading to physical abuse.

Children are dependent on the food their parents prepare or stock in the kitchen cupboards. The only time that blood-sugar escalations and slumps can be controlled is during the preparation of the meal. Once a child is full of foods to which s/he is either allergy-sensitive or hypo/hyper-reactive it is impossible to self-control behavior. This statement is so important that for the benefit of all children who are punished for behavior they can not possibly be held responsible for, we are compelled to say it again. *Once a child is full of foods to which s/he is either allergy-sensitive or hypo/hyper-reactive, it is impossible to self-control behavior.*

Learning disabilities and behavior problems encompass enough research material and examples to fill dozens of books, but we feel certain that whatever the variables, an improved diet can't do anything but help. Parents are still the most powerful influence in their children's lives. Good eating habits, like good morals, will be tested, but when durability is proven they will be returned to, held steadfast and passed on to the next generation. So don't gamble with your child's future. Start now to provide the best possible raw materials for building and maintaining a sound, healthy body and mind.

The suggestions listed below have helped us deal with children's learning and emotional problems. Be patient and loving and realize that there are many parents experiencing the same feelings you have had or are having now. We understand and sympathize with your situation and we know that these are positive ways to deal with it effectively. Good Luck!

An inch of gold will not buy a moment of time. — *Chinese Proverb*

WHAT YOU CAN DO WITH PROBLEM SPROUTS

1. Find other parents who are implementing improved diet for behavior control. Share experiences, provide moral support and exchange recipes.
2. Never single one child out and try to change his/her diet or lifestyle. The whole family will benefit, both physically and emotionally, when they all work together to help their special family member.
3. Reduce television viewing time, as children are affected by the sound vibrations, the radiation, the rapid image transference, the light-dark contrasts and may become either lethargic or hyper after prolonged periods of viewing.
4. Make bedrooms conducive to relaxation. Daytime rest is often disturbed by the busy-ness of decor or toys. Restful colors are blues, browns, beige, soft yellows and greens. Check ventilation; indoor pollution is often worse than outdoor. Never use aerosol sprays to make a child's room smell fresh. Open a window instead.
5. Check into lighting used in the classroom. Long exposure to flourescent lighting can have adverse effects on adults, which are intensified in children — contributing to headaches, visual problems and hyperactivity. Read John Ott's *Health and Light.*
6. Evaluate hyperactive or allergy drugs carefully before you concede to using them as therapy. Chemical drugs may have physical side-effects, not to mention the possible future emotional implications of years of dependency. Many cough medicines, aspirins, vitamins and other over-the-counter medications contain sugar, artificial flavors and colors. Avoid these, also, and see *Nothing New; Tried and True* for some herbal substitutes.
7. Begin the day with a relaxed breakfast; complex carbohydrates plus complete protein equals a receptive learner. Send a high protein snack (nuts, cheese, seeds, sprouts) for the mid-morning slump — with teacher's approval.
8. Be sure you're following all the suggestions in this book for improved diet, label reading, increased exercise, complete chewing, relaxation, self-confidence through accomplishment, family recreation, fresh air and sunshine and a balance of work, play, prayer and rest.
9. Enlist your child's cooperation in keeping a diet diary. (Teachers may be willing to help at school.) Note all foods, liquids, drugs, behavior changes, physical activities and academic difficulties. Keep the communication lines open so your child will tell you how s/he feels after eating certain foods. The key to self-responsibility is understanding the correlation between what goes into the body and how it makes the body feel. Make it into a game of discovery.
10. Don't miss *Improving Your Child's Behavior Chemistry* by Dr. Lendon Smith, who has long recommended the removal of refined starches, especially sugar, from the diets of ALL children. In a humorous yet sensitive way, Dr. Smith transmits compassionate understanding along with sound medical advice.
11. A Hair Analysis, the simple procedure of testing hair for levels of minerals in body tissues, may detect a basic, underlying problem. Toxic levels of minerals like lead, cadmium, copper and aluminum are often found in hyperactive, learning disabled and/or delinquent children. For more information, contact: Mineralab, 22455 Maple Court, Hayward, CA. 94541.
12. Children need routine and structure in their daily living activities. If your child is in an open classroom (with learning stations that require a great deal of responsibility and independence) see that s/he receives equal time in a one-to-one directed program that requires very short periods for each task and hands-on experiences in order to increase retention and develop confidence through completion of work.
13. Set up a schedule in your home for your pre-school child's learning and development in preparation for the school experience. Short periods of time spent on creative play — art, blocks, music, puzzles; for directed learning — tying shoes, card sewing, follow-the-dots, counting; for exercise — running, jumping, climbing, balancing, playing catch; and for rest — listening to music, stories, deep relaxation breathing and simple yoga exercises will provide a semblance of structure and an outlet for energies, while introducing the familiar classroom routine. Keep the schedule regular. Vary activities within

each area but keep the same time of day and amount of time for the learning activity constant. Any foreseen changes in routine can be discussed and prepared for in advance.

14. **In his book** *Why Your Child is Hyperactive,* **Dr. Ben Feingold cautions against synthetic dyes and chemical additives while introducing the dangers of salicylates in natural foods. His diet is rigid (though we don't understand why he permits chocolate and sugar) and effective as is evidenced by the network of enthusiastic Feingold Families across the nation.**
15. **Give your child opportunities at home for spontaneous play. Art and music exploration are excellent means for releasing pent-up energy and emotions, while increasing creativity and self-expression. Through rhythm — dance, marching, clapping, playing an instrument and/or singing — a child may be able to, literally act out, sing out, stomp out, etc., anger, resentment, frustration and other feelings.**
16. **Children create emotionally, intellectually and artistically. Their art work is often illustrative of their deepest feelings and as such deserve your attention. Through paints, crayons, collage or clay, young children demonstrate the reality of their mind and emotions but not necessarily the reality of outward appearance. Therefore, encourage conversations about their artwork, being very careful not to criticize or suggest how it "should" look or what color it "should" be. Respect a child's desire for privacy if s/he doesn't want to share feelings about artwork. The very fact that it is** *done* **may mean that there is no longer a need to relate to that subject.**
17. **For more information about understanding and appreciation of children's art, send a stamped, self-addressed envelope and your inquiry to: Karyn Martin Kuri, 6342 Santa Caterina, Citrus Heights, CA. 95601. Also read,** *Art as Therapy With Children,* **by Edith Kramer.**
18. **A warm (not hot!) bath is very calming. Of course, stay with your young child.**
19. **Speak in positive terms to children (and everyone, for that matter). Instead of saying, "You're** *not* **going anywhere because you** *didn't* **make your bed," try saying, "When your bed is made, you may go outside." Crime, violence, schizophrenia, neurotic aberrations and physical ailments of all kinds are manifestations of negative energy. Replace the negative with positive energy, and you help to develop self-esteem.**
20. **If you are tempted to give your child aspirin, laxatives or other over-the-counter drugs, first consider natural alternatives.**
21. **Above all, keep the home atmosphere as relaxed and accepting as possible. Lil' Sprouts grow best in a climate that is filled with happiness and love.**

While we consider when to begin it becomes too late. *Latin Proverb*

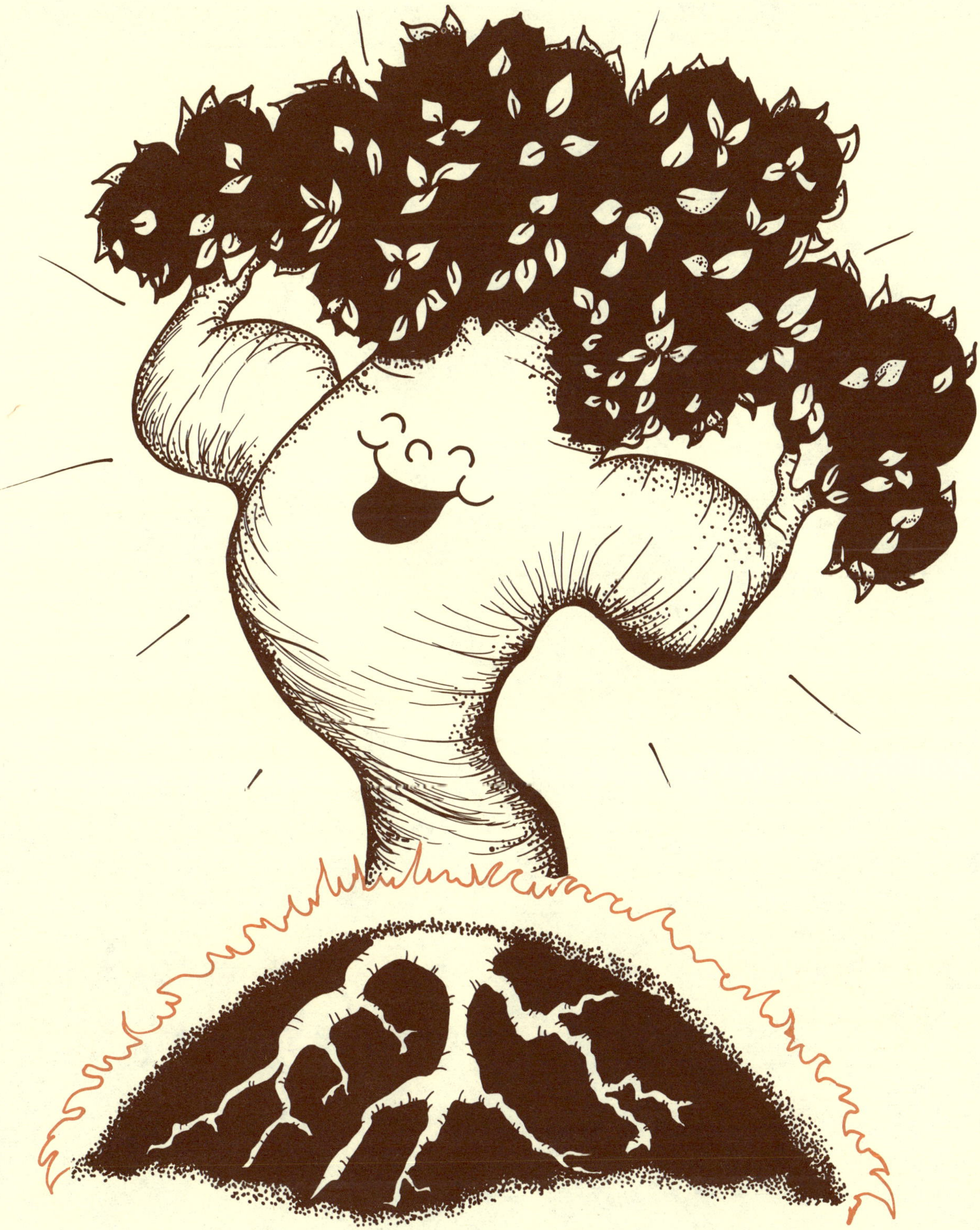

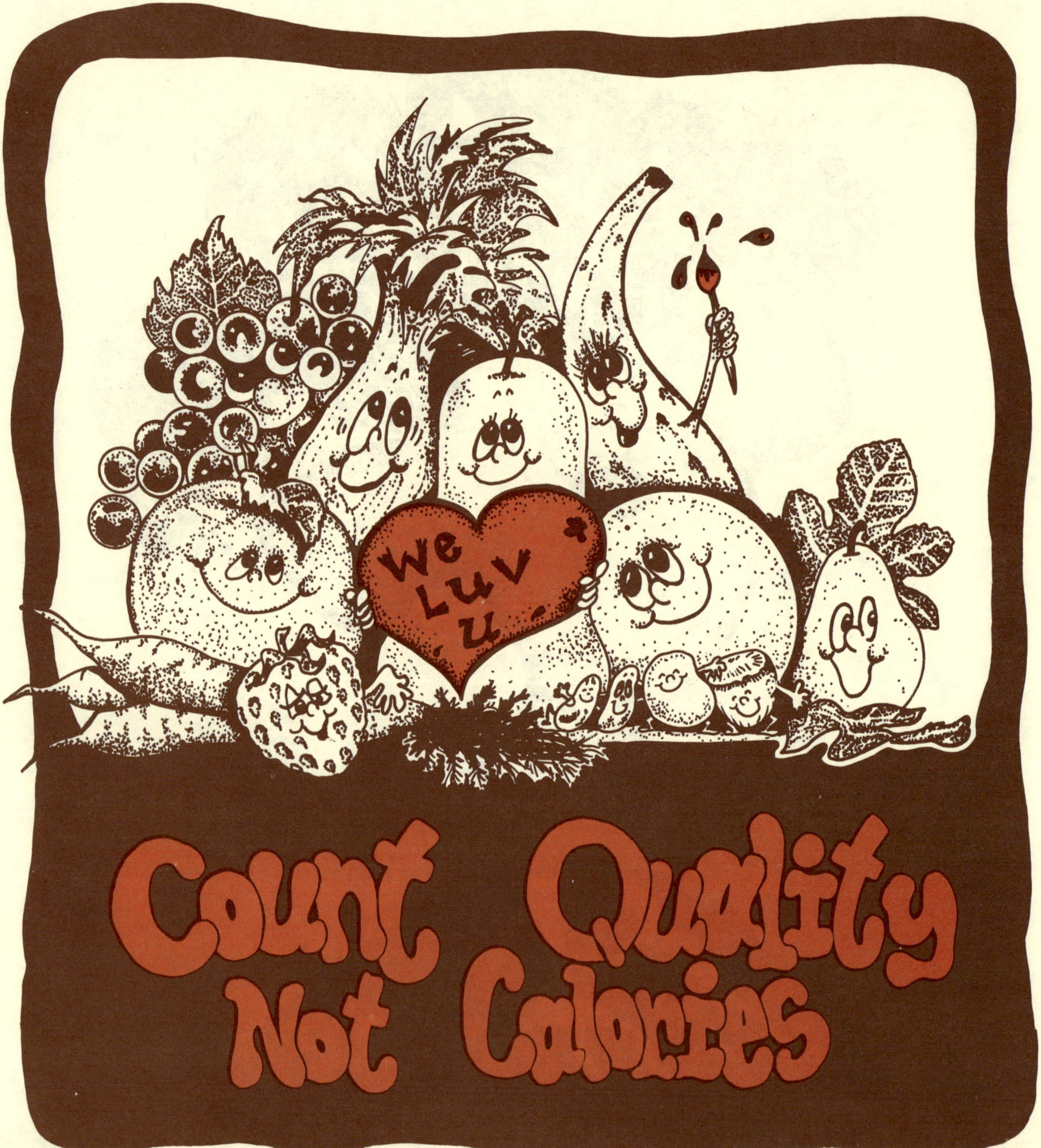
We LUV U
Count Quality
Not Calories

Count Quality; Not Calories

Normal Weight: Mission Impossible?

We Love Your Body, brains to bladder
Taller, shorter, thinner, fatter,
The calories you needn't count
In greater or lesser amount,
It's the nutrition and energy that matter!

Although tricks and gimmicks may work for a few, the majority of quick-weight-loss-fad-diet authors know full well the scope of the obesity problem and have capitalized nicely at the expense of a disappointed, still-over-weight and more-depressed-than-ever segment of our society.

A diet is not something you go *on* with the intention of eventually going *off.* Diet is what you eat and drink every day, every meal, every snack, for all of your life. It is the conscientious decision you make every time you open your mouth for the purpose of consuming food. Your diet is an assortment and variety of foods that you, and you alone, choose to ingest for better or worse, in sickness and health, through thick and through thin, until death do you part. It is an accumulation of habits that begin at birth, are learned, and therefore can be changed.

We are all creatures dependent on food for our survival, and common sense tells us that the quality of the food we eat will have a direct effect on the quality of the life we live. Generations of strong and robust people maintained normal weight on fresh, wholesome, natural food long before scientists discovered and labeled nutrients or calories. They ate what God made available to them, without altering or destroying the food's inherent body-building qualities. Providing, growing and preparing food were often laborious tasks which guaranteed that vigorous exercise would be part of their lifestyle.

Tipping the Scales

Today, obesity is America's Number One health problem. An estimated eighty million people are more than 20% overweight and as many as 75% of adult Americans are carrying around as much as ten extra pounds. Excess weight is associated with heart and vascular diseases, back and foot problems, a higher incidence of breast cancer in women, surgery complications and slow recovery, diabetes, sedentary living, skin allergies and irritations, varicose veins and constipation, just to name a few.

For years, ladies' magazines have been the vehicle for the food industry's ploy to reassure millions of women that the way to a man's heart is through his stomach. Not only are the magazines chock full of advertisements, but the very articles and accompanying photographs are all designed to sell the advertisers' products. It's time we recognize that those beautiful, rich, enticing goodies (often associated with families, holidays and love) are nothing more than the blatant peddling of heart-attack food. Even the articles on dieting are so full of coffee, diet colas, no-calorie, synthetic, fake, phony food that they cannot be recommended as beneficial to health.

Validated insurance statistics confirm that the slim person lives longer than the obese or even, slightly overweight person. Perhaps weight problems are not caused specifically by over-eating as much as by insufficient training in the judgment of food selection. Consider how many hours the breadwinner works to make the money to purchase the groceries. Yet, in comparison, how many hours do we spend learning how to buy food and feed ourselves to the best benefit of our health? Unless you are a home economics major, the answer may be that relatively few hours are devoted to nutrition education.

But a change is taking place in the hearts and minds of people all over the world. Indeed, *you* are part of that change. You are taking responsibility for the condition of your own (and your family's) health. You are to be commended for your forthrightness and courage. We hope that your experiences with change will be as pleasant and rewarding as ours have been.

Food! What is it? What's in it?

Whole, raw foods contain protein, carbohydrates, fats, water, vitamins, minerals, enzymes, chemicals, cellulose, distinct flavors and calories, all designed by The Master Craftsman to provide our bodies with everything necessary to begin life and continue the miraculous process of regeneration.

Processed food, on the other hand, started out as the above, but has been modified — often more than once. Heat is probably the first offender, destroying all enzymes and some vitamins and minerals, altering flavor and appearance, and breaking down texture. In an attempt to restore desirability to processed food, a myriad of chemicals may be added in the form of: preservatives, anti-oxidants, emulsifiers, stabilizers, flavor enhancers, coloring agents, sweeteners, bleaching agents, sequestriants, humectants, thickeners, firming clarifying, curing, foaming, anti-foaming and anti-caking products. The resultant "food" is usually high in empty calories that provide only spurts of energy followed by insatiable hunger and nervous tension.

Of course the food we select is only one of the keys that open doors to normal weight. Equally important factors are: improving digestion, recognizing and dealing with stress and increasing daily exercise.

Plan a Relaxed Meal

"Digest (v. di jest', di-; n. di' jest) v.t. 1. physiol. To change food chemically in the alimentary canal into material suitable for assimilation by the body." Sounds simple enough, yet it is one of the most complex functions of the human anatomy. Fifty percent of digestion takes place in the mouth *if* we chew our food well. Many people gulp down huge meals, but due to inadequate chewing, suffer from gas and distention caused by undigested food fermenting in the intestines. When we eat small portions of food and chew properly, digestion is complete, absorption is thorough, and we are satisfied with less.

There are no gimmicks to losing excess weight, but if any one factor can have the most beneficial effect on a weight loss program, it would have to be learning to eat slowly and chew, chew, chew! Food is the crude fuel; our bodies, the refineries. Only by thorough chewing and complete digestion can we expect our fuel supply to enable us to operate at maximum efficiency.

A Diet Diary — For Personal Insight

Despite the saying that fat people are happy people, severe mental and emotional stress often accompanies obesity. It is futile to try to establish the order of occurrence — does fat cause stress or does stress cause fat — for we will only be faced with the same old chicken or egg routine. Instead, think of weight control as a twin sister and heir-apparent to mind control.

Before you can be in command of your own mind, and therefore your own body, you must know yourself. You will be surprised how much you can learn about your inner person by using a diet diary. In just one week of keeping notes, you can begin to identify certain foods, as well as certain conditions that affect the way you feel. When in tune with your emotions, you will be able to control your eating habits and your weight.

In short time you will correlate the intrinsic connection between physical and mental well-being, thus you will need to write less and less as you become more and more sensitive to your needs. Just remember, you *learned* all of the habits that you have today. *Unlearning,* or change, is more of a challenge, but you will be better equipped to meet and surpass goals if you judiciously keep a diet diary.

DIET DIARY

On the left page, RECORD:

1. What you ate
2. Raw or cooked
3. Natural or processed
4. Quantity
5. Time of day; time allotted
6. At home or restaurant
7. Alone or with someone
8. Around smokers/heavy pollution
9. Supplements taken
10. Type of exercise

On the right page, EVALUATE:

1. How you feel
2. The pace of your day
3. Meditation/rest
4. Schedule; regular or interrupted
5. Attitude during preparation and eating
6. Non-food related emotions or events
7. Physical discomforts: gas, heartburn, constipation, diarrhea, etc.
8. Reactions, such as: lethargy, hyper-activity, insomnia, etc.

Make Calories Work for You

When we remember that a calorie is a measurement of heat, not of weight, then we can put food intake versus energy output into perspective. As long as the heat energy expended (movement) *matches* the heat energy consumed (calories from food) a person's weight will remain constant. When the heat energy expended is *less* than the heat energy consumed, a gain in weight results and when the heat energy expended is *more* than the heat energy consumed, a loss of weight will occur.

It doesn't make sense to eliminate such foods as avocados, dates, bananas, nuts, seeds and cheeses (as many dieters do) just because of their calorie count. Eating the widest variety of foods available is the best insurance for obtaining the diverse nutrients necessary for maintaining the highest level of energy.

Rather than scrupulously counting calories, why not take advantage of naturally high complex carbohydrate food and *do* something with those power-packed calories? Bike, hike, run, skate, swim, dance; whatever turns you on. Do it with vigor and vitality, knowing that you are burning, not only the calories consumed at the most recent meal, but some that have been stored over the years, as well!

If the discipline of calisthenics, jogging or exercise classes is too much for you, then allow yourself extra time to *walk.* Walk everywhere you can. Park several blocks from where you work or shop, and walk. Plan to meet a friend in the park and walk. Walk to school, to church, to the grocery store; walk to a garage sale, to pick up the newspaper; use any excuse you can think of to walk, but *walk* every day.

Walking is the ultimate exercise. By stimulating every muscle and organ in the body, walking promotes better breathing, digestion, circulation and elimination. A brisk walk in the early morning is a grand way to start your day. Try it for one week and keep track of how different you feel. The over-all glow that emanates from deep within, will be the only motivation you'll need to wake up and do it again the next day, and the next . . . and your body will love you for it!

WHAT YOU CAN DO

1. **Determine quality of food by using the least processed, closest to natural product available. Let your body be the "food processor" it was designed to be, then go out and burn those calories with productive activity!**
2. **Allow at least twenty minutes to chew your next meal. If you finish before twenty minutes, just sit there and wait until the time is up. Soon you will be able to train yourself to slow down, chew, relax and enjoy your food.**
3. **Dim the lights and play soft music during the dinner hour. Make a point of taking a few deep relaxation breaths before, during and after a meal.**
4. **Initiate pleasant conversation during meals; avoid the common practice of using the dinner hour to air complaints, scold, punish or hash over the world situation.**
5. **If you have only five minutes in which to eat, then eat only five minutes' worth of food. More would only remain undigested.**
6. **If you are unable to control your emotions, just don't eat. You'll survive fine with a glass of fruit or vegetable juice, which requires very little digestion. Wait until you calm down, to eat.**
7. **Call your program a "health gain" instead of a "weight loss" method; the idea of "losing" implies giving something up and you may subconsciously want that part of yourself (the lost weight) back.**
8. **Never miss a chance to exercise. A healthy body absorbs positive energy and releases negative energy during exercise; at the same time your body becomes more shapely, your mind becomes more at peace.**
9. **Bicycle to work; climb stairs instead of using the elevator. Run around the block on your break. Stop at the local Y or fitness center after work and play racketball. Get the whole family involved in organized activity.**
10. **Do not confuse hunger with tension, boredom or loneliness. Keep your diet diary with you at all times so you can see in black and white how your emotions affect your eating habits and vice-versa.**
11. **Be polite, but firmly refuse food that you know will upset your body chemistry and put you back where you once were. If your hostess is offended because you** *don't* **eat her chocolate mousse, that's her hang-up. If you get a splitting headache later because you** *do* **eat the rich dessert, you have sacrificed your well-being for what the hostess would call courtesy; for what we would call condescension.**
12. **Use your mirror instead of your scale, to indicate how you're shaping up. Exercise develops muscle and muscle weighs more than fat. You may stay the same weight for weeks, yet fit better into your clothes. The scales may deceive, but the full-length mirror never lies!**
13. **Eradicate idleness. Convert spare time into energy-expending activities. Take a fitness class at the Y. Be a volunteer — any kind of volunteer. Participate in community theater, adult education or local politics. Find an art form that makes you happy and chances are that you can make it profitable too!**

Balancing the Scales

The goal, of course, should not be to reduce weight to the point of skin and bones just to look smashing in the latest fashions. The aim is to develop a sensible diet, forever, that furnishes sufficient nutrition for growth or maintenance and provides for pleasant and peaceful mealtimes.

A definite physiological change takes place when food intake is reduced for the purpose of losing weight. The mental attitude must correspondingly change from one of sacrifice and deprivation to one of self-accomplishment. When you strive to improve general health, weight-loss will be a welcome side effect rather than the main ambition, and the most noticeable balance will be in your personality, not in your scales.

Mission Accomplished!

Like the vine that appears to be growing out of nowhere through the tiny, insignificant cracks in the concrete wall, a health program thrives on hidden determination. We would like to pass along a Formula for Determination shared with us by our seventy-year-old friend, Victor Croxton. He is one of the many wise and wonderful senior citizens that we cherish for having never relinquished the Mother Earth Spirit — special people, who through their reverence for humanity and respect for Nature radiate the kind of health and happiness that we admire and look forward to in our own retirement years.

In Victor's words, "You can accomplish ANYTHING you want to IF:

1. *You have the burning desire to do it*
2. *You have the proper tools to do it*
3. *You do it and do it and do it and do it!"*

This book is intended to provide you with the proper tools. You must furnish the burning desire and the stick-to-it-ive-ness. We are certain that if you follow a natural diet and back-to-Nature program for three months, you will want to follow it for the rest of your life.

As your weight normalizes and your shape improves, *you* will be the only incentive you need to continue your new lifestyle. Then, instead of praying for help to get yourself together, you will thank God and praise Him daily for this magnificent handiwork, your body, that He has created and given you the responsibility for keeping fit for His purpose. Soon you will discover new areas of interest, new possibilities in your life, new doors, and you will have a key for every one of them!

Do You Work?

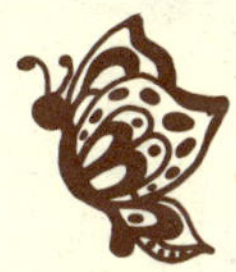

How often am I, a homemaker, asked this dynamite question?
"Do you work?" is a query loaded with an underlying suggestion.
That if I am not a part of the bring-home-a-paycheck-force,
My value as a human being has less worth. That's absurd, of course!

For being a person, wife, mother, maid, nurse, secretary, chauffeur and cook,
Provides a world of working experience, why, I could write a book . . .
To manage a household effectively requires systematic organization
More complex than the business world's computerized automation.

Six a.m.; jog two miles, do yoga postures and facial, get family up by seven —
Prepare the breakfast, pack lunches, clean house, attend a meeting by eleven.
Sing Randy to sleep, refinish chest of drawers, shape the loaves and bake the bread.
Weed the garden, dry forty pounds of fruit, for my class, have three chapters read.

Take Wendy & Matt to the Y, Dan & Chris to the track, and return by four-o-eight.
Pick up Mona at the gym, drop Heidi off at work, drive carefully, now don't be late.
Purchase a week's supply of groceries with the last $10.00 in the hat.
I challenge any executive efficiency expert to perform a miracle like that!

Now slice and dice and steam and cream, make a healthy dinner they'll all adore.
Just once I'd like to call in sick or protest with sign in hand: "I'll cook no more."
If everyone cooperates, in half an hour we'll have some chow.
"Is it really going to take that long? C'mon Mom, we're hungry NOW!"

As my man arrives home, I remember some silly thing I read just the day before,
It had to do with a bubble bath and greeting him in cellophane at the door!
Instead, my clothes are rumpled and sweaty and my hair goes every which way,
But he doesn't notice, he just kisses my sticky cheek and says, "Hi, how was your day?"

Now all the kids are sound asleep, it's peace and quiet time for me,
To sew a blouse, tie macrame, or write some poetry.
I curl up cozily near the wood stove to contemplate life on this good earth,
And I chuckle as I glance at the paperback, borrowed from a friend,
Titled: How to Get Paid What You're Really Worth!

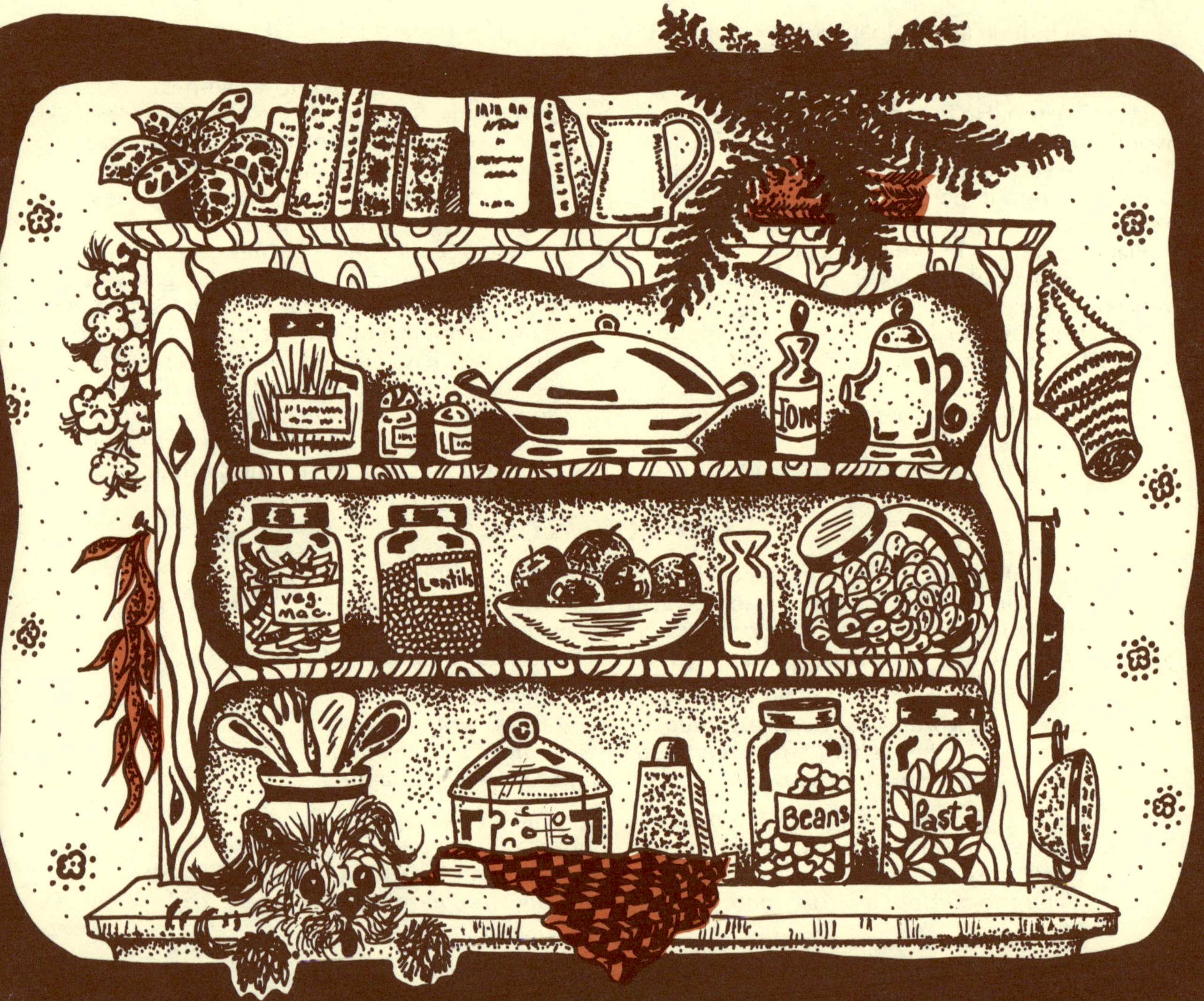

Purchasing Power

Purchasing Power

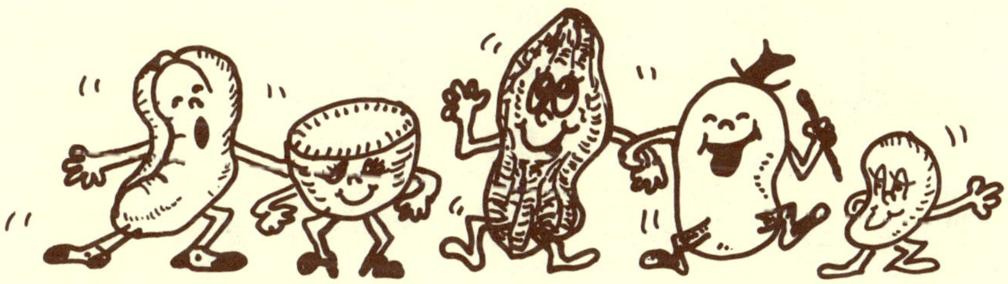

Diet Horizons - -
A Categorization of Today's Diets

Within the realm of dietary patterns, malnutrition can occur at any level, but more commonly occurs at the extreme ends of the spectrum. (See chart on following page.) A typical Junk Food or Basic Four Processed diet may work for the first ten or twenty years, but it becomes increasingly difficult for the body to maintain and repair cells with continuous use of poor building materials. Gradually the body weakens and becomes vulnerable; diseases invade like weeds in an untended garden, strangling the vital forces that are relied upon to maintain and regenerate life.

Focus your attention on the Basic Four Unprocessed level of the chart and note that it is positive, practical, economical and provides ample variety for taste, texture and appearance as well as biochemical sufficiency. It is Nature's original menu and we are grateful that in spite of Man's meddling temperament, these foods endure.

Where Are You Now? What is Your Goal?

Bear in mind that the diets described on the chart, ranging from Basic Four Processed to Vegan, are all biochemically sufficient. In other words, they will support life. It is up to the individual, however, to determine if the goal should be merely sufficient, or optimum, health. We are convinced that if you will conscientiously try the suggestions that are outlined in this book, for at least three months, you will be so "together" that you will never settle for "typical" again.

CAUTION: You may be susceptible to such name-calling as "Health-Food-Nut" by your junk-food-junkie-friends; "Health-Fanatic" by your relatives; "Food-Faddist" by your former doctor; "Weird-Wife" by your helpless husband or "Heartless-Husband" by your exhausted wife; and "Mad-Misguided-Mom" by your kids. Disregard their teasing and realize that they are insanely jealous because you look so great, you're working circles around them, and they all know that sooner or later they are going to have to admit that you are right.

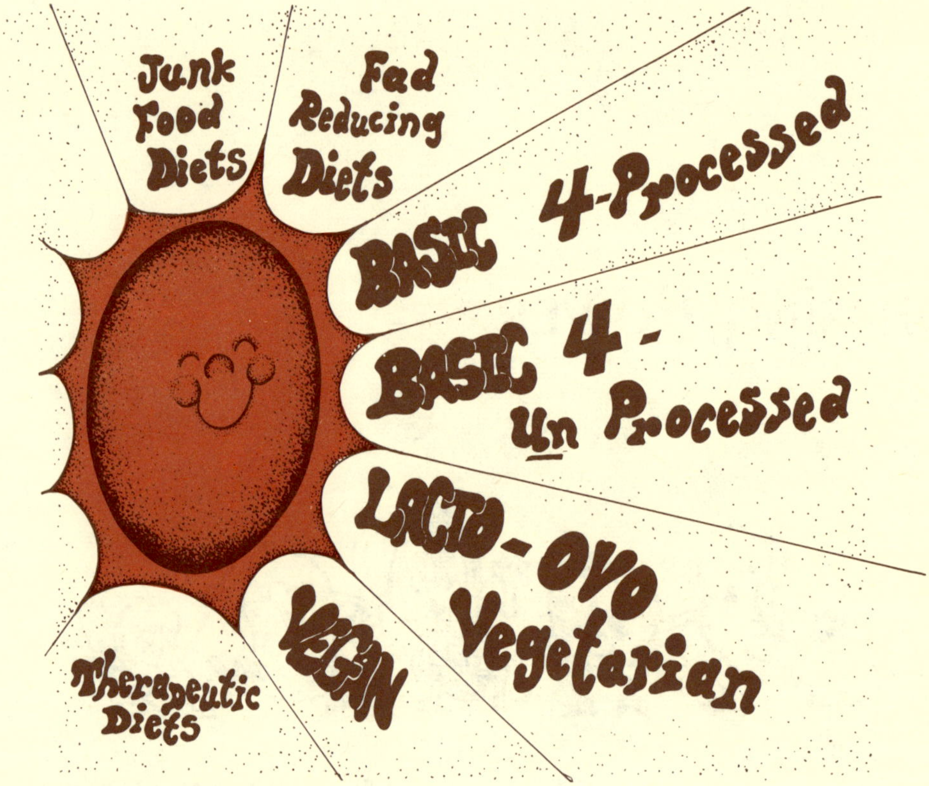

Key to Diet Horizons Chart

JUNK FOOD DIET: Includes all of the chemically flavored, dyed, preserved and French-fried American fare. It contains approximately 40% fat, 40% refined starches and sugars, 20% protein (100 grams — about twice as much as required). Fast food establishments and processing companies prepare meals leaving consumers with restricted choice and lack of ingredient and nutritional information. Emphasis is on eye appeal, quantity and convenience, while quality, digestibility and nutritive value take a back seat.

FAD REDUCING DIETS: Promote the books and fortify the authors' wallets, but most are biochemically insufficient. Fat, starch, protein and/or calories are often eliminated or unbalanced. Emphasis is on losing weight and counting calories to the exclusion of long-term health effects. Artificially sweetened foods are promoted at ridiculous prices, again with complete disregard to possible future risks. Coffee, black tea and diet soft drinks are encouraged and labeled "free foods." Common sense is left by the roadside in favor of the low calorie route.

BASIC 4 PROCESSED DIET: Is the seemingly adequate diet of the average supermarket shopper, who believes that "fortified" is as good as the real thing; whose purchase of each new product is based largely on curiosity or media advertisements; who considers convenience, cost and nutrition, in that order; who rationalizes that one item from each food group constitutes a "complete and balanced meal"; and who, though budget-minded, seldom realizes that one-third of the packaged-food dollar is spent on advertising and packaging. That's $1,000 out of an average yearly food budget of $3,000.

BASIC 4 UN PROCESSED DIET: Is a whole foods diet with the widest choice and most personal responsibility for purchasing, storing and preparing food to retain nutrients. Foods

DIET HORIZONS

JUNK FOOD DIET: greasy french fries, white bun hamburgers-hot-dogs, carbonated beverages, milk-less shakes, over-cooked, re-heated, cafeteria-style food, frozen T.V. dinners, pot pies, desserts, candy, etc.

FAD REDUCING DIETS: coffee, black tea, diet soft drinks, straight alcoholic drinks, hi-protein liquid diet packages, instant breakfast drinks and bars, low-cal gelatins, the gamut of high-priced, artificially sweetened and flavored products, specialty breads, one-food emphasis (eggs, grapefruit, turkey), fat-free foods, sugarless gum and mints, expensive brand-name weight reducer dinners.

BASIC 4 — PROCESSED DIET: fortified dry cereals, toaster-poppers, non-cholesterol imitation frozen meats and eggs, TVP meat extenders, canned and packaged soups, salad dressings and seasoning mixes, dinners-in-a-package, pre-breaded fish sticks, treated cheese spreads, over-salted, bagged pretzels and chips, canned, salty vegetables, treated frozen potatoes, canned spaghetti, ravioli, macaroni and cheese, canned fruit drinks and juices, cake and dessert mixes, packaged pastries, hydrogenated peanut butter, ice creams, white pastas, bologna and other lunch meats.

BASIC 4 — UN PROCESSED DIET: unadulterated meat, fish and poultry, fresh fruits and vegetables, whole grain breads, dried legumes, whole grains, raw nuts and seeds, sprouts, plain yogurt, kefir, natural hard cheeses, farm fresh eggs, certified raw milk, untreated honey, vegetable and whole grain pastas, fresh-pressed juices, cold-pressed oils, unhydrogenated peanut butter.

LACTO-OVO VEGETARIAN DIET: Same as Basic 4 — UN Processed, with the elimination of meat, fish and poultry.

VEGAN DIET: Same as Basic 4 — UN Processed, but excludes ALL animal products.

THERAPEUTIC DIETS: Sproutarian (all seeds, beans and nuts are sprouted); Fruitarian (all organic fresh fruits); Vitarian (excludes seeds, nuts and grains); Totally Raw (nothing cooked); Mucousless (no meat, eggs, dairy products, grains, fats, legumes or nuts); Macrobiotic (stresses spiritual qualities of certain foods, emphasizing personal balance of yin-yang forces with ultimate goal of grains only plus some liquid).

---

are purchased fresh and unprocessed whenever possible; dry foods are purchased in bulk, then divided with friends or properly stored for future use. Consumer educates self as to source of food and growing conditions, while remaining independent of advertising and flashy packaging. Personal awareness of food and its relation to health often entices home gardening; diet usually is comprised of 20% fat, 70% complex carbohydrates and 10% protein.

LACTO-OVO VEGETARIAN DIET: Eliminates meat; protein obtained by combining milk, cheeses, eggs and yogurt with bean, grain and nut dishes. Increased consciousness in food selection and method of preparation promotes more raw, home-grown foods and intense respect for the human body, the planet and all life. Often motivated by ethics, health, religion or economics, the person becomes more ecology-minded and peace-oriented.

VEGAN DIET: Omits all animal products. Many supplement diet with Vitamin B-12. This diet requires advanced knowledge of gardening, nutrition and food combining and involves tremendous commitment of time, energy and dedication to Mother Earth. It is an ethical, non-violent, total lifestyle which is admirable and certainly a goal to work toward, but not practical for all.

THERAPEUTIC DIETS: Include Fruitarian, Sproutarian, Vitarian, Macrobiotic, Mucousless and Totally Raw. These self-limiting diets are usually undertaken for short periods of time as a therapeutic aid in recovering from disease, shock, surgery, or coming off a long fast. Reserved for highly motivated and dedicated persons of esoteric discipline, these diets require ideal conditions and a Garden-of-Eden environment. They are excellent body tonics for a brief time, yet not meant to be a sustaining diet.

First and Foremost

Changing to a whole foods diet means buying your foods as close to the condition in which they were grown as possible. The routine of buying convenience food may be just that — a convenient routine. But routines can change. Picture a mother in a supermarket telling her child that she would like to make a cake from scratch. The curious child may respond, "Okay, but where do we find the package of scratch?" The new whole foods routine may seem a little overwhelming at first, but taken one step at a time, will prove to be worthwhile. Do the best you can and remember that each step will lead you that much closer to your goal.

An important aspect of choosing whole foods over processed is that you have some control over what happens to the food. When you prepare a double recipe of pizza or ice cream, you do not concoct a batch of chemicals to flavor, color and preserve the extras that you plan to freeze and use within a few months. But the purchase price of frozen pizza and commercial ice cream includes, among others, the addition of butylated hydroxytoluene and sodium carboxymethylcellulose respectively, because they may sit in a warehouse, grocery or home freezer for a year or more.

The producers of commercial products are concerned about marketing, distribution and profit. *That* is what the convenience food business is all about. In our kitchens, we are concerned first and foremost about quality and nutrition, then about taste and appearance. We know, however, that the most nutritious foods will be enjoyed only if they please the eye and delight the palate, which can be done without synthetic dyes and flavors or chemical preservatives. *That* is what this book is all about.

Maybe the Label is Natural

Due to increased competition from the natural foods industries, name-brand manufacturers are increasing their production and advertisement of preservative-free foods. When the art work on the front of a packaged food displays a crock of honey, a dish of butter, a sheaf of wheat and the word "natural" in bold type on all four sides of the box, be suspicious. Read the ingredient list carefully and don't be conned by the semantics of advertising. The word "natural" as used by the processed food industry may just mean anything that is derived from food.

When we refer to natural throughout this book, we mean those foods which have not been physically abused by modern technology — the whole pineapple, the whole potato, the whole grain, etc., OR those foods which use a minimum amount of processing with chemical-free ingredients, such as bread with whole grain flour, ice cream with real milk and unfiltered, unheated honey; and nuts and seeds that have not been bleached, oil-roasted and salted.

Other acceptable processes include hulling, cutting, drying or rolling (as with grains), in some cases pre-steaming to retard enzyme action, and home canning, drying and freezing. Oats that have dried fruit and raw nuts added are still natural, but oats "improved" with brown sugar, enriched flour and vanillan have lost their natural classification.

Most natural foods are found in plain packages or bulk containers so you can bag them yourself. They are not backed by millions of dollars in advertising and are, therefore, seldom seen on commercials during children's television programs. In our opinion, the most ridiculous and dominant ads are for the least natural foods; they intimidate and emotion-motivate the American homemaker to purchase worthless products. When you are insulted by certain ads, write letters to the manufacturers and simply refuse to purchase their merchandise. Insist that, if they want your business, they change their advertising format as well as their product.

Your Safe-Deposit Box

Consider home storage of food as an investment. Buy in bulk, treat with care and reap benefits in the future. Purchase wholesale whenever you can, dividing with a friend or a group of friends for more variety. A "safe-deposit box" in the form of an extra refrigerator can be purchased second hand and will pay for itself the first year.

For example, you may buy fifty pounds of walnuts for 75¢ a pound in October; shell and store them, refrigerated, to use gradually over the year. Next August, when shelled walnuts are selling for $4.00 a pound (with no indication of where they've been stored all year), your own walnuts, including cold storage, are only costing you $.95 a pound. You can call shelling nuts hard work or you can gather your family 'round a toasty fire, serve some hot mulled cider and shell nuts while you share fellowship — a dividend that cannot be measured in terms of dollars and cents.

Whether you identify it as a pantry, a storeroom or a vault, the cool, dark cupboards or room you select to store bulk beans, grains, nuts, seeds, herbs, dried foods, unopened oils and home-canned goods, will serve as a trusty reservoir for items that might otherwise require a special trip to town. Storing food saves time and gasoline and helps you to avoid inflationary prices. If you maintain a cache of flours, shelled nuts, opened oils, cheese and eggs in your extra refrigerator, the only foods you will need to purchase on a regular basis are fresh dairy products and the fresh fruits and vegetables that you don't grow yourself.

Beans, whole grain pastas and seeds for sprouting, can be decoratively displayed, out of direct light, in recycled glass jars. Be sure to label *everything*. Lani once cooked for an hour what she thought was wild rice. Only the ghastly odor and Stan's memory saved them from dining on grass seed!

We spend money for nice clothes that wear out, we buy a new car only to have it depreciate in value, but when we invest wisely in whole food for future health, it's like having money in the bank . . . only safer.

Closer to the Source

COMMUNITY FOOD CO-OPS & FARMERS' MARKETS are springing up all over the country. In a Co-Op, you work a certain number of hours each month in exchange for a discount on groceries. A farmers' market is usually not as fancy as a supermarket and this is to your advantage. Both places can provide you with most of your produce, juices, yogurt starter, kefir, certified raw dairy products, grains, beans, nuts, seeds, herbs, flours, chapatis, pita breads, dried fruit and whole wheat 'n' honey baked goods. They will often allow you to bulk order for a small fee.

LOCATE ORIGINAL FOOD SOURCES by scouting around your community. The choices are good, prices are better and the new friendships developed are the best part of being one's own middleperson. Find a bakery or friend who bakes whole grain breads. Look for a creamery that makes fresh butter and undyed cheeses. Buy certified, raw milk from a local farmer or dairy. Purchase eggs from a friend whose hens are free to peck and scratch for food.

HEALTH STORES sell vitamins and food supplements, and are a good source of many food supplies. Get to know the proprietor and ask for case prices and a mail-out of specials. There are a growing number of companies that are concerned about marketing quality foods which contain a minimum of additives and you will usually see them in a health food store first.

GROCERY STORES are often a good source of fresh produce. So, relax, you can still visit the friendly checkers at your local stores when you stop in to pick up such items as olives, chilis, pineapple in its own juice, tomato paste, paper products and other items which may not be available elsewhere. Introduce yourself to the produce person and ask to be called in the event that ripe produce is in danger of spoiling over the weekend. This kind of friendship could keep your freezer cold and your food dehydrator warm all year long.

Wherever you do your shopping, have the confidence to ignore flashy advertising, the courage to make the sometimes awkward changes, and the assurance that the benefits will balance the time and effort involved. The law of supply and demand is regulated by our buying habits. When we use our purchasing power to increase demand for whole food, then more and more quality products will become available. You can be an activist without being a revolutionary. You can be a consumer without being consumed!

It is better to debate a question without settling it than to settle it without debating it.
Joseph Joubert

WHAT YOU CAN DO

1. At your own pace, discard, dump, reduce consumption of, refuse to buy more of, or recycle the following:
   CHOCOLATE is high in fat and sodium, requires five times its weight in sweetener to be palatable and contains caffeine, theobromine and limited nutrients. Substitute carob powder. (See *P.S. Stone-Age Food for Space-Age People.*)
   CARBONATED BEVERAGES include dietetic as well as regular, also fruit-flavored drinks. Use fresh pressed juices and perrier water or make smoothies instead.
   PROCESSED CHEESES and dyed, flavored cheese spreads can be replaced with Jack, raw milk cheddar, farmer's, feta, bleu, ricotta, hard parmesan or reliable cottage. Make home-style spreads with two kinds of shredded cheese, some cottage or ricotta and herbs.
   PROCESSED MEATS contain sodium nitrates and nitrites, artificial color and flavor and are made from some of the most fatty and undesirable parts of the animal. These include bacon, ham, frankfurters and luncheon meats and meat spreads. (See *Labor of Love Lunches* for sandwich filling ideas.)
   THE WHITES are MSG, salt, shortening, flour and sugar and are so prevalent that we have devoted the entire next chapter to their misuse.
2. Now you can begin to stock your pantry with some of the following items:
   BEANS: small red, lentils, split peas, garbanzos, pintos, soy, mung, adzuki.
   GRAINS: brown rice, oats, millet, bulgur, wheatberries, pearl barley, soy grits, buckwheat, rye.
   SEEDS: sesame, alfalfa, radish, cabbage, chia, celery, dill, sunflower, flax, pumpkin.
   RAW NUTS: almonds, walnuts, cashews, filberts, pecans, brazils, peanuts (a true legume), coconut, pine nut.
   FLOURS: soy, whole wheat pastry, stoneground whole wheat, rye, buckwheat, whole corn meal, rice, potato, barley, millet, wheat germ, bran, arrowroot.
   SWEETENERS: raw, unfiltered honey, unsulphured molasses, sorghum, real maple syrup, date sugar, powdered barley malt, dried fruit, homemade jams and jellies.
   SEASONINGS: low-sodium vegetable powders, kelp, sea salt, cayenne, tamari-soy sauce, basil, chili powder, nutritional and smoked yeast, and a variety of herbs.
   MISCELLANEOUS: carob powder, protein powders, non-instant powdered milk, cold-pressed oils, cider vinegar, whole grain or vegetable pastas, old-fashioned peanut butter and spices.
3. Spoil your produce with TLC. Unless you grow everything, it is next to impossible to know the exact origin or growing method of every fruit or vegetable you eat, but follow these suggestions for the best purchase and care of produce:
   PLAN your meals around in-season fruits and vegetables and then select the freshest possible produce. If you grow your own, pick either in the early morning or the late evening, but not in the heat of the day. Immediately refrigerate both garden and market produce.
   PREPARE produce for eating by washing quickly and thoroughly. Do not cut or shred until just before preparation time.
   EAT veggies raw about 75% of the time; protect color, flavor and nutrients by steaming briefly, sauteeing or crock-pot cooking, where nutrients remain in the broth. (See *Kitchen Keys* for further information.)
   STORE leftover veggies in glass jars with lids in the refrigerator. The kids can see them clearly and will devour them for snacks, or you can use them in tomorrow's lunch or salad. If you store leftovers in opaque plastic containers you may forget to use them while they are still fresh.
   SAVE any water left over from vegetable cooking for soups and stews. Diane once recommended to a friend that she use her vegetable-cooking water to nourish her plants. She forgot to mention that she uses no salt in the cooking of the veggies. Her friend used salt and all her plants died. Maybe people should listen to plants as well as talk to them.
4. Be sure to read *P.S. Stone-Age Food for Space-Age People,* page 242, which further defines most of the whole foods that are mentioned throughout this book.

A Nationwide Goal

The U.S. Senate Select Committee on Nutrition and Human Needs published an outline for Dietary Goals in January, 1977, backed by such prominent Senators as Hubert Humphrey, George McGovern, Robert Dole, and Charles Percy. This was challenged by certain industries with vested interests, but received over-all support from a majority of farmers, food retailers, government officials, scientists, and consumer advocates, as well as endorsement from many nutritionists, health educators and members of the medical professions.

The purpose of the report was to more accurately inform the general public of the relationship between eating habits and the development of disease. This has resulted in an increased awareness of nutrition and a healthy curiosity for learning more about how food affects the body. The news media now have frequent articles and exposes regarding the latest developments in the areas of health, diet, exercise, nutrition, and chemical pollution of air, water, soil, and food.

Though we may be conditioned to consume highly questionable foods, we should all make some effort to incorporate the Committee's recommendations in our food selection and preparation. The following recommendations are nearly identical to the Basic Four Unprocessed Diet segment of the Diet Horizons Chart:

1. Increase consumption of fruits and vegetables and whole grains.
2. Decrease consumption of meat and increase consumption of poultry and fish.
3. Decrease consumption of foods high in fat and partially substitute poly-unsaturated fat for saturated fat.
4. Substitute non-fat milk for whole milk.
5. Decrease consumption of butterfat, eggs and other high cholesterol sources.
6. Decrease consumption of sugar and foods high in sugar content.
7. Decrease consumption of salt and foods high in salt content.

In the past, persons who were wise enough to avoid instant convenience foods and put these dietary principles into effect for natural living and healing were adversely labeled "health food nuts." They are to be commended, not ridiculed, for practicing for a lifetime what the public is just now beginning to accept as valid: that Nature designed the best diet.

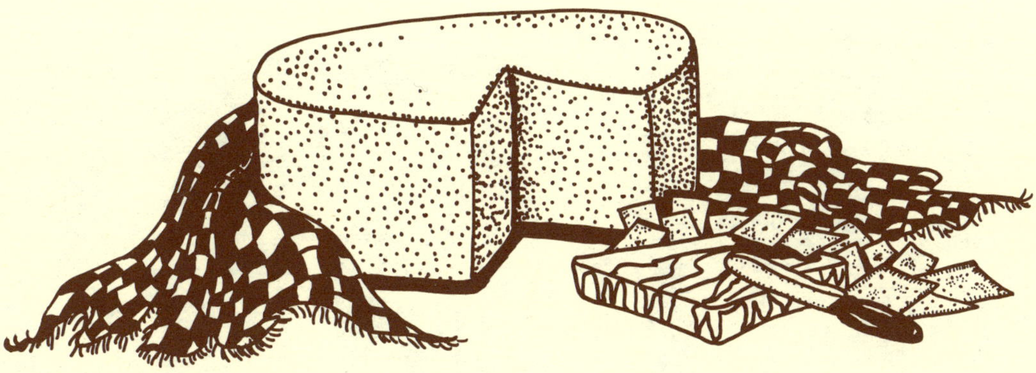

The journey of a thousand miles starts with a single step. *Chinese Proverb*

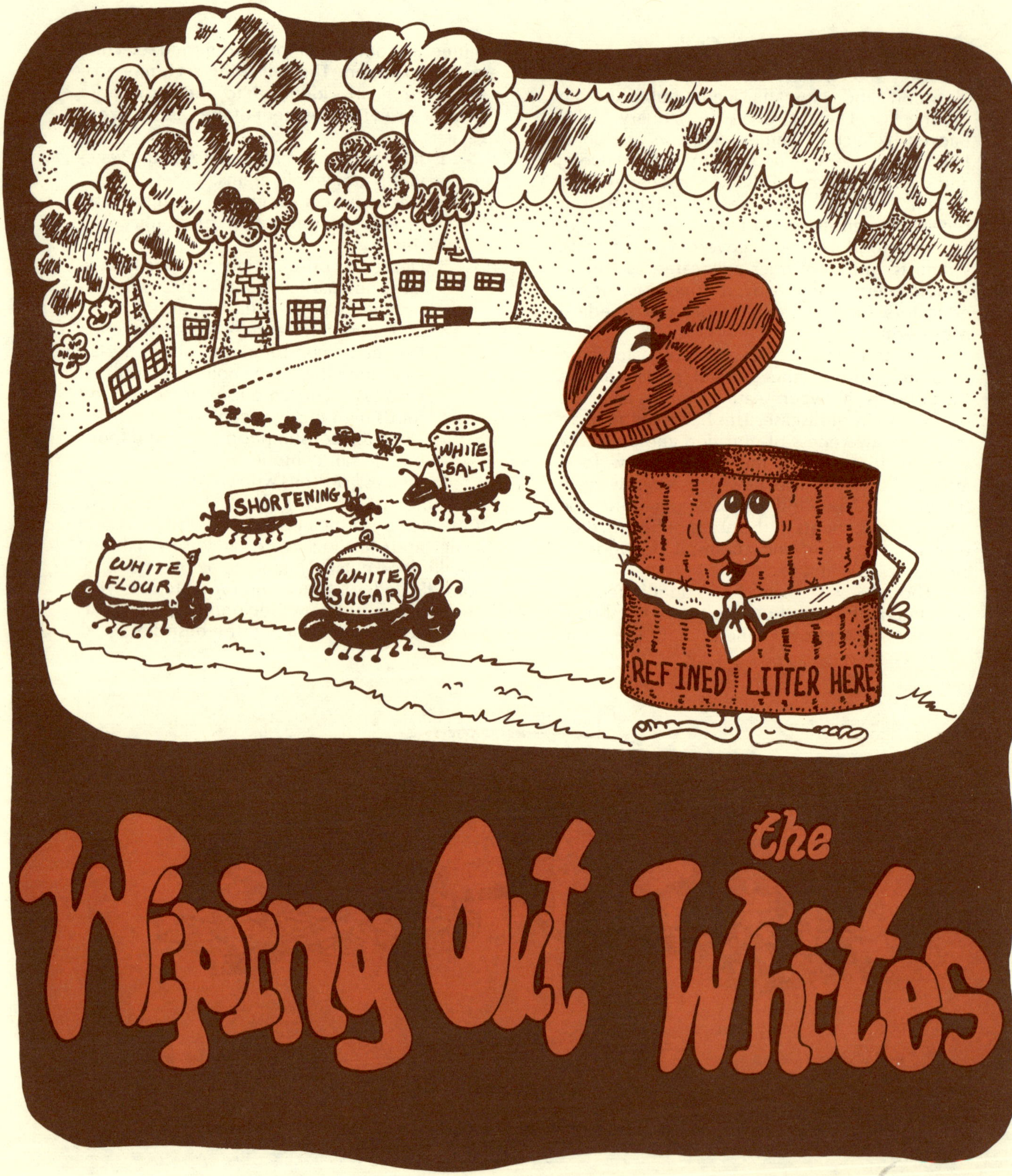

Wiping Out the Whites

Wiping Out The Whites

Fast Food Mania

In our highly technological society
We fear there is little sobriety.
As we become participants in the human rat race,
Our demands for "fast food" increase their pace.

We need to have pre-prepared food that won't spoil,
That can be zapped with a microwave; wrapped in foil,
And taken wherever we're running, to be eaten.
But this kind of food is really cheatin'.

It's cheatin' our bodies of good nutrition,
Yet few of us stop on our own volition.
We like the convenience. What time it saves!
Yet all it does is make us slaves

Slaves to the modern food processing plants,
Slaves to the advertisers' million dollar chants.
Our minds boggle at the newest "sure winner."
Our children scream, "Get Zonkies for dinner!"

Concession stands are big offenders,
Though perhaps the worst are machines without vendors,
That silently sit there awaiting our change,
Then noisily shoot out the snacks. Well, it's strange,

How people are so willing to sacrifice.
If it's FAST, they're ready to pay any price.
It's "instant" rice instead of a whole grain dish,
And great big macs rather than broiled fish.

It's chips and soda pop, gum and candy,
When fresh fruit and juices are so plentiful and handy.
Now, you ask what's so bad about food that's fast?
If we told you all the facts you'd be truly aghast!

For instant, colorful, prepackaged junk
Is laced with ingredients that would make us flunk

A test to describe and identify.
Why, we can't even pronounce them, hard as we try!

There's artificial colors, flavors and preservatives,
Emulsifiers, stabilizers; that's being conservative.
Sugar and salt — used in most foods as fillers
Even though ol' Doc admits they can be killers.

Let's look at a typical fast foods' meal,
Then you decide if it's for "real."
A hot dog with sodium nitrite and red dye;
Potatoes-first frozen-then in rancid oil, deep fried.

A cola with caramel, sacharrine and caffeine,
Or a shake without any milk or ice cream.
Mix all in your stomach — to say the least,
Your meal is a genuine chemical feast.

Now the top five diseases, plaguing our nation,
Are diseases of modern civilization.
Non-existent in primitive African tribes
Who don't eat red meat, chew tobacco or imbibe.

Who don't consume sugar, white flour or salt.
That's great for them, but where lies the fault?
Our ancestors' ancestors' food was still pure,
Unadulterated and NOT instant, that's for sure.

Their vegetables and fruits were fresh and unsprayed.
Their whole grain bread was freshly made.
Their method of preservation was to dry by the sun,
Rather than load food with chemicals by the ton.

But since the Industrial Revolution,
Our food has undergone fast evolution.
Rapid progress explains our increased pollution;
We worry and fret over a possible solution.

While our bodies' adjustments are gradual and slow,
The synthetic carcinogen list seems to grow,
So, become a label reader; to the managers announce,
That you refuse to buy what you can't pronounce.

Demand that your produce is fresh from the farm.
Anything canned or boxed might cause harm.
For a good diet, eat food with living vibrations,
Unladen with chemicals under investigation.

Eat whole foods prepared with T.L.C.
The extra time is worth it, you will see.
Once-deadened taste buds will bloom and flower;
You'll zippity-doo-da through your day with new power.

"The proof is in the puddin'" as the old adage goes,
And that proof is when you feel good — from your head to your toes.
From the beginning to the end — and all through the middle,
REAL food is much too big to belittle!

Good Intentions

The refining of the "whites" — salt, shortening, sugar and flour — was originally intended to make a wider variety of products available to a larger segment of society. Since spoiled food benefits neither the producer not the consumer, great pains were taken to remove anything from packaged food that could cause spoilage.

At first the purpose was legitimate and we doubt that any thought was given to the loss of the life-force or nutrients by removing selected parts of the whole food. But today we know better. We know that the whites are unnecessarily used in processed foods as fillers and to satisfy taste addictions, mostly of sweet and salty. Chemicals are added to flavor, color, stabilize, emulsify or preserve the product in order to make it last as long as possible on the grocery shelves or in home cupboards.

Unfortunately, highly processed foods containing the whites and chemical additives are all too prevalent in fast food establishments, cafeterias and vending machines, where the criterion is to feed the largest number of people for the least amount of money. The health of the patron is rarely considered.

Famous professionals with impressive titles receive exorbitant sums to publicly promote the safety and validity of the whites, while debunking the entire natural food movement as quackery. These vested interests are quick to indicate that sugar provides energy, enriched flour is just as good as whole grain, and fortified cold cereals — regardless of sugar content — meet the government's standards for a complete and balanced meal. (When served with milk, fruit, eggs and toast, *anything* would meet the standards!)

Though our hearts told us otherwise, there was a time when we listened to these obscure statements because they were tidy, expedient and spoken with authority. Today is different. Today we know we have a choice. We do our own research, we set our own standards and we trust our own intelligence. We hope that this chapter will spur you to explore a more complete history of the whites. *Sugar Blues* by William Dufty is a great place to begin.

Salt — Licking the Problem

Research indicates that excess sodium contributes to high blood pressure, a disease once reserved for the elderly, but now diagnosed in young adults, children and even babies. Sodium silico-aluminate, an unnecessary chemical, is added to make the salt free-flowing. Why wait until you have to be put on a low-salt or salt-free diet? Have the entire family cut down now as a preventative. Although we include minimum amounts of sea salt in our recipes, we hope that as your tastebuds adjust, you will decrease the amount of salt and increase the amount of herbs and spices.

WHAT YOU CAN DO

1. **Observe for one week the number of foods you serve which list salt as an ingredient. Try to differentiate between a food's flavor and mere saltiness.**
2. **Replace table salt with three parts kelp granules to one part sea salt. Both are rich in minerals and kelp is a good natural source of iodine.**
3. **During periods of high humidity, add a few grains of rice to your sea salt/kelp shaker to prevent caking.**
4. **Make some Gomazio (twelve parts toasted, crushed, sesame seeds to one part sea salt), keep it on your dining table and use it in place of salt.**
5. **Recycle old salt. Use it to clean your cast iron skillets. Just sprinkle in a teaspoon of salt and rub with a paper towel. Voila! Clean and ready to use again. (See** ***Holiday Harmony*** **for other ideas on salt recycling.)**

MSG — The Sly One

Monosodium glutamate is a flavor enhancer produced from wheat or corn gluten, or from sugar-beet by-products, all common allergens. Not only does MSG enhance flavor and preserve color, it also has anti-oxidant properties; thus possessing a remarkable ability to disguise poor quality food. As little as one-fourth teaspoonful can trigger an adverse reaction in sensitive individuals. MSG was removed from most baby food in 1969 by public pressure, after tests showed brain and eye damage to new-born mice.

Beatrice Trum Hunter, in *Consumer Beware!*, states that since 1972, more than 40 million pounds of MSG have been poured into American foodstuffs each year, an unbelievable figure that is expected to double in our lifetime. Over 10,000 different processed food products contain MSG and most restaurants use it lavishly to help their food taste better. Dormant taste buds can be revived and taught to enjoy the old-fashioned succulence of old-fashioned food, without the addition of MSG.

WHAT YOU CAN DO

1. **Experiment with basil, thyme, parsley, cumin, turmeric, tarragon, dill and other herbs and spices which will augment the delicate flavor of the vegetable or grain dish.**
2. **Make your own salad dressings, soups, gravies and mayonnaise from scratch.**
3. **If you eat in restaurants frequently, make an effort to find ones that will honor your request to exclude MSG from your meal. Take your own salad dressing. Better yet, discover a natural foods restaurant, whose proprietors are usually health-conscious and avoid using questionable products.**
4. **Scrutinize labels and deliberately avoid anything that contains MSG, a totally non-essential and highly questionable substance.**

Fats — The Greasy Story

Lard is a solid animal fat, high in cholesterol and low in nutrients, while shortening and margarine are hydrogenated vegetable oils. Hydrogenation is a chemical process that uses high temperatures, hydrogen and nickel or other catalysts to saturate the oil. The result is so unpalatable that it must be bleached, filtered, deodorized, and in some cases, dyed and flavored to make it acceptable. While the finished products — satin smooth shortening and spreadable margarine designed to fool Mother Nature — are certainly convenient, current medical research indicates a need for further studies of the possible effects of prolonged use.

WHAT YOU CAN DO

1. **Substitute cold-pressed, poly-unsaturated oils, such as soy, sunflower, corn, sesame, safflower or olive oil for hydrogenated fats. Refrigerate after opening.**
2. **Use fresh, undyed butter in small quantities to provide some trace minerals and nutrients.**
3. **Replace margarine with SunButterBlend: 2 parts undyed butter mixed with 1 part cold-pressed sunflower oil.**
4. **Make your own nut and seed butters: blenderize nuts or seeds to a fine powder, adding just enough oil to hold together.**
5. **Purchase old-fashioned, stir-before-using, unhydrogenated peanut butter and keep refrigerated.**
6. **Avoid high temperatures and deep-fat frying. Instead, broil, bake, steam or saute'.**
7. **Use shortening to grease bread pans. Oil doesn't work as well.**
8. **Recycle your deep fryer as an extra crock pot or for heating candle wax.**

Sugar — A Spun Tale

Statistics show that sugar consumption is actually dropping, so be on the alert! The sugar industry will be "hyping" sweets more than ever in an effort to increase sales. Don't be a victim of the "sugar provides you with energy" pitch. Get your energy from fresh food, fresh air and exercise.

The refining of sugar involves toxic chemicals and gases which leave the white crystals devoid of vitamins and minerals inherent in the original cane, corn or beet. This crystalline substance — white sugar — has been repeatedly connected to the pitiful condition of teeth, the growing problem of obesity and the awesome increase of diabetes in our society. Yet food manufacturers have added it to nearly everything that is canned or packaged.

Sour Statistics

"Consumer Reports," March, 1978, lists Coffee-Mate as containing 65.4% sugar; Jell-O, 82.6% sugar; and Shake'n Bake-Barbeque Style, 50.9% sugar. "The Journal of Dentistry," Fall 1974, lists King Vitaman with 61.6% sugar and twenty-six other cold cereals with over 40% added sugar. Despite recriminations, the sale of sugary breakfast foods continues to increase. Most of the commercials during Saturday morning television programming promote presweetened cereals, candy bars or artificially colored and flavored drinks. But where are those comical commercial characters when your child is sitting in a dentist's chair? Is it not ironic that, the same person who cheerfully and without reserve, spends good money for junk food, begrudgingly pays the dentist, whose task it is to repair the destruction wrought by those expensive sweets?

Why We're Hooked

Aside from the sheer taste of sugar, what makes it so appealing that we devour 120 pounds per person per year? Propaganda. Billions of dollars in advertising inform us daily of "how $weet it is!" We are trained from the cradle to the grave to win friends and influence people by engaging in sweet tactics. Children are pacified, coaxed, bribed, rewarded, sympathized with and apologized to by means of sweets. Wives, lovers and sweethearts are serenaded with highly sugared chocolates for any and all occasions.

Many children's clubs and athletic programs promote the health and welfare of kids, then obligate them to sell candy in order to keep their club operating. The sponsoring candy companies can easily afford to allow a high return for the organization because they're guaranteed nation-wide sales, low overhead, no salaries and probably a tax deduction for their "contributions" to charity. Even church bake sales spoil the aura of benevolence by contributing more to the sugar industry than they are able to gain locally.

An occasional dessert has its place in our society, and nutritious snacks are of definite value in maintaining even blood sugar levels. But unfortunately, nibble and snack are The American Way, and most nibblers and snackers prefer sugary treats. Is sugar addictive? Try going one solid week without any sugar (including all the hidden stuff like toothpaste). Write down what you experience in terms of mental, physical and emotional reactions. Then compare your symptoms with an ex-smoker's or drug addict's explanation of withdrawal. If truth-in-labeling laws were totally honest, sugar would be listed as an addictive, delayed-action drug.

The Sugar Connection

A stalk of sugar cane one yard long is enough to make only one teaspoon of refined white sugar. A snack of pie, ice cream and soda pop, may be the equivalent of 20 yards of sugar cane! At least the cane contains nutrients, fiber, and due to all the chewing required, would take some time to eat. How long does it take to devour the average dessert? The regrettable side of the story is that a child may be half the size of his/her parent, yet enjoy an equal dessert portion. In terms of body weight, the child ingests *two to four times* as much sugar as the adult.

As far back as 1945, Dr. Weston Price chronicled his lifetime of research into refined diets and their effect on natives who for generations had thrived on whole foods and then succumbed to "American diseases" after consuming modern, imported foods. Dr. Price's book, *Nutrition and Physical Degeneration,* should be at the top of every reading list and available in every library in the world.

While scientists continue to study the effects of excessive sugar and refined foods on our health, many doctors are already prescribing low sugar diets — along with a fitness program and mega-vitamin therapy — for dealing with the modern diseases of hyperactivity, allergies, alcoholism, schizophrenia, body chemistry imbalance and hypoglycemia. The Drs. Lendon Smith, Roger Williams, Elizabeth Rees, Carl Pfeiffer, Emanuel Cheraskin and other open-minded medical pioneers have repeatedly linked our refined diet to these and other degenerative diseases.

State Corrections Training Officer for Washington State Criminal Justice Training Commission, Alexander Schauss, has completed the first controlled study relating diet to delinquency, published in his book, *Diet, Crime and Delinquency.* Another book he authored, *Orthomolecular Treatment of Criminal Offenders,* examines dietary patterns and nutritional intake of chronic delinquents. He rehabilitates juvenile offenders using a bio-chemical-ecological approach.

Barbara Reed, Chief Probation Officer for the Municipal Court of Cuyahoga Falls, Ohio, has captured the attention of hundreds of parole and probation departments throughout the nation as a result of her years of success in treating criminals and delinquents with a low sugar, high protein and fiber diet. These are two pioneers who, through their work and application of a good diet, have proven the relationship of poor diet to anti-social behavior. They have opened new doors by helping young people out of the chains of juvenile delinquency and into a normal life; even those who were once considered hopeless have responded well to their programs.

Meanwhile, many other dedicated professionals in preventive and whole-istic health continue to study the relationship of a high-sugar diet to over-all health, in spite of raised eyebrows and open criticism by their peers. Watch for their up-to-the-minute research and information for they will certainly open more new doors.

Daring ideas are like chessmen moved forward; they may be beaten but they may start a winning game.
Johann Wolfgang von Goethe

WHAT YOU CAN DO

1. **Everything we eat is converted to sugar or "energy," but natural sources, such as fructose and complex carbohydrates allow the body to be the processor. Your body will take what it needs from the whole food; known nutrients as well as unknown; then use the indigestible cellulose to properly and naturally dispose of whatever it doesn't need. We don't know a commercial processor who can measure up to that standard!**
2. **Purchase nothing that has sugar, brown sugar, corn syrup, artificial maple syrup, dextrose, maltose, sucrose, non-nutritive sweetener or any combination of these on the list of ingredients. Refuse to be enticed by eye-catching earth tone boxes. Direct your eye to the label, then go home and make your own.**
3. **Instead of looking for a sugar substitute, learn to savor and distinguish the many subtle flavors of fruits, nuts, seeds and spices; lightly sweet and naturally satisfying.**
4. **When you must sweeten, replace sugar in a recipe with half as much raw, unfiltered honey, or use unsulphured molasses, date sugar, barley malt, or real maple syrup.**
5. **Reduce the natural sweeteners in a recipe, by one teaspoon each time, until you achieve the right delicate sweetness and mellow flavor.**
6. **Suggest to the leaders of youth organizations that they look to sources other than candy for raising funds — yard work, circus, benefit concerts, or selling nuts or useful household items.**

Flour — Sifting Through the Evidence

Before the 1860's and the invention of the steel roller mill, whole grains were consumed by nearly everyone. Only royalty and the very wealthy were able to afford the small amounts of white flour available, because the refining process was time-consuming and costly. Most of the general populace ate coarse, dark bread which became known as "peasant's bread." The roller mill made the separation of the bran, germ and starch of the grain far more rapid and inexpensive, so that a great number of people could afford to emulate the upper classes by switching to refined breads. White flour was assigned a status quo of its own, while the good stuff (the bran and germ) ended up as animal feed.

Enriched Means Robbed

It took half a century to discover that many of the important vitamins, minerals and protein were concentrated in the wheat germ while the bran was an important source of fiber. Yet today's mills continue to separate, refine, and bleach the whole grain. They also scantily enrich the patent flour by returning a few of the twenty to thirty known nutrients removed in processing. Compare this to someone robbing $25.00 from you, then in a moment of remorse, returning $5.00. Would you feel enriched? The powdery dust known as white flour looks clean and pure and has a long shelf life, but it does little to enrich *your* life.

WHAT YOU CAN DO

1. **Read Labels. Many of the whole grain breads on supermarket shelves are deceiving to the novice natural foods shopper. While containing anywhere from 50-100% whole wheat flour, some breads also contain caramel for a brown color, stabilizers or preservatives to increase shelf life, sugar or corn syrup, and a percentage of enriched, unbleached flour.**
2. **Home-baked bread is your best choice. Besides tasting great, it is a warm and gratifying experience to bake bread. Kneading is good exercise, and working with the smooth, elastic dough can even be therapeutic. Rising extra early to bake bread and rolls is also an excellent discipline. If time is a problem, find a reputable baker who doesn't add the "extras," OR trade your expertise in another area for a friend's homemade loaves of whole grain goodness.**
3. **Select cereals that have undergone the least steps in processing. Try multi-grain cereals, made from rolled, cracked or flaked grain combinations of rye, barley, oats and/or wheat, or millet and rice, with chopped nuts or dried fruit sometimes added. Cooking time varies between eight and twenty minutes, but they can be prepared the night before and just reheated for breakfast.**
4. **Use stoneground whole wheat (hard, red, winter) flour for most purposes. For pastries and lighter cakes and shortbreads, try whole wheat pastry (soft, spring) flour; experiment with soy, rye, buckwheat, barley, triticale and oat flours. Rice, millet and potato flours are mild and blend well with other flours. Wheatberries or whole oats, millet, barley or buckwheat groats cook just like rice. They add a rich nutty flavor, whether combined with onions and herbs for a side dish, or fruits and nuts for a dessert.**
5. **Purchase whole grains that have been kept cool, dry and dark and keep them the same way at home. Once grains are ground into flour, they must be refrigerated.**
6. **See** *Holiday Harmony* **for unique ways to recycle white flour and pastas.**

Chemical Coersion

The Delaney Clause of 1958 states that any chemical known to cause cancer in animals may not be deemed safe for use in the human food supply. Yet of the 10,000 plus chemical additives on the market, at this time at least thirteen are known or strongly suspected to be carcinogenic (cancer causing). Though testing appears rigorous, few chemicals warrant the trust we place in them just because they carry Federal Drug Administration (FDA) approval.

By innocently combining some foods and/or drugs, we could be mixing the potentially hazardous chemicals inside our bodies much the same way Dr. Jekyll might have whipped up a mysterious potion. Eating could be a veritable timebomb when we're playing around with unknown substances. Even the FDA's "Generally Regarded As Safe" list apparently isn't. Remember, cyclamates and red dye #2, banned in 1970 and 1976 respectively, rested comfortably under the GRAS security blanket at one time. MSG was on the GRAS list and used in baby food in spite of medical evidence indicating nerve damage to new-born mice. It took hard-working, self-supporting, consumer groups to lay the foundation for the ultimate removal of MSG from baby foods.

Food industries continue to excuse themselves from responsibility for possible side-effects of chemicals by publishing full page, rational-sounding arguments (predominantly in women's magazines) supporting the "need" for chemical additives. *They* reap the benefits ($$$) while *we* assume the risks (???). We have the right to life, liberty and the pursuit of happiness, but apparently not the right to know what's really in our food. Most parents desire to serve their children wholesome food, but in many instances, if the box were shredded, puffed, fortified, then analyzed, it would be as nutritious as the contents.

WHAT YOU CAN DO

1. **Make your own WE/I LOVE YOUR BODY labels, listing all the wholesome ingredients you put into your homemade foods. The conspicuous absence of sugar and chemicals will get your family used to reading natural labels and may provide the tools they need to make intelligent decisions when they're away from home.**
2. **Read** *Consumer Beware!,* **a very informative book by Beatrice Trum Hunter, and an expose' of the food industry's disregard for potential long-term health hazards — an excellent reference book for the novice or seasoned health seeker.**
3. **Order "Chemical Cuisine," a poster from the Center for Science in the Public Interest. This guide lists and defines many common additives in our foods. It suggests those dyes and flavorings to avoid because of poor testing or carcinogenic possibilities; it cautions against additives that may be unsafe and lists some foods they're found in; and names additives, many of them natural, which at this time appear to be safe. Send $1.75 to C.S.P.I., 1755 S Street, N.W., Washington D.C., 20009.**
4. **Commercial ice cream is one of the most synthetic, chemical-laden substances available for human consumption. Make your own or search out the new natural ice creams and frozen yogurts produced by companies who use honey and natural flavorings. Until ice cream companies voluntarily put ingredient labels on their packages, they simply are not to be trusted.**

This cake was prepared in the kitchen of the ____________ family with these wholesome ingredients: stoneground wholewheat flour, fresh grated carrots, cold-pressed sunflower oil, unfiltered clover honey, farm fresh eggs, pure vanilla extract, homemade baking powder, and a cup-that-runneth-over of love.

Take Charge of the Rest of Your Life

No matter what your age, occupation or physical condition, *today* is the day to decide if you want your health in later years to reflect repeated assaults from adulterated food, drugs and chemicals; or to reflect persistent efforts to provide genuine food, combined with vigorous exercise and a positive lifestyle that make junk food and drugs undesirable. Obesity, high blood pressure, hemorrhoids, varicose veins, osteoporosis, diverticulitis and colitis are not communicable diseases. They do not occur as a result of lack of refrigeration, unsanitary conditions, rodent plague, insect bite, improper canning procedures or germs. Though generally associated with aging, these diseases are more likely the consequences of a lifetime of deleterious eating habits, repeated consumption of devalued food and a sedentary existence.

We are creatures of habit, but we can set aside old habits in favor of new when we know that the goal — a full and healthy life — is worth working toward. After we judiciously save money for retirement, shouldn't we maintain our bodies too, so that we can enjoy those retirement years in good health?

The Labels Game

On the following pages are lists of brand-name products and their ingredients, stated exactly as written on their packages, cans, or bottles. Now that you're more likely to be reading labels, play a little Match Game to check your adeptness at deciphering ingredients and additives in common processed foods.

It has been so long since we have purchased processed food that we were appalled at the enormous amount of really unnecessary additives and preservatives poured into expensive "foods" that are just as easy and inexpensive to prepare at home from two or three main ingredients. It's incredible to think that though dehydration is the oldest and safest form of preservation, commercially dehydrated products still contain preservatives.

Realize that chemicals are big business. When nine million pounds of BHT were produced for foods in 1976, according to "Make It Fresh," an article in October's *Prevention* magazine, and 40 million pounds of MSG are dumped annually into foods, as pointed out by Ms. Hunter in *Consumer Beware!*, one can not refute the profits involved. Think of the tons of other chemicals added to our food supply for which there is no published statistical compilation of amounts!

One matter of interest we noted on our label-reading trip through the food market is that many companies are now letting the consumer know the purpose of each chemical, such as "gum tragacanth (for color)," or "glyceryl-abietate (emulsifier)." Is this a mandatory step, provided for the consumer's information? Or is it a voluntary step taken by the processor in hopes that the consumer will no longer question the additive when its use is "understood?"

Play The Labels Game. See if you can match the ingredients with the product. When you try to determine the differences between dog food, baby food and canned dinners, you'll be amazed at the contradictions (and similarities) of ingredients and nutritional value.

THE LABELS GAME

Game 1 — Match Each Brand Name Product with its Set of Ingredients Below

a. a fruit-flavored gelatin (box)
b. an Italian gravy mix (package)
c. a fruit-flavored drink (package)
d. a seasoned barbeque flavored crumb topping for chicken (box)
e. a cream of chicken soup mix (package)
f. a so-called old-fashioned lemonade drink (bottle)
g. orange marshmallow candies, shaped like peanuts (package)
h. a vegetable beef soup mix (package)

Ingredients

1. Ingredients: salt, Hydrolyzed Wheat Protein, Hydrolyzed Cereal Solids, Dehydrated Garlic, Modified Starch, Dehydrated Onion, Mono Sodium Glutamate, Spices, Chicken Fat, Silicon Dioxide (anti-caking agent), artificial flavors, Disodium Guanylate, Disodium Inosinate.
2. Ingredients: sugar, gelatin, adipic acid, disodium phosphate, fumaric acid, artificial color, natural flavor with BHA, artificial flavor.
3. Ingredients: sugar, modified cornstarch, salt, tomato powder, brown sugar, partially hydrogenated soybean, cottonseed and palm oils, whey (from milk), spices, gum tragacanth (vegetable gum thickener), citric and malic acids (for tartness), beet powder (for color), Dextrin (from corn), paprika and extractives of paprika (for color), Mono Sodium Glutamate (flavor enhancer), distilled vinegar, dextrose (corn sugar), artificial flavor, garlic powder, yeast, artificial color, natural flavor, onion powder, hydrolyzed vegetable protein (for flavor).
4. Ingredients: enriched egg noodle product, natural flavors, dehydrated vegetables (potatoes, carrots, green beans and onion powder), wheat flour, salt, dried corn syrup, Mono Sodium Glutamate (flavor enhancer), sugar, dehydrated beef, isolated soy protein, potato starch, caramel color, vegetable gum, cornstarch, hydrogenated vegetable oil (contains one or more of the following oils: cottonseed, soybean, palm), garlic, dehydrated, dehydrated parsley — spices.
5. Ingredients: water, nutritive sweetener (sugar and/or corn sweetener), citric acid (for tartness), sodium citrate (controls acidity), gum acacia (vegetable gum-provides body), vitamin C, sodium benzoate and potassium sorbate (preservatives), glycerylabietate (emulsifier), natural flavorings, sodium metabisulfite (preservative), triethyl citrate, triglycerides, dioctyl sodium sulfosuccinate (stabilizer), artificial color, BHA (preserves freshness), ascorbyl palmitate (emulsifier).
6. Ingredients: sugar, citric acid (for tartness), mono calcium phosphate (controls acidity), natural and artificial flavors, artificial color and Vitamin C.
7. Ingredients: sugar, corn syrup, gelatin, artificial flavor and artificial color.
8. Ingredients: spray dried hydrogenated coconut oil, modified food starch, dried corn syrup, natural flavors, salt, whey solids, MSG (flavor enhancer), dehydrated chicken, non-fat milk solids, vegetable gum, dehydrated onions, buttermilk solids, dehydrated parsley, oleoresin turmeric, disodium inosinate and disodium guanylate (flavor enchancer).

Answers: a2, b1, c6, d3, e8, f5, g7, h4.

Game 2 — Match Each Brand Name Product with its Set of Ingredients Below

i. a loaf of white bread (plastic-wrapped)
j. a chocolate fudge frosting mix (box)
k. a devil's food cake mix (box)
l. a dry cereal (box)
m. individually wrapped chocolate cream pastries (box)
n. a green goddess salad dressing (bottle)
o. a dietetic vanilla flavored pudding mix (box)
p. a whipped topping mix (box)

Ingredients

9. Ingredients: sugar and dextrose, enriched bleached flour, partially hydrogenated soybean oil, cocoa processed with alkali, leavening (baking soda, dicalcium phosphate, sodium aluminum phosphate, mono-calcium phosphate), propylene glycol monoesters, modified food starch, iodized salt, mono and diglycerides, cellulose gum, artificial flavors, soy protein isolate, dried whey solids, artificial coloring.
10. Ingredients: modified corn starch, potassium chloride, carrageenan, artificial flavor, 0.38% calcium saccharin, a non-nutritive artificial sweetener which should be used only by persons who must restrict their intake of ordinary sweets. 25 mg. saccharin per serving and artificial color.
11. Ingredients: sugar, whey, animal and/or vegetable shortening (may contain one or more of the following: partially hydrogenated beef tallow, soybean oil, coconut oil, palm kernel, cottonseed oil, palm oil, lard, with mono and diglycerides), enriched bleached flour (niacin, iron, thiamine mononitrate, mono-calcium phosphate), salt, soy flour, eggs, artificial flavor, carboxy methyl cellulose, lecithin, agar.
12. Ingredients: sugar, dried corn syrup, cocoa, animal and/or vegetable shortening (contains one or more of the following partially hydrogenated fats: soybean oil, cottonseed oil, beef tallow, palm oil, and/or lard), with freshness preserved by BHA and BHT, wheat starch, salt, artificial flavor, mono and diglycerides, polysorbate 60, sodium caseinate.
13. Ingredients: degermed yellow corn meal, sugar, cocoa processed with alkali, corn syrup, natural cocoa, salt, malted milk, coconut oil, corn starch, guar gum, artificial and natural flavors, carrageenan, sodium phosphate, sodium ascorbate (Vitamin C), calcium carbonate, niacin, iron, Vitamin A, Vitamin B6, Vitamins B12, B1, B2, and D2.

14. Ingredients: sugar, hydrogenated palm kernel oil, propylene glycol monostearate (emulsifiers for uniform blending of oil), corn syrup solids, sodium caseinate (a protein), whey (from milk), artificial flavor, sodium silico-aluminate (prevents caking), hydroxylated soybean lecithin and acetylated monoglycerides (emulsifiers), BHA and citric acid (preservatives), and artificial color.
15. Ingredients: enriched flour (flour, barley malt, potassium bromate, niacin, iron, thiamine, mononitrate, riboflavin (B Vitamins), water, corn syrup, soy oil, yeast, salt, corn flour, mono-calcium phosphate, sodium stearoyl-2-lactylate, soy flour, ammonium sulfate, calcium peroxide, calcium iodate, potassium iodate.
16. Ingredients: soybean oil, water, vinegar, sugar, sour cream, artificial sour cream, salt, spices, anchovy paste, Xanthan gum, polysorbate 60 and algin derivatives for consistency, dehydrated shallots, dehydrated onions, potassium sorbate and calcium disodium EDTA to preserve freshness, FD & C Yellow #5 and other artificial colors.

Answers: i15, j12, k9, l13, m11, n16, o10, p14.

Game 3 — Match Each Brand Name Product with its Set of Ingredients Below

a. a high meat beef dinner for babies (jar)
b. a roast beef spread for people (can)
c. a vegetable and beef dinner for babies (jar)
d. a high-protein dog food (can)
e. a chicken flavored dog food (can)
f. a beef ravioli dinner for people (can)

Following Are Ingredients for Two Dog Foods, Two Canned Meat Dinners and Two Baby Foods. Can You Tell the Difference? Compare Nutrition.

HINT: Two of the products say 100% natural, nutritious, no preservatives, no artificial color on their labels.
Two of the products say NO added salt, sugar, preservatives, artificial flavors or colors, MSG, or flavor enhancers.
Two of the products make no claims to naturalness or nutrition.

1. Ingredients: roast beef, water, hydrolyzed vegetable protein, salt, calcium reduced dried skim milk, modified food starch, lactose, onion powder, MSG, natural flavorings, sugar, cysteine hydrocholoride, disodium inosinate, disodium guanylate.
2. Ingredients: water, carrots, beef, rice flour, tomato puree, potatoes, wheat flour, green split peas, potato solids, rice, onion and torula yeast.
3. Ingredients: whole eggs, liver, chicken by-products, cracked yellow corn, soybean meal, wheat millrun, chicken parts, wheat germ meal, fish, meat and bone meal, soybean oil, beef by-products.
4. Ingredients: water, enriched wheat flour, beef, carrots, cooked beef, sugar, corn starch, cracker meal, modified food starch, salt, soy protein concentrate, cheddar cheese, textured vegetable protein (soy flour, soy protein isolate, caramel color), hydrolyzed plant protein, dehydrated onions, caramel color, citric acid, natural flavorings and oleoresin paprika.
5. Ingredients: water (added for processing), chicken by-products, liver, whole eggs, cracked yellow corn, soybean meal, chicken parts, wheat millrun, whole dressed chicken, fish, wheat germ meal, meat and bone meal, soy oil.
6. Ingredients: water, beef, rice flour, tomato puree, carrots, wheat flour, potato solids, torula yeast and onion.

Answers: a6, b1, c2, d3, e5, f4.
The dog food is 100% natural.
The baby food contains NO added salt, etc.
The people food makes no claims to naturalness or nutrition.

When your horse is on the brink of a precipice, it is too late to pull in the reins.

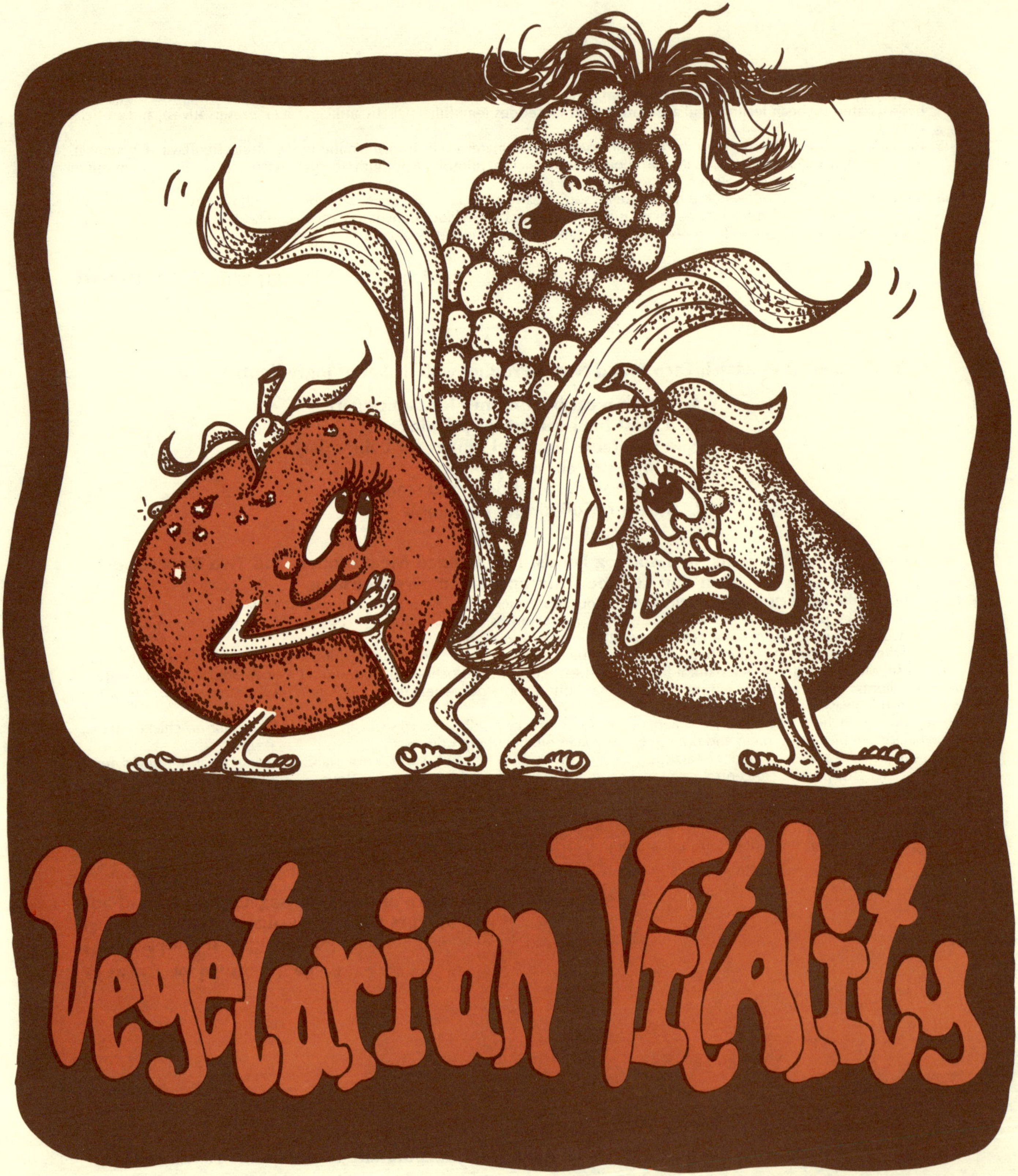
Vegetarian Vitality

Vegetarian Vitality

Vegetarian ABC's

What's a Vegetarian to Eat If Not Meat?

There's Avocados, Artichokes, Asparagus, all green,
Bananas, Berries, Barley . . . and Beans.
We eat Cabbage, Cucumber, Coconut, and Cashews,
Dates and Dried fruit that must be well-chewed.

Eggplant is Elegant, and all Fruit is sublime!
But Garlic and Grains stand the test of time.
We sip Herb teas with raw Honey; eat pure Ice Cream, homemade.
Drink rejuvenating Juices like carrot or lemonade.

There's Kefir, and Kelp, containing minerals from the sea.
Lima beans, Lentils, and other Legumes like split peas.
Millet, Mushrooms and Melons taste great,
And most varieties of raw Nuts are first rate!

Onions, Okra, and Oats are nutritious,
While Pineapples, Peaches and Plums are delicious!
Yes, it's Quality, not Quantity that really count.
So we eat Rice and Raisins in modest amounts.

St. John's bread (that's carob), contains vitamins you need.
For calcium and protein; find these in Seeds.
When you Sprout Sesame, alfalfa and Sunflower,
Without doubt, there's an increase in nutritive power!

How about Spinach, Squash, String beans and Swiss chard?
To prepare them, you steam them; it's not very hard.
Tamari is soy sauce; Tofu, a soy cheese.
We eat Tortillas and Tomatoes as much as we please.
Turmeric, Tahini, Triticale; in English, plain,
They're a seasoning, a butter, and a hybrid grain.

Understand that Vinegar is fine, if it's apple cider.
Whole grain pastas and breads; the selection's Wider,
When you can choose from soy, rye, millet or Wheat.
Whole grain chapatis are also good to eat.
Though labeled "enriched," White flour's deprived.
When fed to rats, they just don't survive.

X-cellent are the food choices for vegetarian cuisine.
If you've read this poem you know what we mean.
Yams are high in Vitamin A,
And Yogurt can be prepared a 100 ways.
Last is Zucchini; it's versatile too.
Now, what and how do we eat? Let's review!

We eat loaves and patties and burgers and roasts,
But there's a big difference, we can proudly boast.
For, instead of dead chickens, pigs, turkeys and cows,
They're made from grains, beans, nuts, veggies — that's how!

So, if you'd like to eat your meals without meat,
You know that it's really no magical feat.
It's healthy, humane, beautiful and cheap.
The food list is endless, as are the bounties you'll reap!

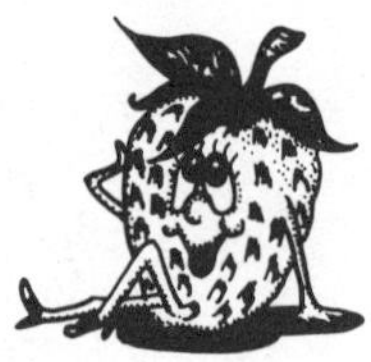

Why Vegetarianism?

A vegetarian diet may be the survival diet of the future. Today, self-motivated, independent people from a variety of lifestyles, age groups, social status and vocations state aesthetic, ecological, physical, economic, ethical and religious reasons for eliminating, or at least reducing their intake of meat. As we become more conscious of the mass starvation and malnutrition in our world as well as the millions of early deaths due to degenerative diseases, we can look to vegetarianism as an economical and nutritious way to feed the masses while conserving fuel, energy, land and money.

It takes ten times more land to raise
the cow
Than to grow the grain it must eat.
So conserve the land; get your protein
first-hand,
Eat the grain instead of the meat.

The term "vegetarian" was coined in 1842 in England. It comes from the Latin word "vegetus," meaning whole, sound, fresh, or lively. The ancient Latin term "homo vegetus" describes a mentally and physically vigorous person. Indeed, this was so of such renowned people as da Vinci, Emerson, Thoreau, Ghandi, George Bernard Shaw, and Dr. Albert Schweitzer — all vegetarians.

An increasing number of marathon runners, long distance bicyclists and other athletes are removing flesh from their diets — discovering that while meat-eating bogged them down; abstaining from meat and eating a high complex carbohydrate, whole foods diet increases energy, lengthens endurance, and accords them a clearer head and lighter body.

A Gas Shortage

Generally a vegetarian diet contains less fat, fewer calories, more fiber and a wider variety of foods. Other long term benefits include lower blood pressure, shorter digestion time, increased energy, stamina, endurance and resistance to disease. A vegetarian rarely experiences gas, indigestion, heartburn, constipation, lethargy, or shot nerves. Instead, most "veggies" have a sense of mental well-being and an overall desire to maintain optimum physical fitness.

You can get more disease from
a sparerib
Than munching on a bug-chewed leaf,
And more nutrition from
sunflower seeds
Than a high-cholesterol beef.

Vegetarian Terminology

A VEGAN eats no animal products, relying entirely on plants for survival.

A LACTO-VEGETARIAN eats a plant-based diet and includes milk products from either goats or cows.

A LACTO-OVO VEGETARIAN supplements a plant-based diet with fresh eggs and dairy products.

A PREDOMINANTLY VEGETARIAN person includes fish and sometimes fowl, making every effort to secure the freshest, least polluted or chemically treated product.

Some rivers are so polluted
You can't eat the fish that
you've caught.
Some beef is so shot with hormones
It'd be safer to just let it rot.

Regrouping the Food Groups

Classroom instruction of the conventional U.S.D.A. Basic Four Food Groups — two Meat, three Dairy, four Bread/Cereal and four Fruit/Vegetable servings daily — is usually accompanied by gorgeous full-color picture posters and handouts. It would seem visually, (the way most children learn) that one-half of our dietary intake should be protein, i.e. meats and dairy products, since these foods account for half the pictures on the posters.

MEAT: While legumes, nuts and seeds are mentioned under proteins, they are relegated to minor and insignificant positions, both verbally and pictorially. First, a huge roast and a thick juicy steak catch your eye, then a fish or a dozen eggs. A few beans and even a peanut or two may be scattered about the protein picture, but for the most part, children never learn of the beneficial combinations of less expensive forms of protein. The child's eye picks up the largest and most pronounced object in the picture and records in the brain: protein equals meat.

There is even a slant on the amount of protein required, as taught in the United States compared to other parts of the world. The WHO, (World Health Organization) recommends 37 grams of protein for an adult male, while the U.S. Recommended Daily Allowance (RDA) is 65 grams for adults and children over four. Is it possible that our "standards" are so much higher simply because we need to keep the economy flowing among the meat and dairy producers? Do we really *need* that much protein? Could the current rise in kidney disease possibly be contributed to by overloading the body with protein so that the kidneys must work double-time to deal with toxic protein by-products?

DAIRY PRODUCTS: In the dairy grouping a child will likely find a picture of cheese, already sliced and wrapped in individual plastic packets, and a carton of cottage cheese sitting next to a carton of milk. But the most colorful — therefore the most remembered — dairy product will be the ice cream, which may be topped with a gooey sauce or a facsimile of fruit. The visual association remains in the brain; the message is duly implanted: ice cream fulfills the quota for a dairy serving. Maybe a hundred years ago when ice cream was real, but not today.

CEREALS AND GRAINS: These are often represented by a loaf of bread (usually white) and a box of common grain, like oats. The picture may include an assortment of white pastas to fill in the scenery much the way they are used to fill out a skimpy meal. Simply because wholesome whole grains do not exist in the pictures, many children grow up never having enjoyed the delightful flavors of buckwheat, bulgur, barley, brown rice or millet.

They associate the word cereal with flashy boxes of cold, crinkled, processed-beyond-recognition grains which provide little more than a trinket in the bottom of the box while zapping their parents' pocketbooks. We can't really blame the cereal industry for marketing air-puffed cereals. After all, if people were willing to pay you for air at the going price of food, wouldn't you start selling it too? Even a few cents worth of added synthetic vitamins, nearly doubles the package price.

FRUITS AND VEGETABLES: Unfortunately, fruits and vegetables are sandwiched together in one U.S.D.A. Basic Four grouping, which insinuates that neither is important enough to have a category of its own. Is this a confirmation to us all that meat, milk and starches are the most prominent, while fruits and vegetables are among the also-ran, foodstuffs? We, as parents of growing children, see a definite need for directing more attention to fruits and vegetables as well as teaching the skills involved in preparing them to provide the most possible nutrients.

Fractured Foods

Conventional nutrition education spends a lot of time talking about whole, nutritious foods, then spends a good share of class activity time preparing high-sugar, high-starch, nutrient-depleted treats. Remember, in teaching children about nutrition, they will learn very little of what we say but nearly all of what they see and help us *do*. The most subtle incongruence of the conventional food groups formation lies in the inference that over-processed-then-fortified foods are equally as nutritious as their whole counterparts. A parent may rationalize that the family's nutritional needs have been met because so many servings of a particular category have been represented in each meal.

For example, lunch may be canned spaghetti, canned green beans, a slice of white bread with margarine, fruit-flavored gelatin and a pint of milk, with a choice of plain or chocolate. (Incidentally, this is not an uncommon selection from school lunch menus across the country.) By food groups, the lunch is believed to provide: spaghetti — one meat, one vegetable (tomato sauce), and one cereal (pasta); green beans — one vegetable; bread — one cereal and one fat; gelatin — one fruit; and of course, one milk serving.

Never mind the fact that the entire meal is so fractured by over-processing that the only nutritional value may be the small amount of synthetic vitamin fortification that must be added in order for the food to legally be called food! Disregard the likelihood that the beans are over-cooked, heavily salted and minus a good share of nutrients that went down the drain with the water; that the amount of meat in a can of spaghetti is not sufficient to meet complete protein needs; and that the gelatin is more sugar than anything else and can not possibly substitute for real fruit.

In reference to chocolate added to milk — can we ignore the studies done by Dr. Hal Huggins, D.D.S. (and reported at the Atlanta Dental Convention, in March, 1977) where animals in the chocolate milk group in Dr. Ralph Steinman's experiment, showed 400% increase in dental caries rate over the 62.5% sugar group and the whole milk group? Of course, there is more to that study than we can go into here. But let it suffice to say that giving children the choice of chocolate milk or fruit-flavored drinks over whole milk is like playing Russian roulette with their teeth. They have no idea of the consequences and therefore, should not be given the responsibility for deciding an issue that could have disastrous effects.

Generally speaking, the U.S.D.A. Basic Four Food Groups are too casual in their implication that all foods — regardless of their processing — are equally as nourishing and safe to the consumer. They also place far too much importance on meat and dairy products, giving the general public a biased viewpoint of what constitutes a healthy diet.

Infinite Possibilities

When meals are prepared at home from foods as close to their natural state as possible, and emphasis is on using a variety of different *kinds* of foods as well as different forms of preparation, there will be no need to rationalize or compartmentalize foods. The nutritional values will be superior when all parts of the food are used, and the whole foods will ensure a balance of complete proteins, carbohydrates, vitamins and minerals, as well as small but necessary amounts of fats.

To meet the body's daily requirements, weekly requirements, even lifelong requirements, foods (nutrients) must be consumed in their whole form. The following Whole Foods Basic Four chart is merely a guideline for a wide variety of menu possibilities and taste sensations. Rather than twenty ways to prepare hamburger — you will have twenty different legumes and grains to combine twenty-times-twenty different ways in conjunction with twenty different vegetables — the possibilities are as exciting as they are endless.

Forwarned, forarmed; to be prepared is half the victory. *Miguel de Cervantes*

WE LOVE YOUR BODY
WHOLE FOODS BASIC FOUR

1. GRAINS, LEGUMES, NUTS & SEEDS:
Five to seven servings daily, including breads.
2. VEGETABLES:
Four servings daily, including dark leafy greens in salads.
3. FRUITS:
Up to four servings daily with at least one raw citrus.
4. DAIRY PRODUCTS & EGGS:
Individual needs differ; children two to four dairy servings daily, adults one to three dairy servings daily. Three to six eggs per week.

(One serving equals one-half cup or eight ounces.)

Limited amounts of natural fats and oils are important "extras" in our diet. Nuts and seeds will provide some; other sources are olives, avocados, cold-pressed oils and fresh butter.

Food Combining for Quality Protein

Protein is necessary in the structure, maintenance and repair of every bone, muscle, hair and cell in the human body. Proteins are composed of building blocks called amino acids. Of the twenty-two amino acids, there are eight that the body cannot produce, but must obtain from outside sources. All eight must be present in the correct proportions for maximum utilization.

While meats and dairy products contain the eight essential amino acids, thus forming a complete protein, fruits, vegetables, nuts and grains usually lack one or more amino acids. Therefore, it becomes desirable to combine a food such as whole grain bread or crackers, which lack the amino acid lysine, with a dish of chili or a bean spread or dip, which is strong in lysine, thereby forming a complete protein. Legumes and grains complement each other beautifully.

Following is a diagram depicting non-meat protein foods and how they can be combined to form complete proteins. The heavier line indicates that *most* varieties in each group complement each other. The thin line shows that *some* varieties in each group combine well to supply the amino acids. NOTE: All dairy products are complete protein. If you choose to avoid dairy products, you will need to be more judicious about protein combinations and may wish to read *Diet for a Small Planet* by Frances Moore Lappe' or *Laurel's Kitchen* by Laurel Robertson.

The price of ham is expensive;
For lamb chops, it's 'out-of-sight.'
That's why I don't feel apprehensive
About having soyburgers tonight.

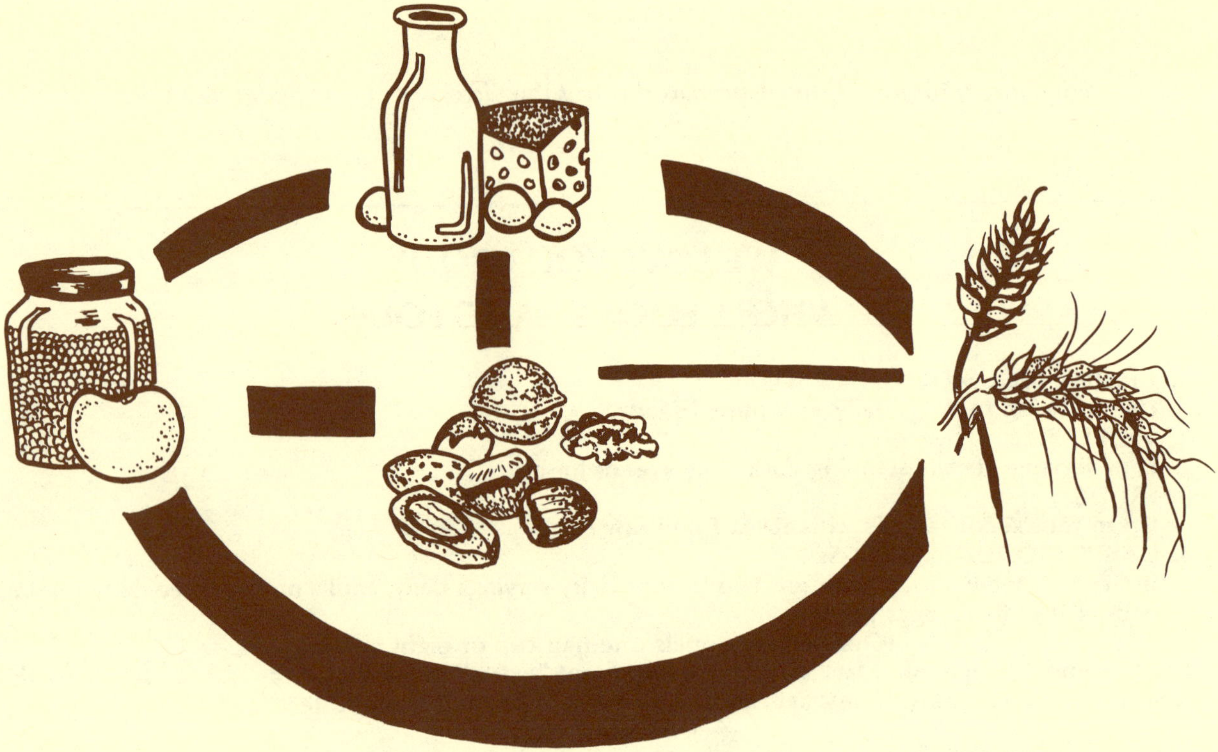

A Safe and Sane Diet

A vegetarian diet is not a sacrificing one! Quite the contrary, it simply means that you opt for an infinite array of whole grains, legumes, nuts and seeds, vegetables and fruits, and eggs and dairy products. Most vegetarians freely choose to adopt this pattern without any negative feelings of limiting their food choices, lifestyles or friends. If you've been advised by a doctor to reduce red meat intake, don't panic. Half the fun is in learning how to combine these foods for the best high quality protein utilization, while treating your tastebuds to some sensational cuisine.

There is nothing fanatical or risky about adhering to a sensible, balanced vegetarian diet. There is, however, a greater spiritual awareness of the oneness of all living things on this planet, and a positive acceptance of the close relationship we have with every living creature. Vegetarianism can be just the beginning of a more perceptive lifestyle in which we re-evaluate our value system, re-educate our educated minds, and re-sensitize our senses about world hunger, natural resource depletion and energy overconsumption.

The law of supply and demand
Is an economic fact of life.
To feed more people on less land,
We must use chopsticks instead of a knife.

As with most of the changes we have made in our effort to live a more natural lifestyle, we chose vegetarianism because it feels good. Listen to your body; give it the right raw materials every day and it will respond with unlimited dividends for a lifetime of good health.

WHAT YOU CAN DO

1. Make changes slowly, start with one or two meatless meals the first week and substitute fish or fowl for red meat at least twice a week.
2. Plan meals so the "main attraction" is a souffle, quiche, chef's salad or hearty soup; then relegate small portions of meat to side dishes. (See *Serendipity Suppers* for vegetarian main dishes.)
3. Have plenty of crisp, crunchy raw vegetables for snacks; and raw salads for mealtime.
4. Take care not to revert to packaged foods to "fill up" the plate as well as the stomach.
5. If your attitude is one of "giving up" meat, you may begin to substitute sweets. But remember, a processed, sweet-toothed vegetarian is in worse shape than a meat-eater!
6. Think of vegetarianism as a positive movement toward reduced heart disease and increased energy levels. With the money you save at the grocery counter, you can buy yourself a good pair of shoes and run for your life!
7. Vegetable scraps — peelings, leaves, stalks — that aren't used in making stock should be added to the compost heap.
8. If you have teen-agers who are reluctant to trade hamburgers and fries for whole grains and veggies, let them read this list of notable stars and athletes who have changed their diets to whole foods and/or vegetarianism. Many magazines feature articles about their lifestyles. Actors and Actresses — Dennis Weaver, Ruby Dee and Ossie Davis, Nick Nolte, Dyan Cannon, Belinda Montgomery, Sandy Dennis, David Carradine, Samantha Eggar, Cloris Leachman, Susan St. James, Susan Richardson (Eight Is Enough), Lynda Carter (Wonder Woman); Comedians — Marty Feldman, Steve Martin, Dick Gregory; Recording Artists — Debby Boone, Tiny Tim, Johnny Rivers, The Captain and Tennille; Athletes — Pete LaCock (Kansas City Royals), Roger Brown, Herb Brown and Ralph Simpson (Detroit Pistons), Jim Keat (Philadelphia Phillies), Bill Walton (San Diego Clippers), Captain Alan Jones, Howard Mudd (S.F. 49ers); Authors — Andrew Weil, David Wallechinsky, Gypsy Boots, Susan Smith Jones (physical fitness instructor at U.C.L.A.).

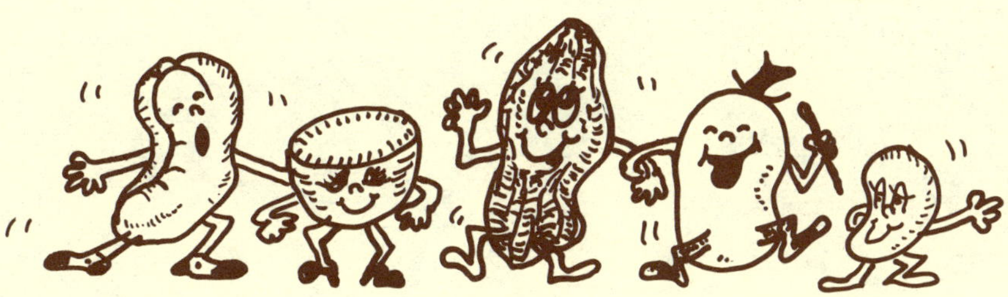

All of the animals except man know that the principle business of life is to enjoy it.

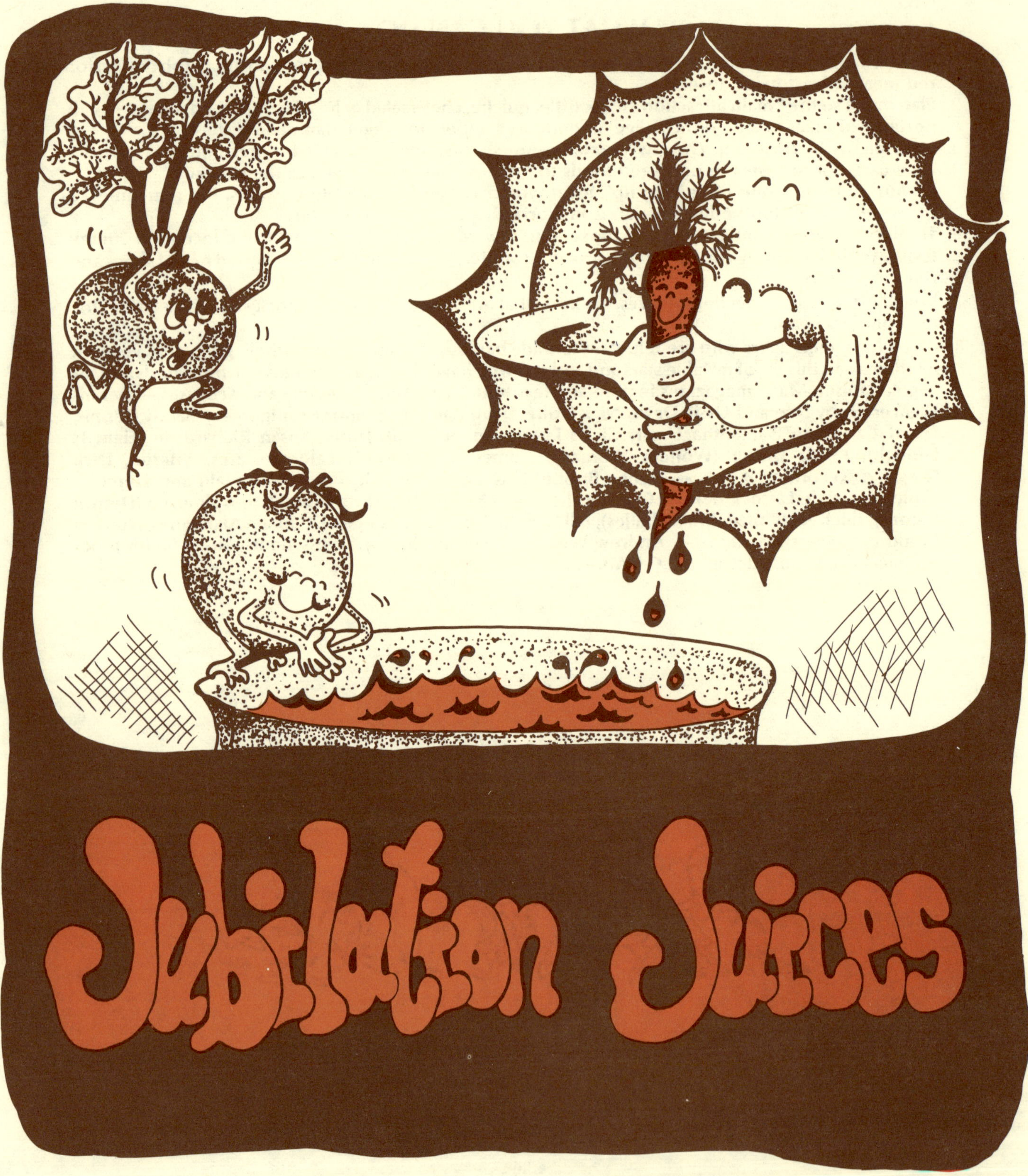

Jubilation Juices

Jubilation Juices

Eat To Live; Don't Live To Eat

Observe the animals for repatterning long lost eating habits. They rarely over-eat, taking just what is necessary for metabolic processes and survival. Wild animals are the ultimate environmentalists, for they eat only that which is natural and uncooked, leaving their habitat free of packages, cans, bottles, and any possibility of forest fires. When sick or injured, an animal will lick its wounds and wisely refuse to eat, so that healing forces and energies are concentrated on the injured areas of the body rather than the digestive processes.

If you can never remember whether to "starve a fever and feed a cold" or "feed a fever and starve a cold," take your cue from the animals. When ill, ignore admonitions from well-meaning friends or relatives who say, "Eat this to keep up your strength." Though the clock may signify mealtime, heed the intelligence of your own body. It will probably say, "I'm very thirsty, but I just don't feel like eating." Listen carefully — Nature has just prescribed a liquid fast.

By Nature's Own Hand . . .

Fasting is an intense, personal experience, involving the entire body. Everyone fasts. You fast from the time you have your last meal or dessert until you break-the-fast in the morning; usually a period of time anywhere from six to twelve hours. After assimilating three meals a day, plus numerous snacks, digestive organs need a rest.

Some people fast strictly for religious reasons, while others fast for cleansing purposes — that is, to rid the body of the accumulation of toxins.

People who are very ill and fast for healing, must do so under close supervision of a professional. Many cases have been documented of persons who were cured of degenerative diseases through fasting. When the body's organs are allowed to rest, then all energies — blood, oxygen and nutrients — are focused in the area that needs repair; a regeneration of cells occurs, and healing can take place. There are fasting clinics in the U.S. and Europe where very ill or obese people may fast and rest and exercise under the constant supervision of trained personnel. Consult a Whole-istic health practitioner for more information on extensive fasting.

Who Should Not Fast?

Diabetics, whether taking oral drugs or injecting insulin, and people with hypoglycemia must keep a continuous "log on the fire." Eating several, small, well-balanced meals keeps body functions running smoothly, and fasting would only disrupt this careful and deliberate scheduling. Therefore, they must be involved in a daily exercise program that will help them maintain peak condition and prevent toxin build-ups.

Pregnant women and nursing mothers should not fast for the obvious reason that they are the lifeline food source for their unborn and newborn babies. Growing children, whose spontaneous play *is* exercise, need not fast, but here again, when ill, they should not be force-fed. If you have a debilitating disease or unstable physical condition, consult your own physician before considering a fast.

The Great Caffeine Fix

Some foods actually have a negative effect on the body and may cause an increased pulse rate. They are stimulants, irritants or stress-makers, and many are addictive. These include common allergens such as red meat, processed cheeses, pasteurized milk, caffeine, chocolate, sugar, drugs, some spices, wheat and corn. Often depression, irritability, hyperactivity and/or headaches occur when these foods are eaten. Similar withdrawal symptoms occur when they are omitted during a fast.

It is ironic that even those people who pay close attention to eating the right kinds of foods, continue to relish their coffee to the bitter end. Even without the potent caffeine, repeated exposure to the body of the exact same substance, day after day after day, can only be harmful. (The adage "an apple a day keeps the doctor away" cannot be taken literally, for the protection comes in eating a wide variety of fruits.) As long as people continue destructive habits, they will counter-act the benefits of good nutrition.

The billions of dollars annually spent on coffee, colas, black teas and chocolate lend support to the power of caffeine addiction. As if stimulating the heartbeat were not enough, caffeine also increases the flow of blood plasma through the kidneys, thus allowing some B-vitamins to be lost in the urine.

Chocolate adds insult to injury by means of theobromine, a central nervous system stimulant, and oxalic acid, a potential inhibitor of calcium absorption. Calcium is Nature's own relaxant. How often are small children coaxed to drink their milk by the addition of highly sweetened chocolate powder, only to be punished later for excited and unruly behavior? The child's conduct may have been nothing more than an uncontrollable reaction to the cup of cocoa.

The only portion of our society that really benefits from the "great caffeine fix" are the producers and marketers of the products — a sad commentary when safe alternatives to the hazardous drinks are available.

Fasting can aid the allergy-sensitive person in determining the foods that are irritating to the system, by introducing one suspected food at a time after at least twelve hours without food, and recording any adverse reactions. Fasting is also an excellent way to break an addiction, whether it be caffeine, cigarettes, alcohol or drugs. If you can survive three days of a juice fast without a coffee break, then you can thrive without it for the rest of your life. Besides saving money, it is incredible how much you can accomplish when you don't waste time on your habit.

A Short Cleansing Juice Fast

Consider the value of a short juice fast to help cleanse your system. Try a one-day fast, once a week for awhile before attempting a three-day fast. Become aware of how your body reacts in a voluntary 24-hour abstinence from food. It is beneficial for a healthy adult to fast once a week for the rest of his/her life.

Drink only water, herbal teas and *fresh* fruit or vegetable juices. Stimulating beverages, including diet drinks are actually more detrimental during a fast. Herbs are therapeutic, medicinal substances from which many drugs are derived. Their use should be researched and their healing qualities respected. Exclusive and repetitious use of the same herb tea can be as harmful as the coffee, cola, cigarette or alcohol habits. (See *Nothing New; Tried and True* for herb tea blends.)

How Will I Feel?

A three-day juice fast is easy to undertake, but, since many people have eaten processed foods and/or excess food much of their lives, three days may not be enough time to feel the benefits of the cleansing processes. Your body will continue to eliminate toxins, and depending upon the degree of toxicity, you might still be feeling the uncomfortable effects of this elimination on the third day. You may experience headaches, dizziness, hunger pains, irritability, or weakness.

Poisons may overload the system as they are quickly sent into the bloodstream for disposal. A coated tongue, body and breath odor, skin eruptions and excessive perspiration are all signs of elimination and should be welcomed and tolerated. If you have a Whole-istic Health Center in your area, you may wish to treat yourself to a colonic, a massage, a sauna or a steam bath. If you diligently exercise and make time for relaxation, you will soon feel light, energetic, and open to the real physical and spiritual powers within you.

Becoming Reacquainted With God

Ultimately, fasting can be looked upon as a true spiritual awakening. Begin with a positive attitude and you will not feel that it is a sacrificial act at all, but an affirmative self-discipline, putting you in control of your body.

Even on a short fast, you will feel closer to the One who created you. You will feel the Spirit in and around you; experience balance; body, mind, and emotions, merged into one centered person. You will radiate joy and vitality, the visible reflection of your aura (life-force or energy field). Freed from concerns about food, you can open yourself completely to this higher level of consciousness. Listen with your heart — you will hear less of the material and more of the spiritual. Contemplate your purpose here, where you're coming from, and where you're going. You will become acutely aware of your capabilities as you connect to and confirm the immense power of God.

If you have already established your directions on this planet, then be assured that your GOOD intentions can lead you to BETTER service when you are in the BEST of health.

WHAT YOU CAN DO

1. **Find a partner. It may be your husband, wife, or a good friend. Whomever you select should share your enthusiasm for the fast and be willing to follow through, and keep in close contact. This is very important!**
2. **Prepare yourselves for fasting two to three days before you begin by reading books and some scriptures about fasting. (I Corin. 7:5; Gen. 1:29; Psalms 35:13; Isaiah 58:3-6; I Kings 19:8; Exodus 34:28; Matthew 6:16-18; Luke 5:33-36; Matthew 4:1-4; Matthew 17:21; Daniel 6:18; Daniel 9:3, and the first Chapter of Daniel).**
3. **Drink at least eight glasses of liquids daily. (See recipes for fasting juices under** *Better Beginnings: Breakfasts.)* **Juices — fresh fruit, vegetable, especially green drinks and clear vegetable broths — will help remove toxins more readily than just plain water, while they help maintain an even blood sugar level. If you tend towards low-blood-sugar, go easy on the fruit juices, diluting with equal parts water.**
4. **Pour your drink into a pretty glass and don't read or work while drinking. Just enjoy the drink! Sip slowly; use a straw if necessary to slow you down; swish liquid around in your mouth, and "chew" it so that the saliva enzymes will aid assimilation.**
5. **You may choose to drink prune juice in the morning if you feel constipated. A warm water and lemon juice enema can be comforting at this time. We shower, brush our teeth, and douche, so we should not balk at the idea of cleansing the colon. Relax; allow one teaspoon lemon juice to a quart of warm water. Relax. In twenty minutes you'll be glad you did.**
6. **Keep a daily record of your liquid intake; how you feel physically, mentally, emotionally; in short, be sensitive to what is going on inside yourself. RECORD. Share feelings with your friend. S/he is probably experiencing many of the same things.**
7. **Support each other. Do not expose yourselves to temptations over which you might not have control, such as an evening with friends where gourmet food will be served.**
8. **Keep busy; plan to hook a rug, weave, macrame', create with clay, sew, paint, or whatever hobby you enjoy most.**
9. **Devote at least fifteen minutes a day for private prayer or meditation, where your mind can be still and you can be open to higher thoughts. Remember, you are drinking nothing but live, fresh, raw liquified food, with the highest nutrients, enzymes, and life force. You will need less sleep, have more energy, and be more sensitive to your surrounding environment. Choose the vibrations you**

want to flow in for upliftment, such as beautiful soft music, a warm bath, a book of devotions, prayer or poetry. Don't hold unkind thoughts in your mind, as these can only cause a conflict and destroy the peace and feeling of well-being that will soon be a part of you.

10. **Make time for a brisk long walk; ride your bike, or do some Hatha-Yoga and deep breathing exercises daily. While it is important to get enough rest and relaxation, it is also imperative to do some exercise to speed up the processes of elimination. Remember, you not only excrete through the bowels and kidneys, but also the skin and lungs, so work up a sweat!**
11. **Shower or bathe daily to wash away wastes that might accumulate in the pores. Use a luffa sponge to briskly rub off dead skin cells and increase circulation to the skin.**
12. **It is important to end your fast gradually. On the first day, when coming off a fast, eat small portions of soft raw vegetables or fruit at one-and-a-half hour intervals, chewing thoroughly. The second day, increase portions of raw vegetables or fruit and eat at two hour intervals. On the third day, have a cooked food at one meal only (like millet or rice), while continuing to drink plenty of liquids. By the fourth day, increase to regular amounts at mealtime, of whole natural foods, and continue to chew thoroughly and relax during meals. Also continue your walk and/or daily exercise.**

Dost thou love life? Then do not squander time; for that is the stuff life is made of.
Benjamin Franklin

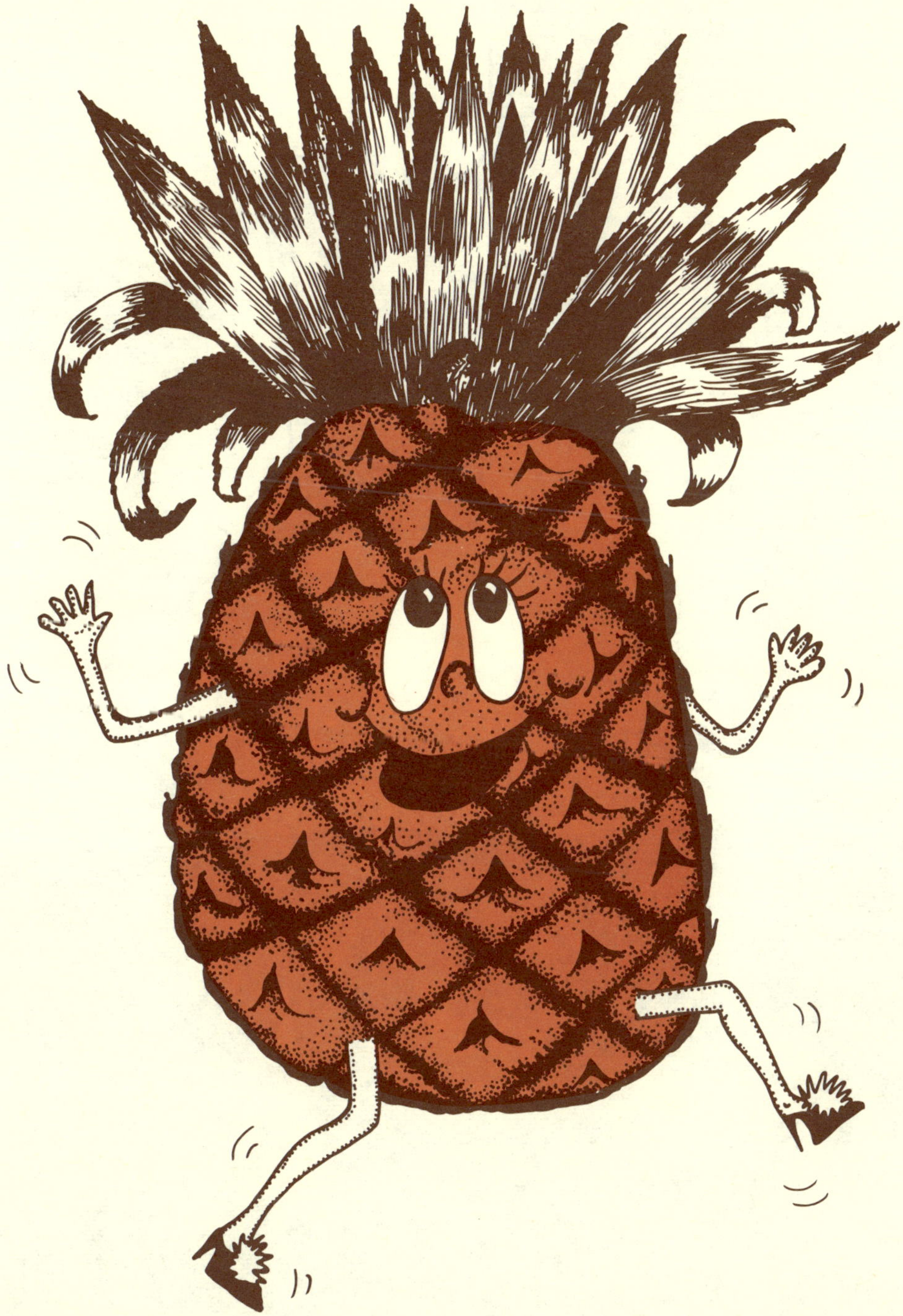

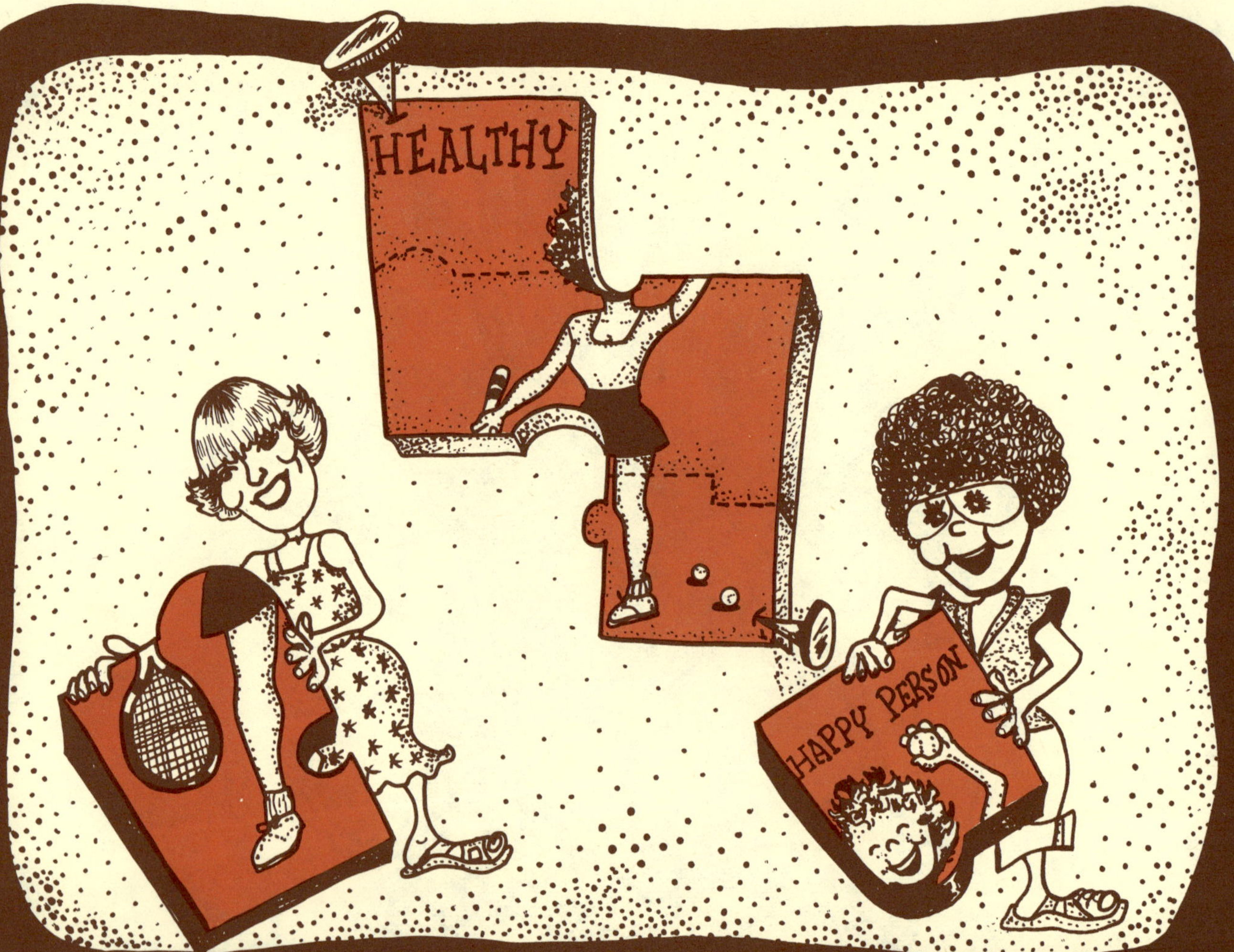

Getting it Together

Getting It Together

Centering

Every human being is a trinity of body, mind and spirit, with each part influencing the whole. Though we all are essentially what we eat, we are also what we think and believe. The foods we include or fail to include in our diets affect not only our physical, but our mental and spiritual persons; and conversely, how we think and feel, affects our well-being.

We can and do attract positives and/or negatives to ourselves, depending upon the thoughts we decide to embrace. When depression, fear and anxiety intrude, we have the ability to repel them. Whatever we send out in thought, word or deed will return; what is given will be received. Like a magnet we can draw delight, gaiety and happiness to our hearts. Having experienced this *joie de vivre,* we can reach out and touch someone close, creating an ever-increasing circle of love. Give love, receive love. Just look around you and see the potential magnitude of this truth — at home and work, with family and friends, in church and the community, and even in international and world relationships. What we visualize will sooner or later externalize in our lives. Jesus said, "By your words ye are justified and by your words ye are condemned."

Whole-istic Health encompasses all of those integral parts that must work together smoothly if we are to maintain the highest degree of whole-body health. No matter how much high test fuel goes into a body, negative emotions of anger, resentment, fear and guilt will create internal chaos until the entire system becomes out of synchronization. When undue stress is placed upon the organs and glands, the result is a body that becomes run down, inefficient, nervous and/or lethargic and which proceeds to age more readily. One cannot expect a change in diet alone to produce total health. It is the combination of a sound diet, a positive outlook and regular exercise that will enable us to become more centered and capable of enjoying life.

A Visual Trip

This Visual-Imagery Game will illustrate the close relationship between the body, mind and spirit; between your diet, your thoughts and your actions.

Before taking this trip, make sure you have fifteen to twenty minutes of undisturbed quiet. Sit in a comfortable position or lie down. Close your eyes. Imagine your destination is a place where you will review all the important, as well as trivial aspects of your life — a place for contemplation and revisions.

Food for the Body

See yourself walking down a path. You arrive at an enormous dumping grounds and there is a large sign in front with your name on it. As you walk through the entrance you stop before another sign. This one says, "Food for the Body." You look at the piles of food on your left; they contain all the junk food you've eaten in your life, all the devitalized, plastic food that has really harmed your body. See the cans of carbonated drinks stacked up in pyramids. Look at the pop bottles lined up like bowling pins. How about the cups of coffee, black tea, cans of beer and other alcoholic beverages? There's a pile of candy bars, piles of instant this and speedy that, frozen pot pies and T.V. dinners, canned soups, luncheon meats, white bread, commercial ice creams, canned sweetened fruits and salted vegetables, artificially colored and flavored drinks, and packaged baked goods. Look at the stacks of aspirin, laxatives, tranquilizers, pain pills, sleeping pills, penicillin. How high does the mound of cigarette cartons go? Visualize it all. Imagine your favorite junk food and how much of it you've eaten throughout your life. Ask yourself, "How, specifically, have these foods and drugs worked *for* me — or *against* me?"

Now, turn around and look at the piles on the right side of the path. Here are heaps of real whole foods that you've consumed in your life. Count all the fresh fruits and vegetables, nuts, seeds, green salads, sprouts, farm fresh eggs, whole grain breads and cereals. How do they compare to those on your left? Have you filled your temple with treasures or trash?

Food for Thought

Walk ahead along the path. Take a few deep breaths. You are coming to another sign. This one says, "Food for Thought." Look to your left. These mounds represent the mental debris, all the negative emotions and thoughts that have occurred throughout your life. Look at the first heap — that's selfishness. There's a large pile of fear, and one of anger. See that mound of envy and jealousy! Other stacks abound — worry, frustration, pride, prejudice, criticism, thoughtlessness — all of which have shaped your life; experiences which have become a reality as a result of early programming and outside influences. Many of these thoughts determined how you have responded to situations and stresses in daily living. For every action there is a reaction. That is the law of Karma. How many of these negative energies have bounced back to you in the form of negative happenings when positive energies could have yielded positive effects?

Now turn around, cross the path and examine the stacks of feelings on your right. These, of course, illustrate the positive thoughts and emotions that have become a part of your character, your philosophy of life, indeed, of all your actions and inter-actions with those around you. First you see a river of unconditional love, with meadows of understanding and compassion on either side. There are numerous heaps of happiness and joy. Charity and kindness. Acceptance and forgiveness. Tenderness and mercy. Examine your mound of confidence and self-esteem! Now, has your mind been filled with enthusiasm or apathy?

Spiritual Storehouse

Move along the path. There is a sign in front of the last set of images that says, "Spiritual Storehouse." On your left it is dark and murky. You don't see any hills. Instead, the soul-hurting aspects of your spiritual life — like doubt, disbelief, depression, cynicism, dispair, closed-minded attachments to doctrinal principles that block your quest for truth and desire to know your God — all have hindered your spiritual growth, weighed you down and have become so heavy that they have created an enormous black hole. This hole contains all forces destructive to the human spirit, a surrender to fate — leaving a lack of purpose and meaning in your life.

Now look at the light-emanating mounds on your right. These piles glow and sparkle. They personify spiritual growth — prayer, meditation, church or worship, uplifting reading material, life and death experiences, traumatic events in your life and in those of loved ones — and how you learned from and responded to these situations. There's a heap of human communication and fellowship. Visualize your spiritual experiences, your encounters with God. Remember when you communed with your Creator at the beach, on a moonlight hike or at a mountain lake. There are stacks of dreams, intuitions, quiet periods of listening and receiving, peace of mind, faith, hope, values, searching for and finding the truth, and a strong unwavering belief. The uplifting qualities of your soul are more brilliant than the black hole is dark. Your spiritual storehouse is full of supplies and savings to draw upon in need. Have you filled it with light or litter?

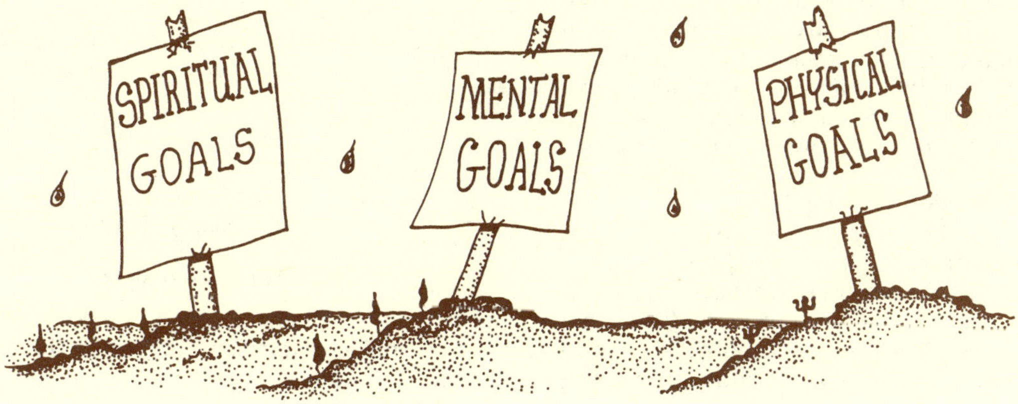

Rebalancing the Triad

Slowly bring yourself to the present and open your eyes. Take a deep breath and stretch. You should have a good idea now of where you've been and how the negatives in your life — whether in body, mind or spirit, work against the positives if they outweigh them, and create an imbalance in this trinity.

So forget the past; it is gone forever, only to be used to gain insight into the future. Today is the time to set new goals and decide how you are going to live the rest of your life. None of us can decide when or even how we're going to die, but we can determine how we're going to live! That is each of our responsibility to ourselves.

Close your eyes once again. Instead of thinking of it as a garbage dump for the past, imagine building rich compost for the future that will nourish the components of the triad and bring them into harmony. Visualize a garden for personal development. Plant one section with "Food for the Body." Project the images of the foods that you *will* be eating, starting today. How bountiful those mounds of good food will be; how vibrant are the life forces and energies emanating from them.

Plant another section of your garden with "Food for Thought." Just imagine all the power in the positive thoughts that is yours for the thinking. Feel the strength in thoughts of love, acceptance and kindness. Give a perfect love and you will receive a perfect love. Observe the delicate balance between the body and the mind.

Sow the rest of your space with the seeds from your "Spiritual Storehouse" making certain to include a surplus of faith, conviction and trust. Surround the entire garden with an aura of sunlight and energy from which you will ultimately harvest growth and awareness. Your goals and means for attaining them lie within you. Just as a fertile compost enriches the worn soil, your spiritual storehouse seems to replenish a weary mind and body and germinate new life. This "internal garden" can only thrive when you weed out the negative vibrations and thus reap the rewards of a full and balanced life. When you nourish your body with whole foods, your mind with confident thoughts and affirmations and your spirit with God's love you will bloom where you are planted.

We may make our plans, but God has the last word. *Proverbs 16:1*

Getting It Together

We must preserve the harmony of our inner gardens (body-mind-spirit). Constructive thoughts reduce stress and create alpha waves in the brain, thus making it easier to "roll with the punches." By thinking and acting positively in a given situation, every-day frustrations become challenges that re-direct our attitudes — toward others as well as ourselves — into productive, successful modes of living.

If we can live each day by the moment and trust that each circumstance will be guided by the Supreme Being, then we have begun to focus on the simple joys and pleasures that surround us. We can be appreciative and grateful for our blessings and ignore the distresses that are constantly present to disrupt each day should we permit them.

The painter advances canvas and oils to the level of fine art by means of practice. The musician enhances a superb instrument and a first quality composition through diligent practice. We, too, can enrich every facet of our lives — individually and collectively — by daily practice of whole-istic living.

When we Get It Together within, we will all radiate the vitality, happiness and serenity that every body, mind and spirit was created to reflect.

What lies behind us and what lies before us are tiny matters compared to what lies within us.

Ralph Waldo Emerson

Your Own Space

Better than average health requires a personal commitment. If you've been taught that thinking of yourself first is selfish, then please reconsider. God said, "Love your neighbor as yourself." You cannot fully love or care for another human being until you fully love and care for yourself. In spite of daily pressures and stress, you must be relaxed and centered, in order to be of any value to those you love.

WHAT YOU CAN DO

1. **Devote time to your hobby or develop a new interest.**
2. **Select a book from a wide variety listed in** *Inspiration For Independence* **to further enlighten yourself nutritionally, emotionally and spiritually.**
3. **Write a poem or compose a song; create a short story; write a letter to someone you love; or write an apology to resolve a conflict and release tensions you both may be feeling.**
4. **Make lists — shopping, repair, or goals. List-making can relieve your mind of trivia and clear it for more important thinking.**
5. **Treat yourself to an herbal bath. (See** *Nothing New; Tried and True* **for recipes.)**
6. **Keep a jump rope handy to jump off that excess nervous energy, let loose those built-up tensions or renovate your supply of energy. Put on a foot-stomping, John Denver record and jump for joy.**
7. **Lie on a slantboard for a few minutes; do the shoulderstand for several seconds, or stand on your head against a wall. You will replenish the blood supply to your brain and take a load off the extra pumping your heart does all day defying gravity. (Work into these positions gradually if you have a history of high blood pressure.)**
8. **Find the quietest place in your environment to do some stretching and deep relaxation breathing exercises. This will relieve anxiety, calm the mind and emotions, and provide you with quiet time for prayer.**

Sun Salutation

You can begin every day with a few salutations to the sun. When done properly this exercises every muscle, joint and organ in the body, and when accompanied by correct breathing, is a complete stretching, toning and relaxation exercise. Each sun salute consists of twelve separate positions (see picture). Begin at "one o'clock," placing hands in prayer position, hold each pose three seconds for the first round, two seconds the second round and do the third set in one continuous, slow motion.

Do you need proof of God? Does one light a torch to see the sun? Oriental Wisdom

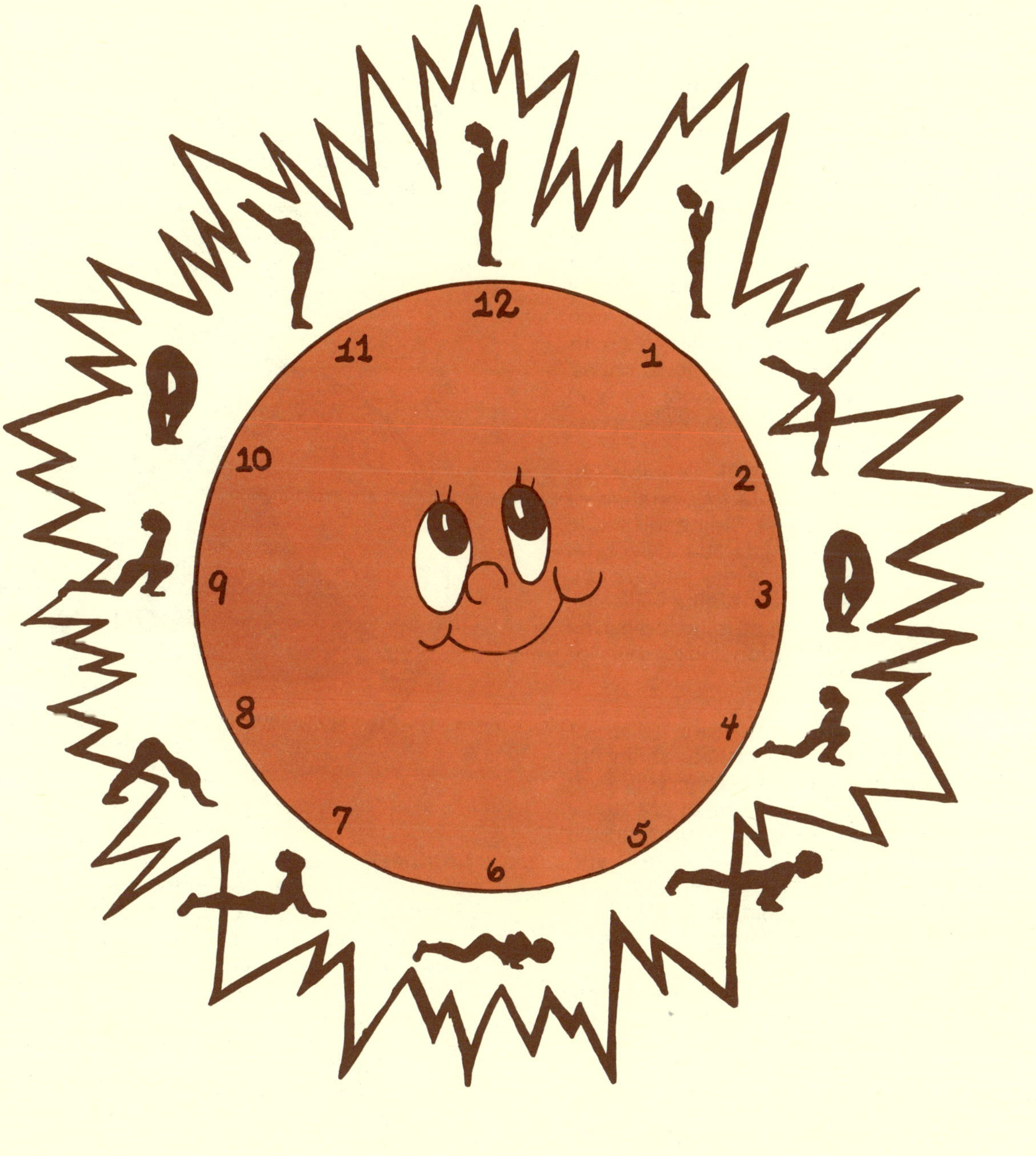

Sun Salutation

Take a slow, deep breath through the nostrils and exhale at position one. As you continue around the clock inhale for positions two, four, seven, nine and eleven. Exhale during positions three, six, eight, ten and twelve. Retain your breath while holding body in a push-up for position five. Keep in mind that there is an inhalation whenever the body is stretched out and back, and an exhalation whenever the body is curled down and forward.

In positions two and eleven, arms are in a V and buttocks should be tight; in positions three and ten, keep knees straight and relax head, shoulders, neck and arms; in four (left leg forward, right leg back) and nine (right leg forward, left leg back), stretch chin toward ceiling and place palms flat on the floor at each side of the front foot — stretching back leg to its maximum. In position six, touch toes, knees, chest and forehead to the floor. As you complete the round with position twelve, relax and breathe normally.

Practice and soon you'll be able to coordinate the breathing with the duration of each position in the exercise. Doing this salute upon awakening will stimulate and invigorate, limbering you for the day ahead, while a round or two of this exercise in the evening will calm, relax and center your body and mind, preparing you for further relaxation exercises or meditation.

Stretching

Animals have an instinctive ability to completely release tension. Have you ever observed a cat stretching? Before, or just after a feline naps, it engages in a long, leisurely stretch of the body, with back arched, paws spread, and a yawn that extends all facial muscles. This single exercise stretches and strengthens every limb and joint of an animal widely recognized for its agility.

You, too, can enjoy that feeling of being lithe and limber, by first stretching, then totally relaxing each muscle. Loosen or remove any tight clothing, glasses or jewelry. Then lie on your back with arms and legs slightly out from your torso.

Close eyes, breathe in deeply through your nose and raise arms over your head. Holding your breath, stretch — really stretch — from head to toe, tensing all the muscles and extending hands and feet to your greatest length.

After a few seconds, exhale slowly through your nose and at the same time, bring arms forward and down again to your sides. Now inhale deeply to the count of six, hold for four and exhale slowly through the nostrils to a count of eight. Repeat three times, all the while imagining as you inhale that energy is flowing throughout your body, and that each exhalation is forcing out pent-up emotions and tensions.

This exercise is equally effective as a relaxing method to induce sleep, or as a stimulating technique to begin your day.

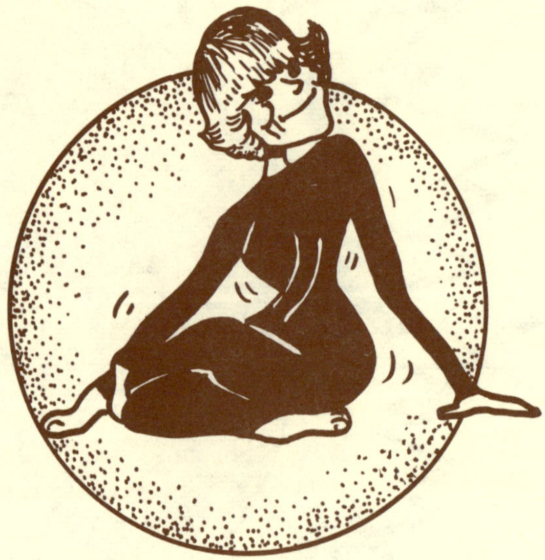

Relaxing

Kneel, rest buttocks on heels, place your hands, fingers extended, on knees. Yawn and stretch your facial muscles. Extend your tongue and hold while simultaneously widening your eyes. (Your neck muscles should be taut.) Now relax.

Rotate your eyes without moving your head, then relax eyelids and keep them comfortably closed. Now roll your head slowly, and in an exaggerated motion, to the left, then forward and down, to the right, and around the back, in a full circle. Reverse. Observe the feeling of relaxation you are already experiencing in and around your neck.

In order to relax your entire body, lie on your back with arms and legs slightly out from the sides of your torso. Begin with the toes; stretch, tense and tighten them, then let them go limp. Follow this same procedure for the ankles, calves, knees, thighs, abdomen, chest and shoulders. Now stretch, tighten, then relax fingers, hands and arms. (You can record and play back your own instructions; speak very softly and slowly when you record, for maximum effect.)

You may begin to feel lighter as you become more aware of the steady beating of your heart. Observe the rhythm of your breathing as the miracle of respiration quietly takes place. When you inhale, feel the life-force vibrations enter your body and as you exhale, notice how you release the tensions.

Concentrate only on what you are doing. Don't let your mind be interrupted with worrisome thoughts and unresolved problems. You will soon guide yourself into a serene and tranquil state.

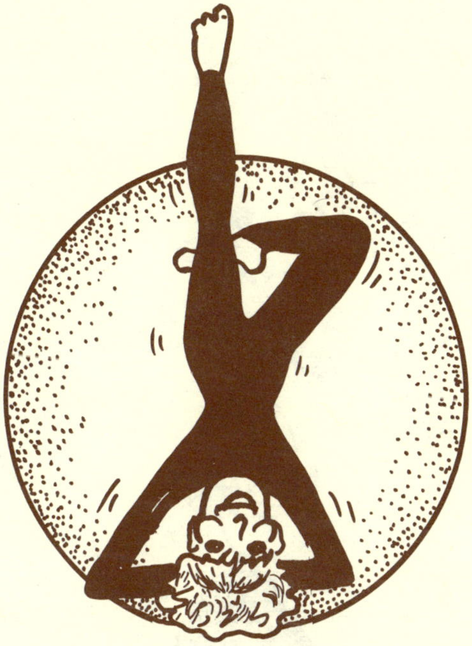

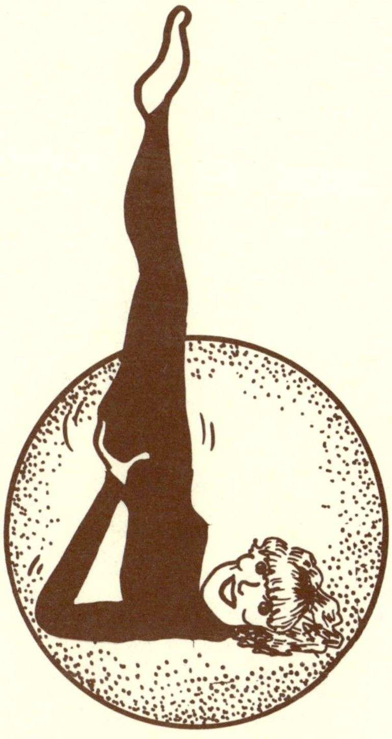

Meditating

You are now ready for ten minutes of silent meditation if you so desire. Some people feel that this practice is non-Christian, or belongs strictly to the East Indian yogi. We feel it belongs to anyone who yearns to become more closely in touch with God.

One prays when one feels a need to give thanks or to ask for help. One can meditate (which is a passive form of prayer without words or thought) whenever there is a wish to communicate with the Creator. By freeing the intellect from conscious thoughts, one can clear the mind and open the channels to receive positive guidance; to tune in to God's wavelength and genuinely *listen*.

Sit quietly in a crossed-legged position in a semi-dark, quiet room, palms face up and resting on your knees. Close your eyes and try to paint a mental picture of a single, solitary, bright light. If this is difficult at first, you might place a single, lit candle or a flower in front of you and concentrate only on the qualities and properties of that object.

Sometimes it takes a painful experience to make us change our ways. Proverbs 20:30

Breathe steadily and deeply, but don't concentrate on breathing. Don't ask for or think about anything. Let the answers come to you from within. There will be no limit to the inspiration and positive concepts that will flow into you when you are receptive to them. Anxieties will disappear, problems will diminish in size, and fresh solutions will come to you. When this happens be thankful that you were able to take *time* to really hear and, beginning today, put into practice the messages that you have received.

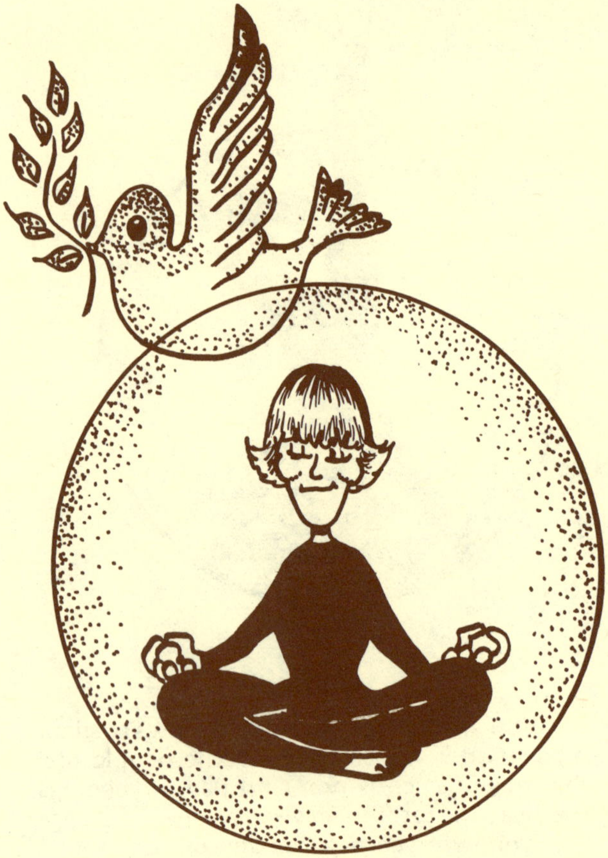

For every thing there is a season, and a time for every purpose under the heaven. *Ecclesiastes 3:1*

There's a Time

There's a time for work, a time for play
A time to listen and a time to pray.
There's a time to give, a time to receive.
A time to question and a time to believe.

There's a time to be quiet and a time to talk
A time to relax and a time to walk.
There's time for fellowship, time to be alone
Time to move out and a time to come home.

There's a time to be serious and a time to clown
A time to be up and a time to be down.
Sometimes we lose and sometimes we win
So turn that frown upside down into a grin.

There's a time to be happy, a time for tears
A time for hope and a time for fears.
No matter the age, no matter the gender
In everyone's life, there's time to be tender.

There's a time to argue, a time to agree
Though we sometimes are captive, we want to be free.
There's a time for satisfaction, a time for desire
We might try to set goals just a little bit higher.

There's a time to be patient, to realize
That after every sunset comes a sunrise.
There's a time to be born and a time to die.
Whatever the time, only God knows why.

There's a time for kind words, a time for a song
A time to feel weak, a time to feel strong.
There's a time when we're ill, a time when we're healthy
We may be poor in possessions, but in blessings, wealthy.

There's a time for the sunshine, a time for the shade
If life hands you a lemon, just make lemonade.
It's been said every cloud has a silver lining
Behind every storm the sun's always shining.

Into all our life comes a little pain
But there's always a rainbow after the rain.
There's time to be daring and to take that chance
A time to rejoice and a time to dance.

For everything there is a season
But when, or why, only God knows the reason.
Whatever you do, make time and space in your day
Life's too short and precious to waste it away.

Everything in the past is beyond retrieving
What the future holds, we're not yet receiving
But the present is within our grasp — it is NOW
So live for each moment; then show a friend how.

And soon from your heart you'll notice a glow
When the Creator's life-force flows into your soul.
As your body interweaves with spirit and mind
The patterns in God's tapestry will be easy to find.

To thine own self be true in whatever you choose
Be positive; have faith, and you'll never lose.
For God has a plan — a time and a place
For each individual in the whole human race.

He wants to create a heaven on earth
Joy in our hearts, a time for rebirth.
But how can we experience this peace from above?
The answer comes from within — it's love.

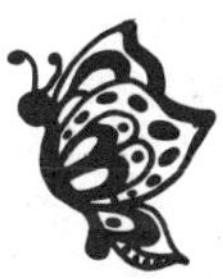

Hidden Beauty

Beauty is like a ray of light. From its beginning, concealed inside a protective covering, beauty radiates a subtle glow toward an undefined destination. Beauty is internal and has little to do with the position of cheekbones or with chest measurements. You may think your features lack symmetry or your shape is shapeless or you are just plain *plain.* But if your skin is clear and clean, your eyes sparkle and your smile is genuine, then you are truly beautiful.

Let's face it, first impressions count and the way you look and feel has a definite effect on your personality. The face (skin, eyes, teeth and expression) can reveal, not only general physical condition, but a great deal about attitudes and character. American Indians once diagnosed illness by reading the facial lines. The quality of the diet, the intensity of the exercise program and the ability to remain centered in a crisis, all seem to manifest themselves in our skin.

The skin is our largest, most sensitive organ, covering approximately nineteen square feet. This veneer may well be our most revealing organ, reflecting the condition of the unseen (thus, often neglected) internal organs. When a skin break-out occurs, the tendency is to conceal the blemish — pack it with a commercial cover-up and hide the inelegant evidence while ignoring the cause of the problem. Indeed, the health of the skin is dependent on the quality of the blood which nourishes the whole body, so consider *any* skin or scalp irritation a barometer of general health, and heed Nature's most obvious warning signal.

Think of the importance of good digestion and ample exercise in relation to the strength and flexibility of muscles and organs, including our skin. Inasmuch as the condition of the skin is often a direct indicator of the condition of the intestinal tract, the same factors responsible for muscle tone and the health of the digestive organs will also affect the skin.

If the large intestine is overloaded or clogged with decaying matter, the by-products (toxins) will search for a way out of the system, usually via the skin. This is clearly an internal problem that no amount of topically applied medications or make-up can be expected to remedy. Only through a diet high in nutrients and fiber from whole foods, coupled with an aerobic exercise program (encourages the release of toxins through sweating) can a sluggish system be opened to the renewed vitality that allows natural beauty to radiate from within.

The Great Cosmetic Cover-Up

Besides the poisons that enter into the body by means of ingested food, drugs and the inhalation of polluted air, there are some toxic assaults that are deliberately applied in the form of highly chemicalized commercial beauty aids. In her 1966 book, *Cosmetics: Trick or Treat?,* Toni Stabile reveals the inadequate testing and lack of concern for appropriate labeling by the cosmetic industry. Labeling laws have improved since then, though appear more clear to the scientific world than to the lay people for whom they were intended. Those who take the time to read the labels seldom understand what they're reading and continue to use a possibly *still* hazardous product, assuming that because the ingredients appear on the label, the contents are automatically harmless.

The seven billion dollars that Ms. Stabile attributed to consumer spending on grooming aids has probably doubled by now with a high percentage of teenagers supporting that industry. The ugly part of the "ravishing beauty" portrayal of cosmetic commercials is the belief they have fostered that good looks, popularity and security are things that you can roll on, smooth on, spray on or paint on.

Beneath the Aphrodite appearance, caustic grooming aids may be responsible for health problems ranging anywhere from minor skin irritation to severe and irreparable eye damage to hideous disfigurement to cancer. Yet an inventory of the average bathroom cabinet will show an array of comely spray cans and jars and bottles of notions and lotions and potions with absolutely no indication of the sources or safety of the ingredients. Do people heed (or even *notice)* the warnings on the label that relieve the manufacturer of responsibility for injuries from the potentially dangerous substance?

At the first sign of skin irritation — itching, rash, flaking, a pimple, boil or any other sensitivity—immediately examine the diet of the last two days and continue to write relevant notations in your diet diary. Then, instead of buying a two ounce jar of commercial or prescription chemicals costing $4.95, (that's $39.60 a pound!) head for the nearest farmers' market and fill your basket with fresh fruits and vegetables and some of the food products that make up the recipes for facials and skin toners in *Nothing New; Tried and True* that are safe for your insides as well as your skin.

Glands Take the Blame

An area of internal health that directly affects the skin is the endocrine gland system, which is responsible for the production and secretion of powerful chemical substances called hormones, that regulate growth and reproduction. When we think of endocrine glands, it is easy to form a picture in our minds of little isolated globules of tissue performing designated duties, like so many parts of a machine. Actually, they are more complex (and vulnerable) and not completely understood, even by scientists. Glands are like soldiers, standing guard on growth and development — just waiting to be called into action, prepared to send messages (hormones) into the bloodstream, then return to their posts to protect the reserves.

There are many mysteries surrounding the glandular system, but it is generally agreed in the medical and psychological communities that the functions of the glands are regulated, to a degree, by the emotions. Of course optimum general health is paramount to both glandular and emotional health, signifying once again, the complex inter-relationship of physical and mental health. This may explain the correlation of emotional pressure and hormonal imbalance to teenage acne, but is by no means an *excuse* for the condition nor does it render acne an inevitable teen-stage of life.

We can blame our glands and the stresses of everyday living for poor skin or we can take the responsibility to train ourselves and our children to *deal* with stress as it occurs; to find the best possible solution to a problem and then forget it. If our solution turns out to be a mistake, then we can learn a new lesson and go on.

To dwell on human errors, our own or others, only compounds the stress, which in turn upsets the delicate balance causing our endocrine "soldiers" to embark on a futile mission, releasing negative "messages" into our bloodstream. Added to the internal biochemical reactions are the external signs of stress that effect the skin: tight neck and shoulder muscles, pursed lips, scowling eyes and crouching brows, dandruff, acne, psoriases, hair loss and an endless list of other difficulties.

It takes a tremendous amount of energy to keep up the appearances of being Super-Person. However severe your problem, it is not the end of the world, nor is it worth the very destruction of your health.

Added Enthusiasm Equals Added Time

You would not enjoy listening for hours to a dull speaker, but when a speech is speckled with graphics, demonstrations and audience participation, you can remain surprisingly comfortable. The key to enjoyability is in the *spirit* of the delivery. Similarly, the key to true beauty is found in the vigor with which an individual approaches life, the careful attention paid to the extras and the enthusiasm which emanates a contagious grace and charm.

How many of us look at a gorgeous model's flat abdomen or peaches and cream complexion and think, "I would love to look half that good . . ?" But how many are willing to dedicate the time, attention and enthusiasm to physical fitness that the model must if s/he is to maintain health and, subsequently, beauty? Instead we make excuses.

We could fill this chapter with the excuses we've heard (and used!) but the most frequent are: "I'm not that vain . . .", "I used to look like that before I had children . . .", "My husband/wife likes me just the way I am," or the all-time, four-star, cop-out, "I don't have the *time.*"

Today is the day to make the time. Mac Davis sings it beautifully, "You've got to stop and smell the roses along the way." Start today. If you're a night person, reserve your space in the evening about fifteen minutes before retiring. If you're an early bird, or want to be one, set your alarm fifteen minutes earlier than usual. In the morning and daily thereafter, when you hear that familiar signal turn off the alarm and use your extra quarter hour to do the stretching of every muscle, referred to in this chapter under Centering.

One week from today set your alarm another fifteen minutes early, (night people adjust evening schedule accordingly) and after your stretches, give yourself any of the facials that can be found in the recipe section of *Nothing New; Tried and True.* One week later set your alarm fifteen minutes earlier and follow both the stretching and facial routines, now using the added time for planning your day or making those lists referred to in Your Own Space — WHAT YOU CAN DO. And one week later arise still another fifteen minutes early; stretch, apply facial, then use your extra half-hour to accomplish any of the things you used to think you didn't have the time to do. Now you have the time.

Whether you choose the morning or evening, you have painlessly added one full hour to your day; *you* did it without bribing, without buying any gimmicks and without making any excuses. In one month you have converted your enthusiasm into accomplishments. You have planned and executed productive days, stretched and toned muscles, kept your skin scrupulously clean, energized your entire body and, literally, added years to your life. When you set goals for yourself, there is no limit to WHAT YOU CAN DO — and there is no stopping you now.

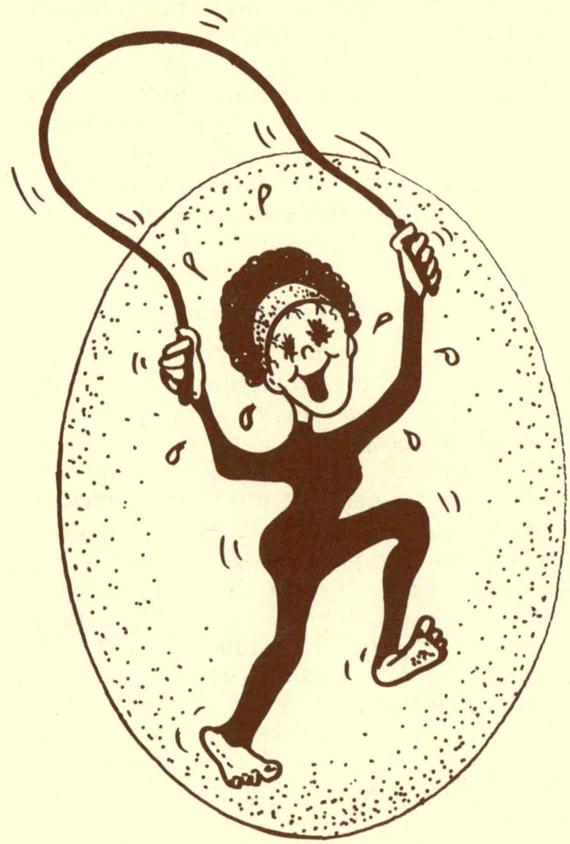

WHAT YOU CAN DO

1. **Pinpoint the specific cause of your stress. Determine what steps you can take to effectively eliminate or solve the problem. If there is truly nothing you can do about a given situation, then you must forget it, or it will control you completely. If, however, you see some possible solutions to your problem, write them down in order of importance and begin action today.**
2. **To relieve pent-up emotions which may cause a negative hormonal chain-reaction:**
   a. **When you feel hurt or sorrowful —** *cry.*
   b. **When you feel frightened —** *scream.*
   c. **When you feel nervous and fidgety —** *move:* **dance, run, climb, jump rope.**
   d. **When you feel angry —** *hit* **a pillow or a punching bag, never a person!**
   e. **When you feel you've been cheated or treated unjustly —** *write* **a letter stating your case. Even if you don't send it, writing will help alleviate your strong feelings.**
   f. **When you feel guilty —** *make restitution.*
3. **No one can upset you without your consent. Withhold your consent in petty situations and reserve your B-vitamins and hormones for the problems that count.**
4. **Stress in itself is not dangerous, it is how you** *handle* **the stress that matters. Great strides have been made just in the last five years in the field of stress management. Check with your county mental health department for help. Read books, attend a class or workshop and learn to deal with problems one at a time so they don't have a chance to build up.**

5. Admit that you are human; if you have tried to cope on your own and it hasn't worked yet, see a counselor. This is by far better than alienating the family you love by bottling your problems inside until you burst.
6. Instead of dwelling on your misfortunes, note that people daily face problems more severe than your own. Volunteer to help the aged, the handicapped, the lonely; in helping others you will automatically help yourself.
7. Each morning when you open your eyes, say, "This is going to be a good day because *I* am going to make it a good day."
8. Smile! You can change your feelings by changing your attitude. When you're smiling you may not get the whole world to smile with you, as the song says, but you're certain to disseminate misery if you scowl, so why not spread around some smiles and happiness instead!

A Do-It-Yourself Puzzle

This chapter has revolved around you and the decisions that you make every day of your life. You are a source of strength for yourself, your family, friends, community and society. You possess the autonomy to learn or unlearn, accept or reject, whatever you choose; to experience failure and go on to experience success. You can let go of old habits and conditioning in favor of a more productive lifestyle and attitude. You are the person who is in control.

Accept the fact that other's opinions are going to be different from yours, but never relinquish your enthusiasm because your opponents are critical, for the only way to avoid criticism is by saying nothing, doing nothing and being nothing.

You are the person who, through your exuberance for life will turn the keys, open the doors and determine your own directions. You are the person who studies each segment of your life — mental, physical, emotional, spiritual — and decides how each seemingly uneven piece will fit into the completed puzzle. You are the person who ultimately will overcome the excuses and thoroughly enjoy life and living each and every glorious day, because *you* are Getting It Together!

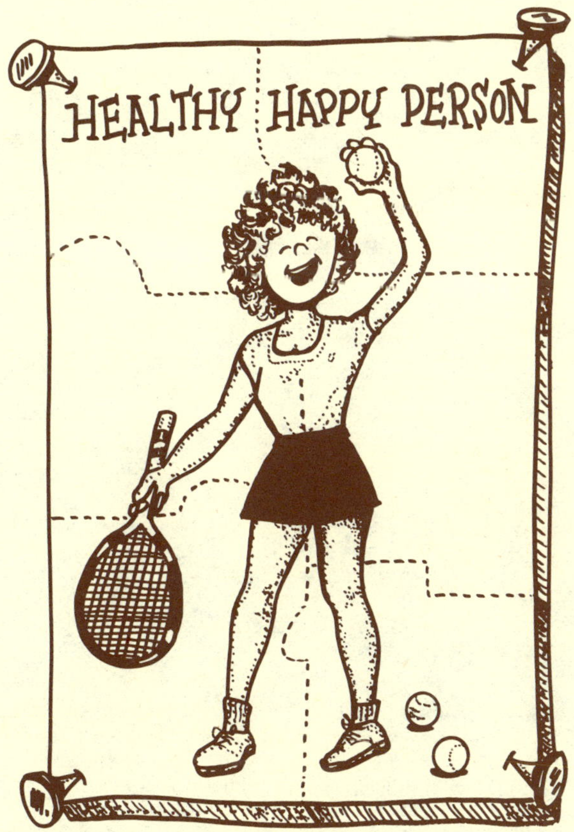

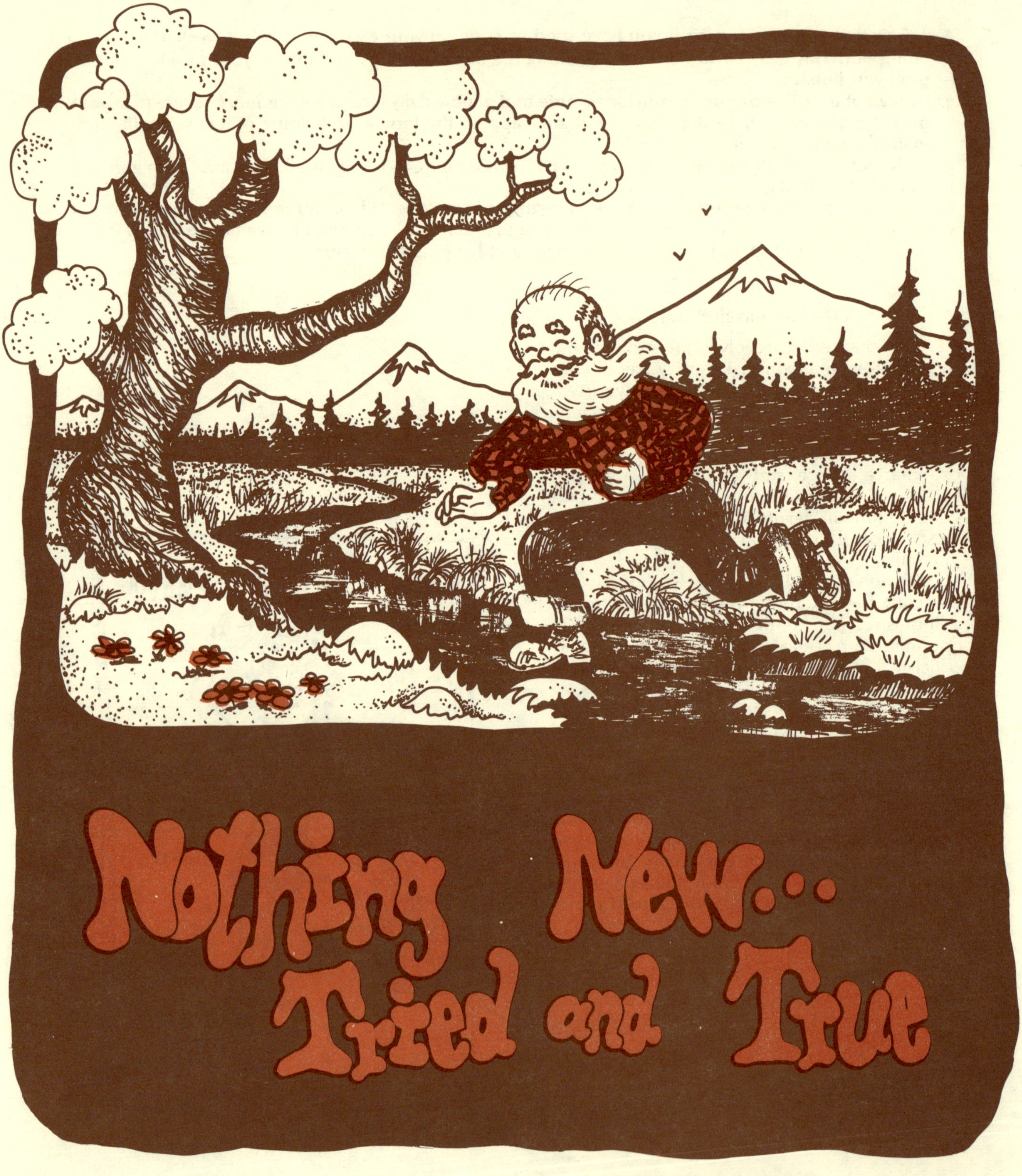
Nothing New...
Tried and True

Nothing New; Tried and True

Full Potential

Psychologists tell us that most people today reach only 5% of their potential. Maybe that is because we are what we eat and only 5% of the typical American diet is worthwhile food. Many animals live ten times their maturation age; yet humans consider themselves fortunate to live only three to four times their age of physical maturity. Might we increase both our life span and our capabilities when we improve our general health and well-being?

Earliest recorded history indicates that our ancestors often lived to be several hundred years of age. Their stone-age diet and common sense approach to survival apparently contributed more to longevity than does our space-age gluttony, gadgetry and greed. The traditions of the centenarians of the Andes in Ecuador, the Hunzukuts of Pakistan, the Abkhasians of Georgia, U.S.S.R. and the barefoot doctors and their people of China, provide most interesting reading and some insight into life without modern technology. They are proof that we can be strong-bodied, clear-minded and at peace with ourselves when we use our native herbs and whole foods sparingly and in harmony with all plant and animal life.

Our eyes have been opened — not just by generations of the long-ago past and isolated cultures — but also by people of our own century and country. They are friends of the earth, who ignore the convenience era and continue the age-old practices of organic gardening, home preservation and resourceful living; in general, refusing to fall prey to mass-fascination with modern technology.

We see today, nearly a century of progress and economic gain that has successfully robbed many people of reverence for and responsibility to our planet. Ask a space-age child where things come from — "Vegetables come from a can at the supermarket; water comes out of a faucet; the sun is something you can see when the pollution isn't too bad; and health is when we take a pill to make us all better."

Yes, technology has given us so much — to take for granted. To our ancient ancestors water, plants, the sun and health were synonymous with life and God. Think how a stone-age child might have responded to those same questions.

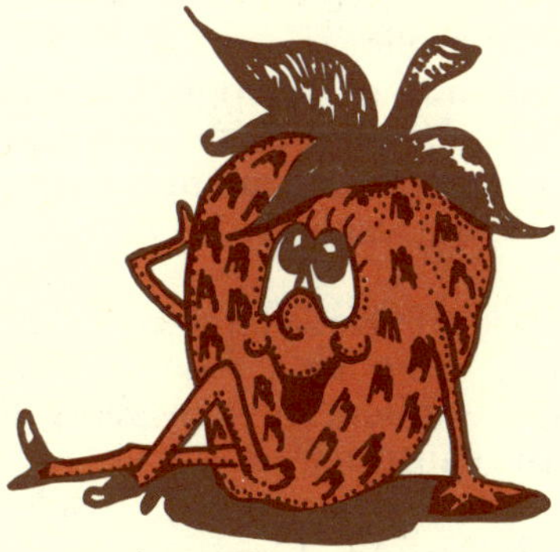

The doctor of the future will give no medicine but will interest his patients in the care of the human frame, in diet and in the cause and prevention of disease. — *Thomas Edison*

Self-Renewal

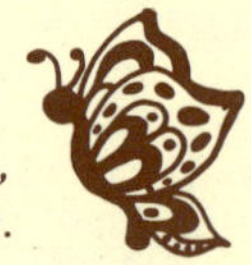

Mother Nature daily performs a silent operation,
The relentless endeaver of physical regeneration.
A series of miracles, each separate and distinct,
Yet, wondrous and inconceivable in the way they all are linked.

From the moment of conception to the end of our mortal days,
We are indescribably spellbound by Her captivating ways.
Her medicines are simple and effective for everyone —
Whole food, rest, air, water and the warmth of Brother Sun.

Within these basic elements are all that we require
To reach our full potential; then others we'll inspire.
So trust in your heart, call it instinct if you will,
Natural living worked in the beginning, it can work for us still.

Household Herbs For Healing and Happiness

The most ancient and traditional methods of medicine include the therapeutic use of herbs. Because we are living in a modernized society where medicine is sophisticated, scientific and analytical, we find it difficult to accept a form of healing based on folklore. Yet herbology, with its emphasis on preventive as well as remedial measures, is the great-grandfather of modern-day miracle drugs. One need not ostracize the medical establishment in order to utilize herbology, for ancient and modern wisdom can complement one another.

Drugs can, however, interfere with the body's normal healing procedures. They tend to force a response or temporarily alleviate a symptom, while neglecting the root cause, and may even antagonize or multiply the problem by leaving toxic residues or causing harmful side-effects.

The Physician's Desk Reference, available at most libraries, is a huge dictionary of prescription drugs. We found, in many cases, that the lists of precautions, adverse reactions, contraindications, warnings and side-effects were longer than the lists of action, composition, indications, administration and dosage. Interesting reading, in light of the reports of billions of dollars spent annually for supposedly *safe* drugs.

While herbs work more slowly than drugs, they are often complete with their own buffers or are used in conjunction with other herbs that combine to aid in the healing process. Because of their complex root systems, (indeed, many herbal preparations *are* roots) herbs often reach for the trace minerals, deep in the soil, that are missed by tuberous or shallow-rooted vegetables. Perhaps these minerals are the "secret" ingredient in herbs, for we know that all the vitamins in the world are of little value without the proper balance of minerals.

The herbologists we have met have been extremely conscientious. They revere our planet and pay tribute to all growing things. They wouldn't inflict a single herb tea repeatedly on their bodies the way many coffee drinkers do, three-five-seven times a day, day after day. They respect herbs for their inherent powers and always remind us that only the body can heal itself; the herbs are merely foods that aid in that process.

The Keys to Delicious Herbal Tea Blends

If you are trying to cut down on coffee or just plain like variety in your beverages, try herbal teas; some for their medicinal value, some for their delightful flavor and some for an excuse to relax and chat with a friend.

Include herbs as companion plants in your garden and experience the joy of drying your own or purchase them from a reputable herb shop. Some major black tea producers are marketing herbal teas, primarily to regain the business they have lost to small herbal co-operatives. Your support of the small herb companies will help ensure their survival and encourage the small business ethic — a practice which is important in other areas as well.

Store dried herbs in airtight containers, *always* label and use within the year. Strengths vary, but one rounded teaspoon of dried herbs to two cups of boiling water is a good, general ratio. Pour the boiling water over herbs that have been placed in a cloth bag, rattan strainer or stainless steel teaball. Allow to steep for five to ten minutes. (Do not allow tea to boil or it will become bitter.) Pour brewed tea into cups for you and your friends; then pour remainder into a thermos and enjoy the delicate flavor at intervals throughout the day. Avoid the use of aluminum pots. Refrigerate any left-over tea and drink cold or save to water plants.

The following tea blends are quite flavorful without additions, but you may want to add fresh lemon juice for vitamin C, honey for sweetness, and/or a cinnamon stick for spice and variety.

Terrific Triple Tea Blends: 2 Parts, 1 Part and To Taste

Papaya Leaf, Lemon Balm and Valerian
Papaya Leaf, Alfalfa Leaf and Wintergreen
Raspberry Leaf, Alfalfa Leaf and Wintergreen
Raspberry Leaf, Lemon Balm and Valerian
Raspberry Leaf, Papaya Leaf and any Mint
Raspberry Leaf, Yarrow and Spearmint
Rose Hips, Comfrey and Licorice Root
Rose Hips, Lemon Balm and a Cinnamon Stick
Alfalfa Leaf, Catnip and Licorice Root
Alfalfa Leaf, Papaya Leaf and Spearmint
Chamomile, Horehound and Licorice Root
Chamomile, Lemon Balm and Spearmint
Comfrey, Hyssop and Fennel
Comfrey, Rose Hips and Licorice Root
Lemon Balm, Comfrey and Goldenseal
Lemon Balm, Rose Hips and Fennel

The Keys to Using Medicinal Herbs

Remember that herbs work more slowly than drugs. They can be potent medicines and in a few cases harmful, even addictive, if misused. Refrain from using the same herb daily for more than two weeks at a time. Do not be foolish enough to use herbs in place of sound medical treatment in cases of obviously severe illness.

All of the properties attributed to the following herbs have been handed down from generation to generation and are never considered "cures," but only lend assistance to the body's own curative powers. Most are acceptable to the average palate, but, we confess, some are ghastly! Adults, as well as children, may be more receptive to the use of medicinal teas if lemon, honey and a cinnamon stick are added for flavor and fun.

Medicinal Herbs and Their Uses

CATNIP: Relieve gas, calm colic, reduce fever.
CAYENNE: Increase circulation, aid digestion, create warmth.
CHAMOMILE: Induce restful sleep, alleviate headache and menstrual cramps.
COMFREY: Soothe ulcers, promote general healing — internal and external.
FENNEL: Increase mother's milk, aid female troubles, relieve gas and colic.
FLAXSEED: Relieve constipation, improve skin; high in nutrients.
GARLIC: Relieve colds, respiratory problems, stimulate digestion, eliminate pinworms, external antiseptic poultice.
GOLDENSEAL: Relieve constipation, nausea, halitosis, itching.
HOREHOUND: Relieve colds, sore throat, coughing, constipation, pinworms.
HYSSOP: Reduce tension, fevers, phlegm, cleanse kidneys and blood.
LEMON BALM: Relieve gas, nausea, menstrual pain and fever.

LICORICE ROOT: Relieve sore throat, coughing, constipation.
PAPAYA LEAF: Aid digestion, calm stomach, cleanse blood.
PARSLEY: Reduce fever, stimulate sluggish system, high in vitamin C.
PEPPERMINT: Aid digestion, relieve colic, fever, strengthen heart.
RASPBERRY LEAF: Relieve discomfort of menstruation, pregnancy, anemia, mouth sores, heartburn and tension.
ROSE HIPS: Relieve cold symptoms, infection; high in vitamin C.
SENNA: Relieve constipation, halitosis, pinworms.
SLIPPERY ELM: Soothe sore throats, ulcers, burns — internally or as a wash.
SPEARMINT: Relieve colic, gas, nausea, soothe weak stomach.
VALERIAN: Sedative for tension, aching muscles, relieve gas, colic, fever.
YARROW: Relieve gas, diarrhea, soothe ulcers, hemorrhoids.
YERBA SANTA: Relieve congestion, sinus and respiratory, ear aches.

The Keys to Herbal Home Remedies

Old-fashioned remedies provide both intrigue and entertainment for the folklore buff. Many are downright ridiculous, but some of the more practical herbal remedies have proven very effective in our effort to cope with every-day disasters, sans over-the-counter drugs.

Not only have the following recipes worked well for us, but the side-effects have been great! Raucous laughter often accompanies a child's reluctance to "take your medicine" when a hand-mirror reflects the faces made before or after the deed is done. Dispensing remedies like garlic and cayenne can be more fun if skits or plays are performed where the audience must "partake of the potion" or "swallow the evidence" in order to facilitate curtain time.

Incidentally, entertainment, in the form of puppet shows, music, stories or role-playing (pretending you are a nurse, etc.) have a profound effect on the ill. Whether it is the pleasure, humor or just plain companionship that promotes healing is unknown, but for certain, the patient whose rest periods are alternated with periods of fun and happiness will recuperate more rapidly than the patient who is both sick *and* lonely or sad.

Home Remedies

GARLIC COLD PREVENTATIVE: To nip colds in the bud — as soon as you feel the first signs of a cold, peel and mince a few cloves of garlic; roll up in a lettuce leaf or slice of toast and chew well. Do this as often as necessary. OR, if you are brave and don't have any meetings in public today, simply chew a clove of garlic like gum and follow up with a shot of cayenne in fresh lemon juice.

GARLIC COUGH SYRUP: Press 1 entire bulb (several cloves) of garlic to exude juice. Mix with equal amount of honey and swallow every hour, allowing mixture to coat throat.

ONION COUGH SYRUP: Quarter 1 small onion into blender. Add 1 T. apple cider vinegar and 2 T. honey. Blend and refrigerate. Take 1 t. hourly or as needed.

SLIPPERY ELM THROAT LOZENGES: Mix 2 T. honey with 2 T. fresh lemon juice. Gradually add ½ cup slippery elm powder, adding more if necessary to make mixture very thick. Refrigerate until firm, then roll into dime-sized lozenges. Dehydrate. Suck on 1 or 2 for sore throat or to coat dry throat while running in cold weather or working in a dusty area.

SORE THROAT GARGLES: To 1 cup hot water, add 1 T. salt OR 1 T. apple cider vinegar OR ½ t. cayenne pepper. Gargle. (Caution: don't swallow the salt water.)

WOUND DISINFECTANT: Mix 1 part salt and 8 parts hot water OR 1 part cayenne and 10 parts hot water OR 1 part garlic juice and 5 parts hot water. Flush wound thoroughly and follow with application of aloe vera gel. VARIATION: Dip wounded area in pure wheat grass juice until bleeding is halted. Apply more juice at intervals with cotton. Expose open wounds to sunlight when practical.

WOUND ANESTHETIC: Numb wound with ice to lessen pain before applying above disinfectants or before removing splinters, insect stinger, or gravel.

MILK SEDATIVE: Heat milk but do not boil; add 1 t. honey and dash ground anise seed per cup of milk. Drink slowly just before bedtime.

TEA SEDATIVE AND BATH: Drink peppermint, catnip, valerian and/or chamomile tea while you relax in a warm (not hot) bath to which a very strong solution of any or all of those same teas — plus some dried orange or lemon peels — has been added.

SOOTHING POULTICES FOR BURNS, CUTS, BITES, STINGS, RASHES: Finely chop fresh comfrey leaf, parsley, eucalyptus, or sweet basil, until you have 2 T. Add a little boiling water and enough slippery elm powder to make a paste. Add any or all of the following: cayenne, garlic, goldenseal or camphor. Apply to tender area, cover with sterile cotton cloth, drink a cup of comfrey tea, relax and rest while the poultice transmits healing nutrients. Change poultice every 2 hours and alternate with applications of aloe vera gel or vitamin E. Expose skin to sunlight when possible.

SALVE FOR CANKER AND COLD SORES: Allow a little homemade yogurt to dehydrate slightly near a warm stove until it is the texture of thick glue. Apply to cold sores, canker sores and cracks in lips. Eat some regular yogurt at hourly intervals to replenish favorable intestinal bacteria and increase B-complex vitamins, which will help heal internally and prevent further lip sores.

SALVE FOR CHAPPED, DRY LIPS: Mash 1 t. avocado OR homemade, unsalted butter with the contents of a 500 I.U. capsule of vitamin E. Apply generously to lips before retiring. For daytime protection: In top of double boiler, melt 2 parts beeswax, 3 parts natural oil (almond, apricot, olive, orange, sesame, etc.), and ½ part camphor. Cool and add contents of 3 500 I.U. capsules of vitamin E. Keep refrigerated.

Medicine That's Easy To Take

At various times in our Motherhood careers, we've tried to spread the rumor,
That when little ones fall and hurt themselves, the key to healing is humor.
When a cut or scratch needs a little something to protect it for awhile,
You can make wearing a band-aid more fun by drawing on a happy smile.

When a child is so sick in bed that those toes won't even wiggle
It's time to get out the puppet show and bring about a giggle.
When you engage in story-telling and zany costume crafts,
You'll find that nothing is quite as contagious as good old-fashioned laughs!

We've witnessed the pain of a bloody bicycle/pavement turn-about
Disappear with the hilarious description of how NOT to do a wheelie burn-out!
"When, in the future on two wheels, you must play the clown,
Remember, love, that what goes up, will abruptly come back down."

Now if the hurt is more serious, like a broken leg in a cast,
Help it heal with a little note that says, "You're sitting still, AT LAST!"
No matter how brief the visit, a hospital can be quite frightful,
Plaster the ward walls with homemade HAPPINESS posters, bright and delightful.

As kids grow a little older, they'll test your mirth-provoking art,
Start looking now, for some amusing ways to repair a broken heart.
It isn't just the children that buffoonery helps to heal,
The aged and bed-ridden blossom, too, from merry-making zeal.

And to save yourself from dog-days, be your own comedienne,
Some clowning around, when you are down, can bring you up again.
You may have met a rare doc who, instead of RX gives a wisecrack,
While you're splitting your side, don't be surprised if you stage an amazing comeback.

For you see, though speaking medically, there's probably no proof,
Healing takes place at an incredible pace in the hands of whimsy and spoof.
We've found that joking, giggling and having a ball can make anyone forget,
Even if just temporarily, the pain or sorrow with which they've met.

Seriousness has its place, of course, but silly, nonsensical, monkey-shines,
Can help a person forget their burden, age is no limit to gibberish and rhymes.
The English language is adaptable to many a riddle and pun,
That will tickle the fancy and funny-bones of just about everyone.

Perhaps if we heard Ho, Ho, Ho's! all the year 'round
We would have peace, health and happiness in each and every town.
For if people in pain can smile, joke and jest,
Their optimism will surely rub off on the rest.

No matter how serious the illness, you can pull out of the strangest places
Little elves whose special task it is to turn frowns into smiling faces.
Yes, the very best medication you'll find, now and forever after,
Is the most valuable medicine known to mankind: uninhibited laughter!

CREATIVE COSMETICS

Medical care is often referred to as health care, but in most cases it is disease care — after the fact. We are glad to see a new resurgence in Whole-istic Health Care: a preventive as well as healing science which places the conscious responsibility for learning about causes and effects of disease on the individual in accordance with the healing practitioner.

An over-all program of improved diet and increased exercise to revitalize a sluggish system will show results almost overnight. But the best program may not be able to counter the side-effects of possibly carcinogenic cosmetics.

Any steps we can take, therefore, to improve the quality and naturalness of the beauty care products we use, is another step in the direction of personal responsibility for our own well-being, appearance and vitality.

Even when the air was fresh and clean, and the only available food-stuffs were wholesome, some help was appreciated to keep the outer surface of skin supple and resistant to the harsh and drying elements. Though the following creative cosmetics may seem strange to our readers, we think many of our beauty-conscious ancestors would be right at home in our bathtubs *and* our refrigerators.

Aloe Vera Plant

The "medicine plant" is not a cactus, as first appearance would indicate. It is a vegetable — a member of the lily family. Easy to grow, needing only occasional watering and organic plant food twice a year, the aloe is probably the most useful natural cosmetic.

Folklore attributes the aloe with properties of external healing of burns, including sunburn, stings and bites, poison oak and ivy, cuts and abrasions, eczema and other rashes, while more recent research has found aloe vera gel to be effective in reducing sensitivity of skin to irradiation.

Chewing the skin of the aloe vera leaf like gum is said to eliminate constipation, but it is an act of true grit on the part of your tastebuds! Internal attributes range from the relief of indigestion and ulcers, to alleviating bladder and kidney infections to freedom from aching joints and insomnia.

We have found aloe vera to be generally healing and nourishing for the complexion. Simply cut a one-inch section of an outside leaf, slit in half lengthwise and scrape gel onto a clean saucer; then spread gently onto the desired area of skin and allow to dry. For internal use, blend one part gel with six parts water or juice.

The gel is most effective in plants four or more years old. Many expensive cosmetics use aloe gel, but the plant is the most economical and potent source. Start some plants while your children are young and by the time they are teen-agers, they will have their own supply of safe complexion care. While waiting for your plants to mature, use the bottled gel available in health stores.

Fresh Lemon

Probably 50% of those bottles, cans, jars and tubes in the average medicine cabinet can be replaced by a fresh lemon. Bacteria have a difficult time surviving in an acid atmosphere, so squeezing fresh lemon juice on a wound may sting, but will have the antiseptic effect of some of the stronger commercial preparations, without sending potent bactericides into the bloodstream. Use fresh-squeezed lemon juice for a bleach, a gargle, to comfort a cold, sore throat or a hangover. It's a disinfectant, a hiccup-remedy and a restorer of the acid-mantle to frequently-washed skin or chapped hands. Diarrhea will usually respond to straight lemon juice, but if that's too strong for you, dilute it with warm tea. Don't put fresh lemon juice into boiling water or tea as the heat will destroy the vitamin C content. Entire aisles of drugstores are filled with highly suspect drug and cosmetic preparations designed to temporarily alleviate or mask symptoms. Leave them on the shelves and simply keep a good supply of lemons on hand at all times.

Luffa Sponge

A fibrous fruit of the luffa gourd, sometimes called the dishcloth gourd, luffa can be cooked and eaten when young and tender, but in its mature state is usually dried and used as a filter or a sponge. For the next best thing to your own masseuse, lather a luffa sponge with almond or coconut castile soap, starting from the extremities, gently massage your skin in tiny circular motions.

A luffa is great for removing dead, dry skin and helps improve blood (thus oxygen) flow to all parts of the body. It can be so invigorating that it is recommended that you never begin near the heart, as the stimulation may be too over-powering for some.

Soft sponges are best for your skin, but if you have a stiff one that is too scratchy, simply use it in your kitchen as a handy pot scrubber. Rinsed well and hung to dry after each use, your luffa will last for years.

Slantboard

You can improve circulation and counter the effects of gravity on skin, blood vessels and internal organs with a slantboard. Improvise your slantboard by recycling that ironing board you hid in the back of the closet, thinking you would never use it again. Leave board flattened and raise one end about four inches with some books.

Now plaster your face with any of the Feel-Good-Facials (to follow) and place moist tea bags over your eyes. Lie with feet elevated, allowing arms to fall comfortably to sides. Fold a blanket to form a resting place for your head, which will probably extend beyond the ironing board surface, but avoid using a pillow, which may cause neck cramps.

Take your phone off the hook while you relax on the slantboard so you won't be interrupted by the "jack-rabbit" reflex to answer the phone. Start with three minutes and increase gradually until you can lie down for fifteen minutes without discomfort. Always get up slowly, sit for a few minutes to regulate your blood pressure, then stand in one place until you sense the return of your equilibrium.

Vitamins

That which is good for your entire body, will automatically be good for your skin, including vitamins and minerals. Sometimes a body that has been depleted of nutrients for many years due to processed foods, pollution and built-up residues from medicines, needs a vitamin and mineral "booster."

The nutrients that we have used effectively for improved skin are vitamins A, B-complex, C, D and E, brewer's yeast, plus the mineral, zinc. These should be obtained, whenever possible, from food, but when problems occur that are the result of a particular vitamin deficiency, we prefer taking supplemental vitamins to taking drugs. We have yet to read of a disease that was the result of a drug deficiency!

It is always important to take the vitamin or mineral *along with* a food that naturally contains some of that nutrient, such as vitamin C *with* grapefruit, or multi-minerals *with* fish. This enhances the benefits of both the whole food and the separated nutrient.

For more information about vitamins, be sure to read *Feed Your Kids Right,* by Dr. Lendon Smith. Geared for parents of kids from infancy through adolescence, but including advice that will last a lifetime, Dr. Smith has provided a complete nutritional and vitamin therapy program for prevention of illness and maintenance of good health, minus the harmful side-effects of drugs.

Water

The human body can survive for months without food, but only a few days without water. Water is necessary for all bodily functions and has been used for centuries, through fasting, to relieve and restore a sluggish system. Mineral bathing and drinking waters in various parts of the world have long been renowned for their healing properties.

Try to drink at least five full glasses of water daily. Get some water by drinking vegetable-cooking water, some in the form of tea, some through milk, some from fruits and fill in with plain water, between meals. As long as you are eating foods high in potassium and low in sodium, you needn't worry about water reten-

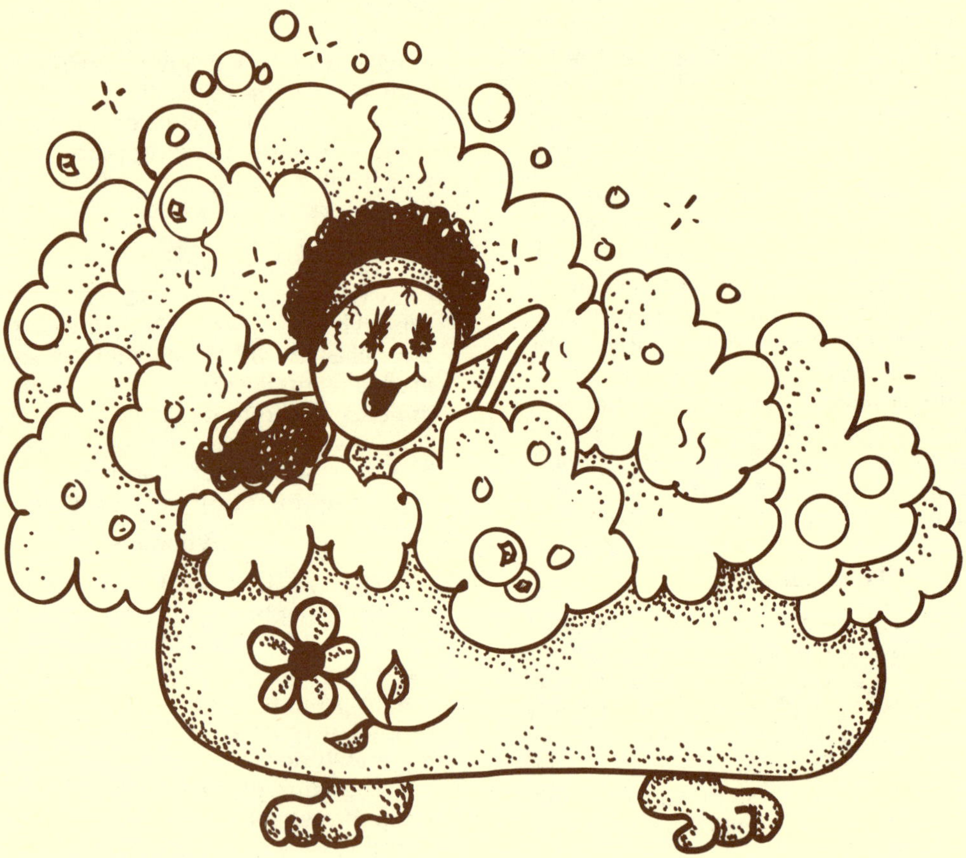

Happy are those who dream dreams and are ready to pay the price to make them come true.
L.J. Cardinal Suenens

tion; in fact, you may notice a definite diuretic effect, as the water flushes toxins from your system.

Externally, a warm bath (98° F.) on an empty stomach is a tremendous sedative and will relax the most nervous person in the most nerve-wracking situation. Granted a quick shower is definitely an energy-conserving way to keep clean, but for special occasions, nothing beats the relaxing herbal/oil bath. Not only will you look and feel terrific, you and the bathroom will both smell delicious!

It has been said that the pre-requisite to being beautiful is being in love. We certainly hope that you are in love every day of your life, but on those days when love doesn't seem to be working for you, try a warm, leisurely, herbal bath.

The Feel-Good-Facial

Some things change over the years, but cleanliness is still next to godliness. Wash your skin with plain, old-fashioned, pure castile soap. Avoid perfumed, dyed and deodorant soaps, as well as detergents and any cleansing agent with hexachlorophene. Because soap is alkaline in nature, and as such will both dry and imbalance the skin, washing should always include a final rinse that replenishes the acid mantle that would otherwise take from four to six hours to be replaced from within.

The *Feel-Good-Facial* method for washing and rinsing involves some perseverence, but the beneficial effects are so obvious that you will be anxious to continue. Before you begin, tie all your hair off your face and brush your teeth until they sparkle.

You will need a large, clean, glass mixing bowl, a towel around your shoulders, one-half of a sterile cotton ball, the oil of your choice, soap, a soft cloth and either fresh lemon juice or apple cider vinegar for the rinse. Now for the part that is going to feel so-o-o good!

Absorb about one-half teaspoon oil (sesame, olive, sunflower) onto the cotton puff and blot gently all over your face and neck. While your skin is elastic, do some facial stretches — form long, exaggerated vowel sounds — A-a-a-a-a, E-e-e-e-e, I-i-i-i-i, O-o-o-o-o, U-u-u-u-u, Ah-h-h-h-h.

Fill the bowl with water as hot as you can stand to put your hands into. Don't be afraid to splash this water directly on your face — if your hands can take it, so can your face. Wet your hands and lather them with soap and, using gentle circular motions, lather your entire face, keeping eyes and mouth closed but not pursed. Take your time, use only your fingertips, for they are the most sensitive. *Never rub* or apply ice to your face. There are tiny capillaries just below the surface that can break and leave permanent, unsightly, red lines, appearing like cracks of lightning on the skin.

Follow your thirty-second lathering with two minutes of splashing of the hot water from the bowl (even when it gets soapy) back onto your face. Pour out the soapy, oily water; rinse bowl and refill with clean, hot water. Splash your face for another full minute. Empty water, rinse bowl and half-fill bowl with tepid water (to close pores), adding up to one Tablespoon fresh lemon juice OR apple cider vinegar. Splash lavishly for one full minute, then pat dry with a soft, absorbant cloth.

Last, and definitely most important, apply a thin layer of healing aloe vera gel to protect the skin from pollution, dust particles and airborne bacteria. Keep hands, telephone receivers, pencils, etc., away from face at all times and avoid going places where you will be exposed to side-stream cigarette smoke.

If your morning routine includes a shower or bath, then do your facial as described but save the final ph-balancing rinse for *after* you are squeaky clean. Triple the amount of rinse and splash all over your body.

Once a week, you may wish to capture an extra fifteen minutes for a *Feel-Good-Sauna*. Prepare a very strong tea from two quarts boiling water and two Tablespoons of any or all of the following herbs: goldenseal, horehound, hyssop, sage, senna, elderflower or fennel seed. Allow tea to steep in large saucepan while you improvise a tent with a large bath towel over your head.

Sit comfortably next to a low table or counter, place your head about five inches above the hot tea, secure the towel to cover any openings and breath deeply for about ten minutes. Follow with a tepid ph-balance rinse to close pores and renew the acid mantle. This mini-sauna is simultaneously relaxing and stimulating. It may be alternated with the *Feel-Good-Scrub,* which has a gritty texture that, literally, removes the outer layer of skin, and therefore, should be done only once a week.

Facial Plasters

Add vitamin E, squeezed from a capsule, to any facial plaster. Vitamin E is said to help regenerate the skin cells and heal blemishes without scars, while it gives a soft appearance to the skin. Apply vitamin E oil around eyes, *very* carefully, to prevent crows feet which result from dry skin. Eggs and yogurt are used for their protein conditioning and the various oils maintain suppleness. Apply facial plaster of your choice liberally to face and neck while you relax on the slantboard or read, or talk on the phone, etc. If plaster is too thin, thicken with a little rice polish.

YOGURT AND CUKES: Liquefy 1 peeled cucumber in blender and gently stir in ¼ cup plain yogurt.
EGG AND POTATO: Cube 1 small potato and liquefy in blender with 1 egg.
LEMON AND BANANA: Blend 1 banana with 1 T. fresh lemon juice and 1 t. sesame oil.
AVOCADO AND HONEY: Mash ½ ripe avocado with 1 t. fresh lemon juice and 1 t. honey.
HONEY AND HONEY: It's sticky! But leaves your skin feeling great!
MAYONNAISE: (See recipe for homemade mayonnaise in *Labor of Love Lunches.)*
EGG AND OIL: Beat 1 egg with 1 t. wheat germ oil.
EGG AND HONEY: Beat 1 egg white until stiff peaks form; add 1 t. honey and fold into beaten yolk.

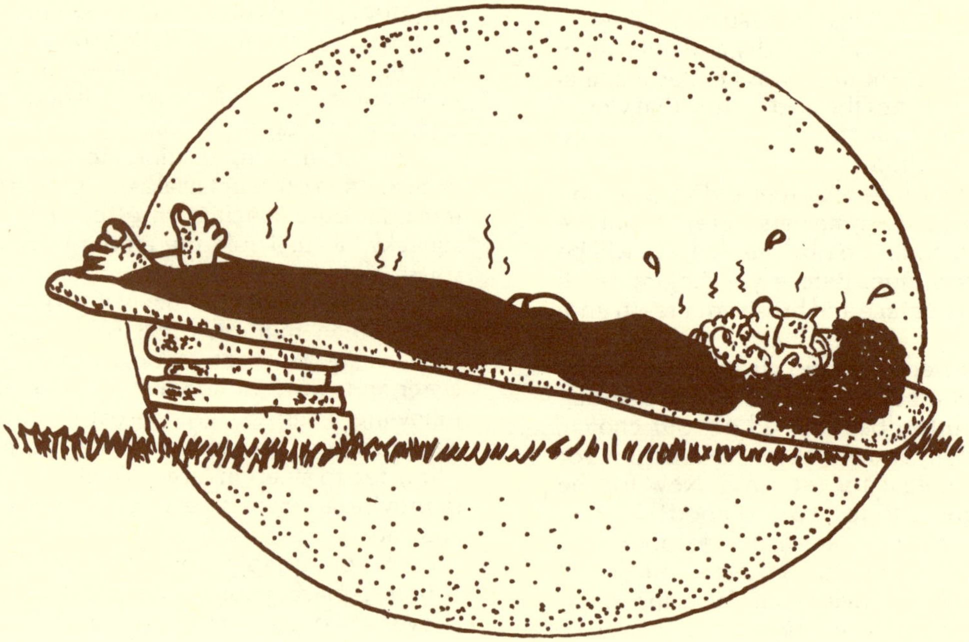

Wrinkles should merely indicate where smiles have been. *Mark Twain*

Facial Scrubs

Use 1 t. of any of these scrubs with the lathering step in the *Feel-Good-Facial.* Massage *ever-so-gently.*

OATMEAL: Blend ¼ cup oatmeal until fine. Add ½ t. cloves and enough orange oil to give a creamy consistency.

CORNMEAL: Mix ¼ cup cornmeal with enough raw milk, cream or plain yogurt to achieve a creamy consistency.

ALMOND: Grind ¼ cup almonds to a fine meal in blender. Add enough fresh pineapple, cantaloupe or papaya juice to form creamy consistency.

All Night Masques

Apply sparingly before retiring, preferably on a night when you are sleeping alone! In the morning, simply eliminate the oil step of your facial. Keep excess refrigerated.

COLD CREAM: Blend equal parts coconut oil, rosewater and lanolin, about 2 T. each. Add about 1,000 I.U. vitamin E if you like.

DREAM CREAM: Mix 2 T. orange oil (or other sweet-smelling oil) with 2,000 I.U. vitamin E.

LECITHIN CREAM: Dissolve 1 T. lecithin granules or powder in 1 T. warm water. Add 1 T. cold-pressed vegetable oil of your choice and blend well.

After Shave Lotions

ALOE VERA GEL: Splash on gel scraped from leaf of aloe plant, or use bottled gel. Refreshing and protective.

CHAMOMILE: Splash on strong infusion of chamomile tea with just a squeeze of fresh lemon juice added.

GINSENG: Splash on strong infusion of ginseng tea to which a little mineral water has been added.

Deodorants

The fact that ingredients are now listed on the side of some commercial deodorants does not guarantee safety. Be very cautious of anti-perspirants. Many work by means of a chemical that inhibits normal secretions of the sweat glands. Sweating is a way to dispose of toxins and regulate body temperature. Blocking this process only aggravates a body odor problem.

BAKING SODA: Simply dust underarm area with additive-free baking soda.

ALOE VERA: Scrape leaf section and apply gel liberally to underarm area, or use bottled gel.

Suntan Lotions

ALOE VERA AND ARTICHOKE JUICE: Actually *any* vegetable-cooking water can be blended with aloe vera gel and smoothed onto entire body to form a protective, vitamin-rich shield against sunburn. If you must be in direct sunlight between the hours of 11:30 a.m. and 3:00 p.m., wear loose, light-colored, cotton clothing and a hat or sun visor.

MAYONNAISE: Beat 1 egg yolk until light and lemon-colored. Slowly beat in 1 cup of corn or olive oil. Whip until thick, then add 1 t. wheat germ oil and 1 t. apple cider vinegar. Mix together thoroughly. Refrigerate unused portion.

Lips and Teeth

HIBISCUS LIP GLOSS: In top of double boiler, melt 2 T. pure beeswax with 2 T. sesame oil and 2 T. almond oil. Cool and add 2,000 I.U. vitamin E, squeezed from capsules. To add color, prepare a very strong infusion of hibiscus tea from ½ cup boiling water and ¼ cup hibiscus flowers. Thoroughly press and drain the flowers and place the dark red liquid in a shallow pan near a warm surface so the excess moisture can evaporate. When the deep red liquid is very thick, add to beeswax mixture, a little at a time, until you reach the desired color. Keep refrigerated.

CALCIUM TOOTH POWDER: Mix equal parts baking soda and powdered calcium OR bone meal. Add a little cinnamon if you wish. Place about 1 t. of this mixture on the palm of your hand; moisten toothbrush and dip into tooth powder. Brush slowly and carefully; rinse thoroughly.

NATURAL TOOTHBRUSH: Boil sections of licorice root until soft. The fibrous texture will scrub teeth as you chew the root pieces. They are not sweet, but give a hint of licorice flavor on your tongue and a refreshing essence to your breath.

BREATH FRESHENERS: Chew cloves or parsley, OR place a dash of ginger on the tip of the tongue.

Eye Care

The most conscientious effort to exercise often neglects the eyes. Move eyes around in their sockets in any manner that feels *strange*. This will exercise muscles that you don't use in everyday activities while strengthening and supporting those you do.

Foods high in vitamin A will help keep your eyes healthy and foods rich in potassium and low in sodium will help rid the body of excess water build-up, preventing a condition called "puffy eyes."

Protect eyes from sunlight by wearing dark glasses or, more important, avoid direct sunlight exposure between the hours of 11:30 a.m. and 3:00 p.m. Evaluate the risks of exposing your eyes to pollutants, such as cigarette smoke, gasoline fumes and factory emissions when planning to attend events and gatherings or even when shopping. Soothe tired, itching, blood-shot eyes with the following compresses:

CUCUMBER: Place 1 thick, juicy slice of cucumber on each eye while you relax every muscle to the instructions of your pre-recorded voice. (See *Getting It Together.)*

POTATOES: Fold raw grated potatoes into 2 cheesecloth bags and apply 1 to each eye. Rest on a slant-board for 15 minutes.

HERBAL TEA: Drink a warm cup of your favorite relaxing tea. Reserve the bags. Lie down on a slantboard with a tea bag on each eye, and relax your entire body, removing all thoughts and "mind pictures" from your head. Consciously feel your eyes "drop" in their sockets.

Foot Care

MAYONNAISE: Massage the bottoms, tops and ankles of your feet with mayonnaise; wrap in cotton or put on all-cotton socks and rest on slantboard. Do not wash; just wipe off excess and enjoy ultra-soft, smooth feet.

BAREFEET: Go barefoot or wear moccasins as often as possible for the ultimate in foot massage. Walking barefoot in the sand will help remove blisters, corns or rough spots on the heels and soles.

REFLEXOLOGY: Borrow from the library or purchase a book on reflexology and learn how to give yourself a foot massage. By improving circulation, stimulating sluggish organs and breaking up crystalline deposits, you will be able to make yourself feel great all over. Put a friend in seventh heaven and give him/her a foot massage.

Hair Care

Sprouted grains, raw seeds and nuts, eggs, fish and all foods high in B vitamins aid in the production of enzymes, hormones and protein for healthy hair and skin. Again, because our scalp is not always visible, there is a tendency toward neglect. Brewer's yeast and eggs have long been added to animal feed to improve hides and hair. They are equally effective for the crowning glory of humans.

Any circumstance which uses up the B-complex vitamins stored in the liver, will contribute to hair and scalp problems. Negative reaction to stressful situations is at the top of the list, but equally important is the over-indulgence of refined sugars and starches, alcohol, animal products, coffee and chocolate — all B-vitamin depleters.

Hair is protein and depends on the ingestion, digestion and assimilation of high quality protein. This is very important because, although red meat is a source of complete protein, it may stay in the intestinal tract for long periods of time, re-releasing toxins and often resulting in incomplete digestion and assimilation. Excessive fat intake from animal products can compound the problem by contributing to extra secretion of sebum. On top of all this, circulation may be sluggish, leaving hair and scalp short of regenerating nutrients and resulting in itching, dandruff and loss of hair.

All of the dietary suggestions in this book are designed to help improve the quality of your blood, while the exercises will ensure that the healthy blood is well-circulated. With these factors working from the inside, hair and scalp deserve only the best and most natural care from the outside.

Brush with a natural bristle brush and comb with a hard rubber or wooden comb. Never touch plastic or metal to your hair or scalp. Use only plain soaps or natural shampoos — no harsh concentrates or detergent shampoo — and always follow with a ph-balancing rinse. Hair spray may make your hairdo last longer, but those tiny particles of chemicals can wreak havoc in your lungs as well as the lungs of anyone who is misfortunate enough to have to breathe the air where you spray. The new pump sprays are an improvement over aerosol cans; however the container change has no bearing on the quality of the chemical ingredients.

Hair Conditioners

YOGURT: Work plain yogurt through your hair, being certain to thoroughly cover the scalp. Massage with fingertips and protect with a shower cap while you exercise. Shampoo and rinse with chamomile tea (for light hair) to which a squeeze of lemon juice has been added.

MAYONNAISE: Massage gently into scalp with fingertips, cover with shower cap and curl up with a good book on self-improvement. Wash thoroughly and follow with a raspberry leaf tea rinse (for dark hair) to which a little apple cider vinegar has been added.

WARM OIL: Warm wheat germ oil or olive oil in a double boiler and massage gently into scalp. Cover with shower cap, plaster face with your choice of facials. Apply tea bags to eyes and relax on slant-board for 15 minutes to nourish the scalp and circulate the blood.

Protein Shampoos

EGG: Mix 1 egg with 1 t. of liquid pure castile soap or shampoo from the health store. Using half of mixture, massage your scalp and shampoo as usual. Rinse and shampoo again with remainder of mixture. Follow with a ph-balancing rinse using your favorite smelling herbal tea to which a little fresh lemon juice or apple cider vinegar has been added.

YOGURT: Mix ¼ cup plain yogurt with 1 t. of liquid pure castile soap or health store shampoo. Use half for first washing and half for second washing. Follow with a rinse of stale beer.

BUTTERMILK: Stir buttermilk, 1 T. at a time, into 1 t. of liquid pure castile soap or health store shampoo to which 2 T. aloe vera gel have been added and blended thoroughly in blender. When consistency is that of yogurt, shampoo as usual. Rinse with your choice of ph-balancing mixtures.

CAUTION: Read labels carefully on commercial shampoos. They may contain just enough natural ingredients to flag "natural" all over the label. In fact, some shampoos are 75% synthetic and some that claim "no tears" contain a chemical that deadens nerve endings so the pain cannot be sensed. Especially investigate baby shampoos carefully!

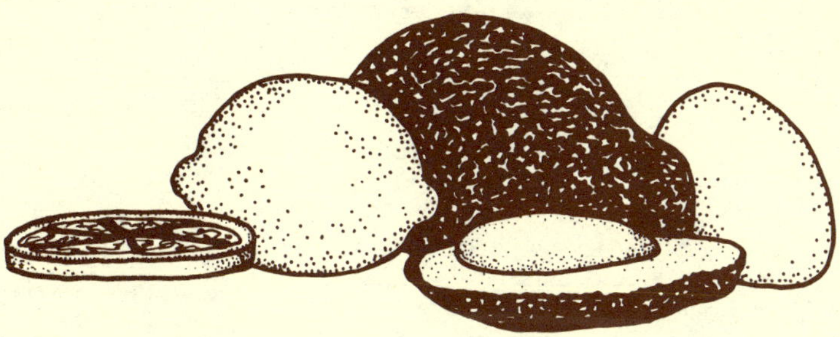

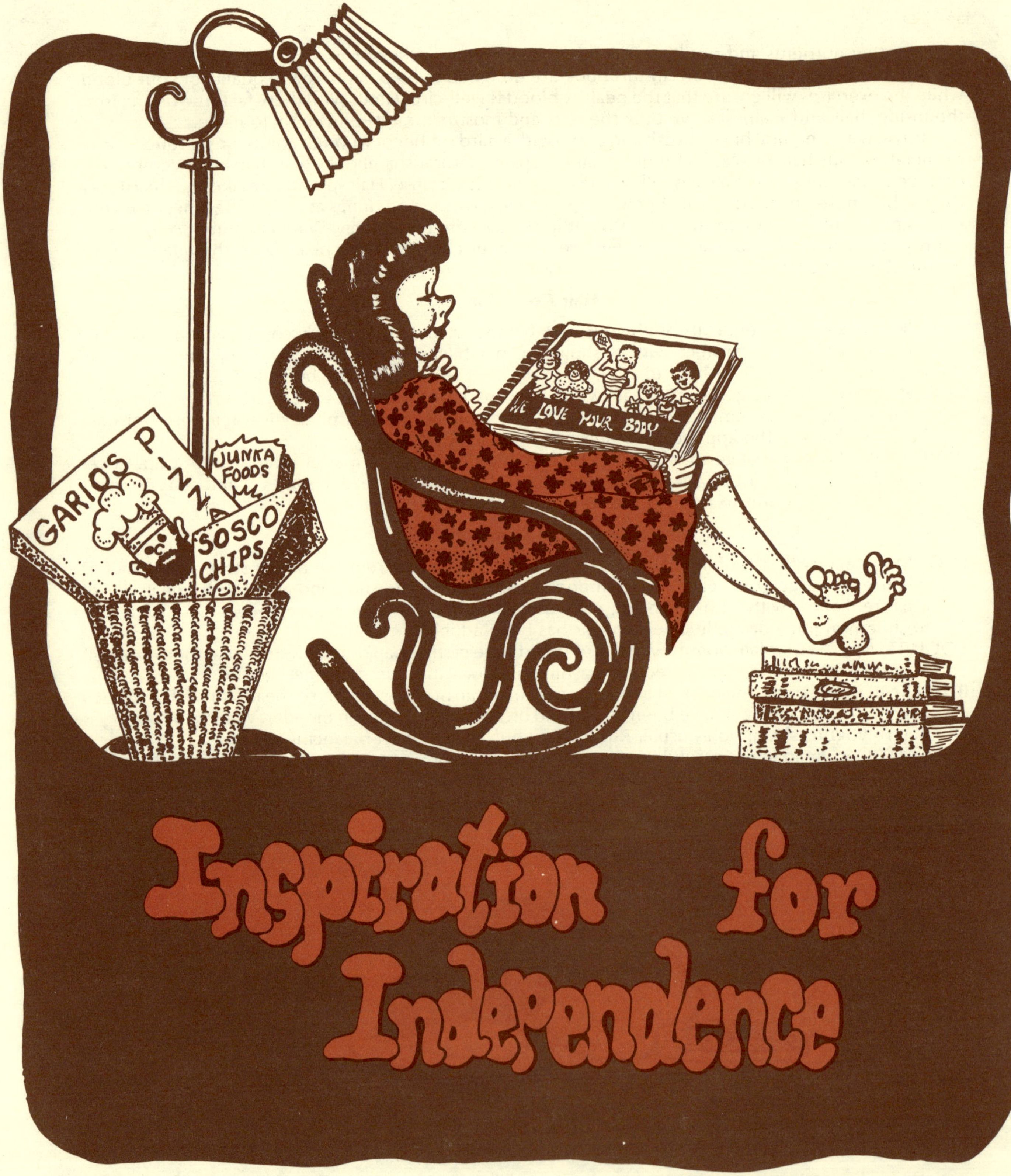

Inspiration for Independence

Inspiration For Independence

Television — Schmellivision!

It takes a mighty powerful force to gradually rearrange
Or transfigure or manipulate or just plain change,
A whole generation of intelligent minds
With neuro-physiological reactions of all kinds:
Confused, spaced-out, dream-walking zombies who've been hypnotized,
Brainwashed, invaded, controlled and mesmerized.

Advertisements flash images that permeate the brain,
In hopes that tomorrow you won't be able to refrain
From purchasing another worthless object you'll likely never use,
But it's made so desirable, you just can't refuse
When your little one says, "Please, I saw it on T.V."
"And EVERYBODY has one — except ME!"

A whole civilization has been excommunicated.
Reading, family games and human conversation, eradicated.
Once, treasured handcrafts were taught to the next generation,
Now our children are victims of sensory deprivation.
We didn't see it coming, it was so cleverly subtle,
Now we must get our young minds out of this muddle.

"Programming" is the problem, we think you'll agree,
Monomania fixation stifles creativity.
Ideals and values are reshaped while sitting blank and unaware,
Crime, debauchery and violence are handled as every-day fare.
Discretion IS possible, some shows we credit and compliment:
News, education, feelings, public interest and sheer enjoyment.

Let's return to at-least-partial-pre-television lifestyle:
Equal time for studies, hobbies, sports and activities, all worthwhile.
Discover new interests or rekindle the old,
There must be some family stories, yet untold.
Dust off the volumes of olden-days photographs,
The fashions alone are good for a few laughs.

Be your own sit-com, play your own quiz shows,
Plant a garden in which memories grow by the rows.
The best way to encourage family members to be creators
Is to write, direct and act in your own live theaters.
Never feel guilty in your cut-down-on-automation endeaver,
For HUMAN communication is the rose that grows forever.

The Perils of Programming

"What you don't know, won't hurt you," is a phrase that could easily have been coined by a powerful figure who wanted the "little people" to remain ignorant of how power is attained. Or it could have been the slogan of a fast food franchise, ensuring the secrecy of questionable business operations, while reaping vast profits from a gullible public.

Regardless of its origin, the statement is false as often as it is true. If you are unable to read or write, you will be hurt in the work-force; if you know little about keeping fit, you will suffer temporary aches and pains that will lead to early aging and chronic ailments in later years; if you do not know how to love, you will miss the greatest joy of life.

What we didn't know earlier in our lives, has hurt us. Heart disease, cancer, diabetes, ulcers and tooth decay, among other physical problems, might have been prevented or at least delayed, had we been better informed. So, in essence, this chapter is our own personal reading list. We hope that the lessons we've learned will inspire you to read, read and read some more; to delve deeper into the world of whole-istic living and to take the time to research controversial issues about which the public sees only the side that Big Brother wants us to see.

Of course this means unearthing things that "we aren't supposed to know" and consequently, "aren't supposed to hurt us." But know we must, if we are to make valid decisions or leave our children equipped to make even more complex decisions in the future.

Hitler (reputed to have been a sugar addict) symbolized the blindness with which people allow themselves to be programmed. Using swastika emblems to give followers a sense of unity; spewing fiery words to implant his beliefs and goals for the "good of the people and the country," he hypnotized them into believing promises he knew would never be kept. Individual freedoms were eliminated and an atmosphere of terror among the people prevailed. History is filled with brazen leaders whose shameless techniques have programmed intelligent people to accept ruthless ideals and then justify their course of action.

We must stop trying to justify poor health by calling it "minor" aches and pains, overweight, lack of energy or nervous tension. We must speak out and refuse to be programmed into mental, spiritual or physical ill-health. We must be grateful for the Beatrice Hunters, the Rachel Carsons, the Ralph Naders and the Michael Jacobsons of the world, who have exposed the other side and found that what we don't know CAN hurt us.

We must continue to read and educate ourselves, being cautious all the while not to believe everything we read on either side of an issue, but to make independent decisions based on the recorded research of others, as well as our own experiences. In Ralph Nader's words, "Everything we're proud of in this country came from people who made waves." For our own benefit and the benefit of future generations — we *must* make waves.

Stay Tuned for a Quiet Commercial

If you are fortunate enough to live near a wilderness area, then you can experience an honest-to-goodness quiet commercial. You can bask in the breathtaking advertisement of Nature; the peace and beauty that echoes between the mountains, rushes downstream and spreads a blanket of tranquility on the valley floor. You will have to listen closely for the chatter of wild animals; they are light on their feet and wish to retain their privacy. Enjoy the serenity, go away relaxed and plan to return in another season, but do not expect the same *program,* for in the wilderness, change is consistent with Nature's laws.

Contrast this to the hustle-bustle of suburbia, where the fluctuations of the stock market, the fashion scene and the latest plastic gimmick direct daily lives. Nature's laws are forever. People who respect and follow them, either because their eyes have been opened by a tragedy or because they just want better over-all health, are labeled "health-nuts." Those who blatantly violate Nature's laws are considered "normal."

Because a single encounter with alcohol, cigarettes or junk food does not kill a "normal" person instantly, they do not worry. They rotely take their aspirin and valium, their heartburn and anti-acid tablets, their no-doze and sleep-ease, their laxative and preparation ouch, and their legal uppers and downers; they pay their medical bills and just keep cruising along, counting on the odds to see them through.

Horizontal, Vertical and Contrast

We are very aware that there are many beautiful, healthy and happy people in between the extremes. In fact we, Lani and Diane, are somewhere in between. We try to obey Nature's laws, but are neither purists nor perfectionists. We are two women living in a complex world, trying to raise our children in a healthy atmosphere, with moral values, independent minds and the tools they will surely need to keep pace with their own generation. We live in a town that has its share of pollution, drugs and other problems, but won't cry "doomsday," for we know that there are alternatives and solutions to every problem and there are too many things in this life worth living for. We have listened to the experiences of enough wise senior citizens to know that we have the best of two worlds: urban and rural, old-fashioned and modern.

Because of electric appliances, we can spend more time with the people we love; because of transportation, we can travel to the wilderness and return refreshed; because of medical science, we can raise our children free of deadly contagious diseases; because of adversity in our lives, we can be grateful for our blessings. Because we have been "normal," we can better appreciate our vitality.

As individuals, we are a balanced contrast. One of us has lived in many parts of the world, one is a hometown girl. One is a professional person, one a homemaker. One is Protestant, one Catholic, one short, blond and one tall, brunette, and on and on.

The point is, that while our hereditary backgrounds and reasons for personal involvement in preventive health are different, our metabolic processes are alike, and basically, the same as yours. We eat, work, play, sleep, walk, talk, pray, cry, smile, hurt, make mistakes and learn, just like most people. We do not pretend to have all the answers. We are not wonder women and aren't insinuating that you should be. Our enthusiasm and zeal come from knowing that we have improved our own little corner of the world. WE LOVE OUR BODIES, and if by spreading our sunshine we help you to love yours, then we have achieved our goal.

And Now a Word From Our Sponsor . . .

About prosperity: There are those who criticize the supporters of the wellness movement because some health enthusiasts have something to sell; vitamins, grain mills, juicers, etc. We don't endorse or sell any brand name products, but in all fairness, we understand why some people do.

If a pianist has a talent that makes people happy and willing to pay to experience the pleasure of beautiful music, then it is only fitting that the artist make a living from music. If a philosopher has an idea, the sharing of which helps people to build self-confidence, fair-mindedness, and genuine compassion for fellow human beings and students are grateful enough for self-improvement to pay for the knowledge, then the teacher has every right to prosper from his/her wisdom. If a once unhealthy person discovers better health through raw juices or vitamin therapy, then s/he has every right to market the idea or product, help others and make a living doing so.

Granted, there are rip-offs. But the real frauds — the ones who are just out to make a fast buck — are the pushers of drugs, pornography, the occult, pesticides and junk food. These are the industries that make their living at someone else's expense. They prey on innocent children, the poor and the insecure. They weasel their way into people's lives under false pretenses and make misleading or downright deceptive claims about their products.

When we catergorize junk food with the above named destructive forces, we are not talking about your neighbors who run the corner deli and serve white bread sandwiches (though we would like to see them try whole wheat!). We're talking about the cold cereal swindle where major universities can receive huge grants in exchange for a prominent M.D.'s vocal support to mothers that children need sugar to start their day. We're also talking about the snack manufacturers who print and distribute free food-service pamphlets to home economic's classes all over the country, full of recipes that use their brand name products. And we're talking about the international industrial corporations marketing hosty-toasties because there's money in junk food.

We're talking about agriculture conglomerates wiping out the small farmer because higher volume means fatter profits; about the tobacco companies that bait family magazines with coupons for free packs of cigarettes in order to hook future customers. And we're talking about the cola companies that unnecessarily add caffeine to their beverages so that young people will unknowingly become addicted to the so-called soft drinks that are potent enough to dissolve nails.

Periodically the newspaper headlines catch our eye, with a caption like, "Health-Food & Vitamin Industries Rip-Off Senior Citizens." We have spoken with many retired people who don't feel cheated when they use vitamins, but could tell you a story or two about sour deals they've received from the medical establishment and the government! So, let's aim those headlines at the appropriate (government subsidized) targets — "Alcohol, Tobacco, Drug and Sugar Industries Rip-Off Humanity!"

We could fill books with similar injustices and promotional propaganda from the already wealthy companies who only stand to profit even more by their advertising ploys. But we don't have to because many other writers already have; that is why it is so important to read, and be informed, in order to make sound decisions based on your own research. The voice of authority is inside *you.*

It's A Crime

"Kids, these days — they've got no respect!"
That's an ancient outcry from the grown-up sect,
Who gripe, point fingers, criticize and complain.
Well, we're tired of hearing fellow adults sing the same old refrain.

Kids don't build the bars, gambling halls or porn shops.
They don't run the sleazy joints where dope pushers make their stops.
They don't organize the occult "religions" that worship devils.
They don't make junk food, colas and candies that screw up blood sugar levels.

Kids don't hoard their wealth while ignoring the poor,
They don't write government bills that spend less on kids, more on war.
They don't give preference to the "beautiful people" and disregard the "average."
They wouldn't consider selling a fellow child into a life of slaverage.

Kids don't sell the guns, knives or books on "how it's done,"
They don't write TV/movie scripts that treat criminals and heroes as one.
They don't bottle the booze, or package the pills
That contribute to a good many of this modern world's ills.

Kids don't blaspheme God or make profanity the common way.
They don't paint the pessimism seen on so many faces today.
They wouldn't take a beautiful body, then photograph it to dehumanize,
For the sake of vanity, sensationalism or financial "enterprise."

Kids don't overcharge, underpay, take graft or monopolize,
They don't politic "for the people" then from vested interests accept a subsidize.
Kids aren't naturally greedy, they wouldn't be spoiled as kings,
If adults wouldn't shower them with materialistic "things."

Kids don't design or publish those full-page ad releases
(Are otherwise good periodicals and newspapers so desperate for sales increases?)
That blatently display smoking, drinking and sex discrimination,
In front of kids who are trying to read or study for information.

Kids don't cheat on taxes, pollute the air or discriminate races,
They don't ask for poverty, ignorance, disease or other disgraces.
They're not born rebellious, belligerent or criminal,
But the messages they receive from adults are often subliminal.

Kids can't have much feeling of esteem or self-worth
If they've been constantly scorned, ridiculed and rejected from birth.
When kids are trapped in a losing situation,
They harbor feelings of vengeance, vindictiveness and retaliation.

How many kids are in trouble today,
Because they never learned to live in a constructive way?
We're only on this planet X number of hours,
Let's teach kids to try to get the most quality from their powers.

Be a leader in 4-H, scouts, the Y or sports programs,
Organize your time to help, you'll find young kids are quite the hams!
You provide the time, incentive, tools, support and just BE there,
They'll do their best to work for themselves as well as those who care.

So the next time you find yourself or a friend complaining about kids today,
Sit down and determine What You Can Do to help; Please, don't delay!
For kids don't stay kids, they become adults in short time,
We must share love and learning NOW if we're to prevent future crime.

WHAT YOU CAN DO

1. **Keep health related books and magazines on end tables, next to the easy chair, in the bathroom, next to the refrigerator or wherever they're likely to be read by other family members.**
2. **Underline important information, especially about hereditary matters, and make comments in the margins of your own books.**
3. **To cut costs of books, borrow from the library, trade around with friends, watch for used book swaps or garage sales, and save up for special reference books or your favorites, with which you are entitled to be stingy and keep on a shelf marked, "Not for Loan!"**
4. **Give books or magazine subscriptions for birthday and Christmas gifts. So many times we have heard people say, "My daughter gave me a book on nutrition and it really got me started!"**
5. **Encourage older children to choose topics on nutrition, physical fitness and environmental issues for class reports; they absorb more when they do their own studying and they learn to evaluate the pros and cons of an issue.**

6. **Hold a non-competitive summer reading program using a chapter of a book or an article from a magazine listed in this chapter to score points. Accumulated points at the end of summer will earn something special: school clothes, concert tickets, hobby supplies, roller skates, etc.**
7. **Join organizations that are geared to the preservation of life and land. If your town doesn't have what you're looking for, put an ad in the paper; you may be surprised at the results. Or bring guest speakers into your present organizations who may help encourage a new health-related program.**
8. **Join a Bible study group. All the information you will ever need for keeping your temple fit for the Spirit is right there, undeniably.**
9. **Whatever you choose to read, read with an open mind and a loving heart and remember that no single person has all the answers and no single key opens all the doors. Take from each book what is of value to you.**
10. **To keep from smothering yourself with one subject, read the same way you would toss a salad: Mix bits of Nutrition with morsels of Inspiration, sprinkle with Exercise, leaf time for Meditation, toss with a tasty dressing of Humor, serve with Awareness and digest only that which is Palatable.**

Our Sources For Independence

The following booklist is not all-inclusive; we continue to keep abreast of new books and would appreciate reader suggestions of books that have been particularly helpful to you. We have not followed every word of advice in every book, nor do we advocate that you do so. We have, however, gained something from each and consider each a source of inspiration and a step toward becoming more independent. We hope that you will never accept pat answers from either side of an issue. Instead, question, research, evaluate; have faith in your own judgment, and plan to *achieve* — whatever your goals may be.

Don't let this bibliography overwhelm you — remember it represents fourteen years of reading by two women very involved in their subjects. To help you decide where to begin, we have placed asterisks in front of the book titles that we consider top priority for the novice.

> *No man can reveal to you ought but that which already lies half asleep in the dawning of your knowledge.*
> *Kahlil Gibran*

Some Keys to Natural Foods Cooking

1. Acciardo, Marcia. **Light Eating for Survival.** Conn.: Omango, 1978.
2. Anderson, Lynn. **Rainbow Farm Cookbook.** New York: Harper and Row, 1973.
3. Brown, Edward Espe. **Tassajara Cooking.** Boulder, Colo.: Shambhala Pub. Inc., 1973.
4. Cottrell, Edyth Young. **The Oats, Peas, Beans and Barley Cookbook.** Santa Barbara: Woodbridge, 1974.
5. Davis, Adelle. **Let's Cook It Right.** New York: Harcourt Brace, 1970.
6. Deadman, Peter and Betteridge, Karen. **Nature's Foods.** New York: Samuel Weiser, Inc., 1977.
7. Duquette, Susan. (Brotherhood of the Sun). **Sunburst Farm Family Cookbook.** Santa Barbara: Woodbridge Press, 1976.
8. Ewald, Ellen Buchman. **Recipes for a Small Planet.** New York: Ballantine, 1973.
9. Feingold, Ben. F., and Feingold, Helene S. **The Feingold Cookbook for Hyperactive Children.** New York: Random House, 1979.
10. Goodwin, Mary T., and Pollen, Gerry. **Creative Food Experiences for Children.** Washington, D.C.: C.S.P.I., 1974.
11. Hagler, Louise, ed. **The Farm Vegetarian Cookbook.** Summertown, Tenn.: The Book Pub. Co., 1978.
12. Hauser, Gaylord. **The Gaylord Hauser Cookbook.** New York: Coward-McCann, Inc., 1946.
13. Hittleman, Richard. **Yoga Natural Foods Cookbook.** New York: Bantam, 1970.

14. Hunter, Beatrice Trum. **The Natural Foods Cookbook.** New York: Harcourt Brace Jovanovich, 1961. (Pyramid Pub., 1977.)
15. Hurd, Frank J. and Hurd, Rosalie. **Ten Talents.** Collegedale, Tenn.: College Press, 1968.
16. Kinderlehrer, Jane. **Confessions of a Sneaky Organic Cook.** New York: Signet, 1972.
17. Kirban, Salem. **How to Eat Your Way Back to Vibrant Health.** Irvine, Calif.: Harvest House, 1977.
18. Kloss, Jethro. **The Back to Eden Cookbook.** Santa Barbara: Woodbridge, 1974.
19. Landgrebe, Gary. **Tofu Goes West.** Palo Alto: Fresh Press, 1978.
20. Lappe', Frances Moore. **Diet for a Small Planet.** New York: Ballantine, 1971.
21. Loewenfeld, Claire and Back, Philippa. **Herbs, Health and Cookery.** New York: Hawthorne Books, Inc., 1967.
22. MacManiman, Gen. **Dry It — You'll Like It!** Fall City, Wash.: MacManiman, Inc., 1974.
23. Martinez, Pam. **Sugarless Cooking.** Issequah, Wash.: Medic Publishing Co., 1977.
24. Robertson, Laurel, Flinders, Carol, and Godfrey, Bronwen. **Laurel's Kitchen.** Berkeley: Nilgiri, 1976.
25. Rogers, Ann. **A Cookbook for Poor Poets (and others).** New York: Charles Scribners and Sons, 1966.
26. Rohrer, Virginia and Rohrer, Norman. **How to Eat Right and Feel Great.** Wheaton, Ill.: Tyndale, 1977.
27. Sloan, Sara. **From Classroom to Cafeteria.** Atlanta, Ga.: S.O.S. Printing, Inc., 1978.
28. Sloan, Sara. **A Guide for Nutra Lunches and Natural Foods.** Atlanta, Ga.: S.O.S. Printing, Inc., 1977.
29. Wallace, James and Wallace, Maureen. **Snackers: The Care and Feeding of.** Seattle, Wash.: Madrona Press, 1978.
30. Whyte, Karen Cross. **The Original Diet.** San Francisco, Calif.: Troubador Press, 1977.

Some Keys to Diet and Exercise

1. Benson, Herbert, M.D. ***The Relaxation Response.** New York: William Morrow, 1975.
2. Bowerman, William J. and Harris, W.E., M.D. **Jogging.** New York: Grosset and Dunlop, 1967.
3. Cooper, Kenneth H., M.D. ***Aerobics.** New York: M. Evans and Co., 1968.
4. Cooper, Kenneth H., M.D. **The New Aerobics.** New York: M. Evans and Co., 1970.
5. Cooper, Mildred and Cooper, Kenneth H., M.D. **Aerobics for Women.** New York: Bantam, 1972.
6. Crenshaw, Mary Ann. **The Natural Way to Super Beauty.** New York: David McKay, 1974.
7. Dechanet, J.M. **Christian Yoga.** New York: Harper and Row, 1972.
8. Folan, Lilias M. ***Lilias Yoga and You.** New York: Bantam, 1976.
9. Hittleman, Richard. ***Richard Hittleman's Yoga — 28 Day Exercise Plan.** New York: Bantam, 1973.
10. Hittleman, Richard L. **Weight Control Through Yoga.** New York: Bantam, 1974.
11. Traven, Beatrice. **The Complete Book of Natural Cosmetics.** New York: Pocket Books, 1976.
12. White, John and Fadiman, James, editors. **Relax.** U.S.A.: The Confucian Press, Inc., 1976.

Some Keys to Nutrition and Health

1. Adams, Ruth and Murray, Frank. **Body, Mind and the B Vitamins.** New York: Larchmont, 1972.
2. Airola, Paavo, N.D., Ph.D. **Are You Confused?** Phoenix, Ariz.: Health Plus, 1977.
3. Airola, Paavo, N.D., Ph.D. **How to Get Well.** Phoenix, Ariz.: Health Plus, 1976.
4. Allison, Linda. ***Blood and Guts — A Working Guide to Your Own Insides.** Boston: Little, Brown and Co., 1976.
5. Ardell, Donald B. ***High Level Wellness.** Emmaus, Pa.: Rodale, 1977.
6. Barton, John E. **Flow Lines to Health.** U.S.A.: Harman Press, 1977.
7. Boston Women's Health Book Collective. **Our Bodies Our Selves.** New York: Simon and Schuster, 1971.
8. Bricklin, Mark. **The Practical Encyclopedia of Natural Healing.** Emmaus, Pa.: Rodale, 1976.
9. Burns, Mary. ***Good For Me!** Boston: Little, Brown and Co., 1978.

10. Cheraskin, Emanuel and Ringsdorf, Jr., W.M. **Diet and Disease.** Emmaus, Pa.: Rodale, 1968.
11. Cheraskin, E., M.D. and Ringsdorf, Jr., W.M. ***Psycho-Dietetics.** New York: Bantam, 1976.
12. Clark, Linda. **A Handbook of Natural Remedies for Common Ailments.** New York: Pocket Books, 1976.
13. Coca, Arthur F., M.D. **The Pulse Test.** New York: Arco Pub. Co., 1959.
14. Coffin, Lewis A., M.D. ***The Grandmother Conspiracy Exposed.** Santa Barbara: Capra, 1974.
15. Cohen, Daniel. **Biorhythms In Your Life.** Greenwich, Conn.: Fawcett Pub., 1976.
16. Cott, Allan. **The Orthomolecular Approach to Learning Disabilities.** San Rafael, Calif.: Academic Pub., 1977.
17. Crook, William G., M.D. **Tracking Down Hidden Food Allergies.** Jackson, Tenn.
18. Crook, William G., M.D. **Can Your Child Read? Is He Hyperactive?** Jackson, Tenn.: Pedicenter Press, 1975.
19. Davies, David. **The Centenarians of the Andes.** New York: Doubleday, 1975.
20. Dufty, William. ***Sugar Blues.** New York: Warner, 1975.
21. Feingold, Ben F., M.D. **Why Your Child Is Hyperactive.** New York: Random House, 1975.
22. Ford, Robert S. **Stale Food vs. Fresh Food.** Pascagaula, Miss.: Magnolia Lab., 1969.
23. Gotzsche, Ann-Lise. **The Flouride Question (panacea or poison?).** New York: Stein and Day Pub., 1975.
24. Gregory, Dick. ***Dick Gregory's Natural Diet for Folks Who Eat: Cookin' With Mother Nature.** New York: Harper and Row, 1973.
25. Hamilton, Frank B., Ph.D. **It's a Gland Life.** U.S.A.: Frank B. Hamilton, 1969.
26. Heritage, Ford., B.S., M.E., Researcher. **Composition and Facts About Foods.** Mokelumne Hill, Calif.: Health Research, 1971.
27. Hoffer, Abram. **Orthomolecular Nutrition.** New Canaan, Conn.: Keats, 1978.
28. Jacobson, Michael. **Nutrition Scoreboard.** New York: Avon, 1975.
29. Kirban, Salem. ***The Getting Back to Nature Diet.** Irvine, Calif.: Harvest House, 1978.
30. Kirschmann, John D., Director, Nutrition Search, Inc. ***Nutrition Almanac.** New York: McGraw-Hill, 1975.
31. Kline, Monte and Strube, Jr., W.P. ***Eat, Drink and Be Ready.** Fort Worth, Texas: Harvest Press, 1977.
32. Larson, Gena. **Better Foods for Better Babies.** New Canaan, Conn.: Pivot Original Health Books, 1972.
33. ***Nature's Big Beautiful Bountiful Feel-Good Book.** By the editors of the Health Quarterly, Nutritional Update and Healthful Living Today. New Canaan, Conn.: Keats, 1977.
34. Page, Melvin E., D.D.S., and Abrams, Jr., H. Leon. **Your Body Is Your Best Doctor.** New Canaan, Conn.: Keats, 1976.
35. Passwater, Richard. **Super-Nutrition.** New York: Pocket Books, 1976.
36. Pfeiffer, Carl C., M.D. **The Schizophrenia's: Yours and Mine.** New York: Pyramid, 1970. Prepared and published by the Professional Committee of the Sch. Foundation of New Jersey.
37. Preston, Robert L. **Healthology — Your Master Key to Perfect Health.** Salt Lake City, Utah: Hawkes, 1977.
38. Price, Weston A. ***Nutrition and Physical Degeneration — a comparison of primitive and modern diets and their effects.** Price-Pottinger Nutrition Foundation. Santa Monica, Calif.: Heritage Press, 1970.
39. Reuben, David, M.D. **The Save Your Life Diet.** New York: Ballantine, 1976.
40. Rodale, J.I. **The Healthy Hunzas.** Emmaus, Pa.: Rodale, 1948.
41. Schauss, Alexander. **Diet, Crime and Delinquency.** San Leandro, Calif.: Parker House Pub. Co., 1980.
42. Schute, Wilfred, with Taub, Harold J. **Vitamin E. for Ailing and Healthy Hearts.** New York: Pyramid House, 1969.
43. Shelton, Herbert M. **Food Combining Made Easy.** San Antonio, Texas: Dr. Shelton's Health School, 1951.
44. Smith, Lendon H., M.D. ***Feed Your Kids Right.** (Dr. Smith's program for your child's total health). New York: McGraw-Hill, 1979.
45. Smith, Lendon H., M.D. ***Improving Your Child's Behavior Chemistry.** Englewood Cliffs, N.J.: Prentice-Hall, 1976.

46. Sussman, Vic. ***The Vegetarian Alternative.** Emmaus, Pa.: Rodale, 1978.
47. Tager, Mark, M.D. and Jennings, Charles. **Whole Person Health Care.** Portland, Ore.: Victoria House, 1978.
48. Thie, John, D.C., with Marks, Mary. **Touch For Health . . . A practical Guide to using acupuncture, touch and massage to improve postural balance and reduce physical and mental pain and tension.** Marina del Rey, Calif.: DeVorss and Co., Pub., 1973.
49. Watson, George. **Nutrition and Your Mind — The Psychochemical Response.** New York: Harper and Row, 1972.
50. Wigmore, Ann, D.D., N.D. **Be Your Own Doctor.** New York: Hemisphere Press.
51. Wigmore, Ann. **Healthy Children, Nature's Way.** Boston, Mass.: Hippocrates Health Institute.
52. Wigmore, Ann. ***Why Suffer?** New York: Hemisphere Press, 1964.
53. Williams, Roger J., M.D. **Nutrition Against Disease.** New York: Pitman, 1971.
54. Williams, Roger J., M.D. ***The Wonderful World Within You.** New York: Bantam, 1977.
55. Yudkin, John. ***Sweet and Dangerous.** New York: Bantam, 1973.

Some Keys to Consumer Education and Environmental Concerns

1. Altman, Nathaniel. **Eating for Life.** Wheaton, Ill.: Quest, 1977.
2. Brodeur, Paul. **The Zapping of America. (Microwaves, their deadly risk and the cover-up).** New York: Norton, 1977.
3. Carson, Rachel. **The Edge of the Sea.** Boston, Mass.: Houghton-Mifflin, 1955.
4. Carson, Rachel. ***Silent Spring.** Boston, Mass.: Houghton-Mifflin, 1962.
5. Cousteau, Jacques Yves, with James Dugan. **The Living Sea.** New York: Harper and Row, 1963.
6. Cousteau, Jacques Yves. **Oasis In Space.** New York: World Pub., 1972.
7. Cousteau, Jacques Yves. **The Ocean World of Jacques Cousteau.** Danbury Press, 1973.
8. DeBell, Garrett, editor. **The Environmental Handbook: Prepared for the First National Environmental Teach-In.** New York: Ballantine, 1970.
9. Graham, Frank. ***Since Silent Spring.** Boston, Mass.: Houghton-Mifflin, 1970.
10. Hunter, Beatrice Trum. ***Consumer Beware!** New York: Bantam, 1972.
11. Hur, Robin. **Food Reform: Our Desperate Need.** Austin, Tex.: Heidelberg, 1975.
12. Katz, Deborah, and Goodwin, Mary T., M.P.H. ***Food — Where Nutrition, Politics and Culture Meet — An Activities Guide for Teachers.** Washington, D.C.: C.S.P.I., 1976.
13. Langer, Richard W. **Grow It!** New York: Saturday Review Press, 1972.
14. Lappe', Frances Moore and Collins, Joseph. **Food First: beyond the myth of scarcity.** Boston, Mass.: Houghton-Mifflin, 1977.
15. Lerza, Catherine and Jacobson, Michael. (ed.) **Food for People, Not for Profit.** New York: Ballantine, 1975.
16. Longgood, William. ***The Poisons In Your Food.** New York: Pyramid, 1975.
17. Mander, Jerry. ***Four Arguments for the Elimination of Television.** New York: William Morrow and Co., 1977.
18. Mitchell, John G., with Stallings, Constance L. (eds.) **Ecotactics: The Sierra Club Handbook for Environmental Activists.** New York: Pocket Books, 1970.
19. Organic Gardening and Farming Magazine Staff. ***How to Grow Vegetables and Fruits.** Emmaus, Pa.: Rodale, 1961.
20. Organic Gardening and Farming Magazine Staff. (edited by Carol Stoner.) * **Stocking Up.** Emmaus, Pa.: Rodale, 1973.
21. Ott, John N. ***Health and Light.** Greenwich, Conn.: Devin-Adair, 1973.
22. Reich, Charles A. **The Greening of America.** New York: Random House, 1970.
23. Senate Select Committee on Nutrition and Human Needs. ***Dietary Goals for the United States.** Washington, D.C.: U.S. Senate, February, 1977. GPO No. 052-070-03913-2. (Booklet of dietary goals).

24. Singer, Peter. **Animal Liberation.** New York: New York Review, 1975.
25. Stabile, Toni. **Cosmetics: Trick or Treat?** New York: Hawthorn Books, 1966.
26. Toffler, Alvin. **Eco-Spasm.** New York: Bantam, 1975.
27. Turner, James. **The Chemical Feast.** New York: Grossman Pub., 1970.
28. Vellela, Tony. **Food Co-ops for Small Groups.** New York: Workman Pub. Co., 1975.
29. Whitesides, Thomas. **Defoliation.** New York: Ballantine, 1970.
30. World Hunger Year. **Food and Hunger in the School and Community. (A guide for Action).** Dept. F.M. 27-06 High Street, Fair Lawn, New Jersey, 07410.

Some Keys to Inspiration and Self-Improvement

1. American Bible Society. **Good News Bible.** (Today's English Version). New York: Thomas Nelson, 1976.
2. Bach, Richard. **Jonathan Livingston Seagull.** New York: Macmillan Co., 1973.
3. Bach, Richard. **Illusions.** New York: Dell, 1977.
4. Baker, Samm Sinclair. **Conscious Happiness.** New York: Grosset and Dunlop, 1975.
5. Beardsley, Lou. **A Family Love Story.** Irvine, Calif.: Harvest House, 1975.
6. Briggs, Dorothy. ***Your Child's Self-Esteem.** New York: Doubleday and Co., Inc., 1970.
7. Cammer, Leonard, M.D. **Up From Depression.** New York: Simon and Schuster, 1969.
8. Carlson, Betty. **Your Life Is Worth Living.** Grand Rapids, Mich.: Zondervan Pub., 1962.
9. Carnegie, Dale. **How To Stop Worrying and Start Living.** New York: Simon and Schuster, 1944.
10. Cole, Jim. **The Controllers.** Mill Valley, Calif.: Jim Cole, 1971.
11. Cousins, Norman. ***Anatomy of an Illness.** New York: W.W. Norton and Co., Inc., 1979.
12. Davis, Albert Roy and Rawls, Jr., Walter C. **The Rainbow In Your Hands.** New York: Exposition Press, Inc., 1976.
13. Dyer, Dr. Wayne W. **Your Erroneous Zones.** New York: Funk and Wagnalls, 1976.
14. Eareckson, Joni. **Joni.** New York: Bantam, 1978.
15. Fynn. **Mister God, This Is Anna.** New York: Ballantine, 1976.
16. Friedlander, Ira. **Wisdom Stories for the Planet Earth.** New York: Harper and Row, 1973.
17. Gibran, Kahlil. **The Prophet.** New York: Alfred A. Knopf, 1923.
18. Ginott, Dr. Haim G. **Between Parent and Child.** New York: Avon, 1969.
19. Ginott, Dr. Haim G. **Between Parent and Teen-ager.** New York: Avon, 1971.
20. Harris, Thomas A., M.D. **I'm OK, You're OK.** New York: Harper and Row, 1967.
21. Hawken, Paul. **The Magic of Findhorn.** New York: Bantam, 1976.
22. Hendricks, Gay and Wills, Russell. **The Centering Book.** New Jersey: Prentice-Hall, 1975.
23. Herriot, James. **All Creatures Great and Small.** New York: Bantam, 1973.
24. Herriot, James. **All Things Bright and Beautiful.** New York: Bantam, 1974.
25. Herriot, James. **All Things Wise and Wonderful.** New York: Bantam, 1978.
26. Hesse, Hermann. **Siddhartha.** New York: Bantam, 1972.
27. Holmes, Marjorie. **Nobody Else Will Listen.** New York: Bantam, 1974.
28. Holmes, Marjorie. **I've Got to Talk to Somebody, God.** New York: Doubleday, 1968.
29. Howard, Jane. **Families.** New York: Simon and Schuster, 1978.
30. John-Roger. **What Is the Power Within You?** New York: Baraka, 1976.
31. John-Roger. **The Christ Within.** New York: Baraka, 1976.
32. Keene, Leonard. **The Kid Book.** Fort Worth, Texas: Balanced Life Assoc., 1976.
33. Keene, Leonard, **Please Don't Hurt Me.** Fort Worth, Texas: Balanced Life Assoc., 1975.
34. Kuhlman, Kathryn. **I Believe In Miracles.** New York: Prentice-Hall, 1962.
35. Lair, Jess., Ph.D. **I Ain't Much, Baby — But I'm All I've Got.** New York: Doubleday, 1972.
36. Lessor, Richard. **Fuzzies (A Folk Fable).** Niles, Ill.: Argus Communications, 1971.
37. Lewis, C.S. **The Chronicles of Narnia.** New York: Collier, 1970.
38. Link, S.J. Mark. **He Is the Still Point of the Turning World.** Niles, Ill.: Argus Communications, 1971.

39. Link, S.J. Mark. **In the Stillness Is the Dancing.** Niles, Ill.: Argus Communications, 1972.
40. Link, S.J. Mark. **Take Off Your Shoes.** Niles, Ill.: Argus Communications, 1972.
41. Maltz, Maxwell, M.D. **Creative Living for Today.** New York: Pocket Books, 1970.
42. Maltz, Maxwell, M.D. **Psycho-Cybernetics.** New York: Prentice-Hall, 1960.
43. Montgomery, Ruth. **A World Beyond.** New York: Coward, McCann and Geoghegan, Inc., 1971.
44. Newburger, Howard M. and Lee, Marjorie. **Winners and Losers.** New York: David McKay, 1974.
45. O'Neill, Nina and O'Neill, George. **Shifting Gears.** New York: Avon, 1975.
46. Osborne, Cecil G. **The Art of Understanding Yourself.** Grand Rapids, Mich.: Zondervan, 1967.
47. Paulus, Trina. **Hope for the Flowers.** New York: Paulist Press, 1972.
48. Peale, Dr. Norman Vincent. **The Power of Positive Thinking.** New York: Prentice-Hall, 1952.
49. Peterson, Wilford A. **The Art of Living. (series).** New York: Simon and Schuster, 1972.
50. Rogers, Dale Evans. **Time Out Ladies.** Old Tappa, New Jersey: Fleming H. Revell Co., 1966.
51. Rubin, Theodore Isaac, M.D. **The Angry Book.** New York: MacMillan, 1969.
52. Saint-Exupery, Antoine de. **The Little Prince.** New York: Harcourt Brace Jovanovich, 1943.
53. Sandpiper Studios (ed.) **Creeds to Love and Live By.** Boulder, Colo.: Blue Mountain, 1978.
54. Sandweiss, Samuel H., M.D. **Sai Baba — The Holy Man and the Psychiatrist.** San Diego: Birth Day, 1975.
55. Schindler, John, M.D. **How to Live 365 Days a Year.** New York: Prentice-Hall, 1959.
56. Sheehy, Gail. **Passages.** New York: Bantam, 1977.
57. Sherman, Harold. **Know Your Own Mind.** Greenwich, Conn.: Fawcett Pub., 1953.
58. Szekely, Edmond Bordeaux. **The Essene Gospel of Peace.** San Diego, Calif.: Academy Books, 1977.
59. Umphrey, Marjorie. **Getting to Know You.** Irvine, Calif.: Harvest House, 1976.
60. Yogi, Maharishi Mahesh. **The Science of Being and Art of Living.** London W.C.1. George Allan and Unwin Limited, 1963.

Magazines

1. **Bestways.** 466 Foothill Blvd., La Canada, Calif. 91011.
2. **The Daily Word.** Unity Books, Unity Village, Missouri 64065.
3. **Food Moniter.** P.O. Box 1975, Garden City, New York 11530.
4. **Let's Live.** 444 North Larchmont Blvd., Los Angeles, Calif. 90004.
5. **The Mother Earth News.** 105 Stoney Mountain Road, Hendersonville, North Carolina 28739.
6. **Organic Gardening.** 33 East Minor St., Emmaus, Pa. 18049.
7. **Prevention.** 33 East Minor St., Emmaus, Pa. 18049.
8. **Runner.** P.O. Box 2731, Boulder, Colo. 80321.
9. **The Vegetarian Times.** 41 East 42nd Street, Suite 921, New York, New York 10017.
10. **Well-Being.** 41 East 42nd Street, Suite 921, New York, New York 10017.

* **ALIVE, Canadian Journal of Health and Nutrition,** Box 67333, Vancouver, B.C., Canada V5W 3TI

Organizations

1. Center for Science in the Public Interest (C.S.P.I.), Director, Michael Jacobson. (CSPI Nutrition Action Magazine; CSPI Reports), 1755 S. Street N.W., Washington, D.C. 20009.
2. Developmental Disabilities Prevention Center, Inc., 843 E. Main Street #201, Medford, Oregon 97501.
3. Friends of the Earth, 529 Commercial Street, San Francisco, Calif. 94111.
4. Greenpeace, 811 N.W. 23rd, Portland, Ore. 97210.
5. The Hunger Project, P.O. Box 789, San Francisco, Calif. 94101.
6. National Feingold Association, 759 National Press Building, Washington, D.C. 20045.
7. North American Vegetarian Society, 501 Old Harding Highway, Malaga, New Jersey 08328. (Send 25¢ for a copy of Facts of Vegetarianism).
8. Oxfam America, 302 Columbus Ave., Boston, Mass. 02116.
9. Parents for Better Nutrition, 33 North Central, Room 200, Medford, Oregon 97501. Director, Thelma Thompson.
10. WHY? (World Hunger Year), P.O. Box 1975, Garden City, New York 11530.

BROTHERHOOD

A rabbi spoke with the Lord about Heaven and Hell. "I will show you Hell," said the Lord and they went into a room which had a large pot of stew in the middle. The smell was delicious and around the pot sat people who were famished and desperate. All were holding spoons with very long handles which reached to the pot, but because the handles of the spoons were longer than their arms, it was impossible to get the stew back into their mouths. Their suffering was terrible.

"Now I will show you Heaven," said the Lord, and they went into an identical room. There was the same pot of stew and the people had the same identical spoons, but they were well-nourished, talking and happy. At first the rabbi did not understand. "It is simple," said the Lord. "You see, they have learned to feed each other."

Give a man a fish and he eats for a day.
Teach him how to fish and he eats for a lifetime.

O Lord, we are what we eat
O Lord, we are what we think
O Lord, we are what we do.
May our food lead to health
May our thoughts lead to love
May our actions lead to peace
And happiness for all beings.

Marc Dake

All things bright and beautiful
All creatures great and small
All things wise and wonderful
The Lord God made them all.

Cecil Frances Alexander

For health and strength and daily bread
We praise Thy name O Lord.

Give us this day

The Lord is good to me
And so I thank the Lord
For giving me, the things I need
The sun and rain and the apple seed
The Lord is good to me.

Come, Lord Jesus, be our guest.
Let this good food to us be blessed.
Amen

ONE SET OF FOOTPRINTS

One night a man had a dream. He dreamed he was walking along the beach with the Lord. Across the sky flashed scenes from his life. For each scene he noticed two sets of footprints in the sand — one belonging to him and the other to the Lord. When the last scene had flashed before him, he looked back at the footprints and noticed that many times along the path there was only one set of footprints in the sand. He also noticed that this happened during the lowest and saddest times of his life.

This really bothered him and he questioned the Lord, "Lord, you said that once I decided to follow you, you would walk all the way, but I noticed that during the most troublesome times of my life, there was only one set of footprints. I don't understand why when I needed you most, you deserted me."

The Lord replied, "My precious, precious child, I love you and would never leave you. During your times of trial and suffering when you see only one set of footprints, it was then that I carried you."

our daily bread

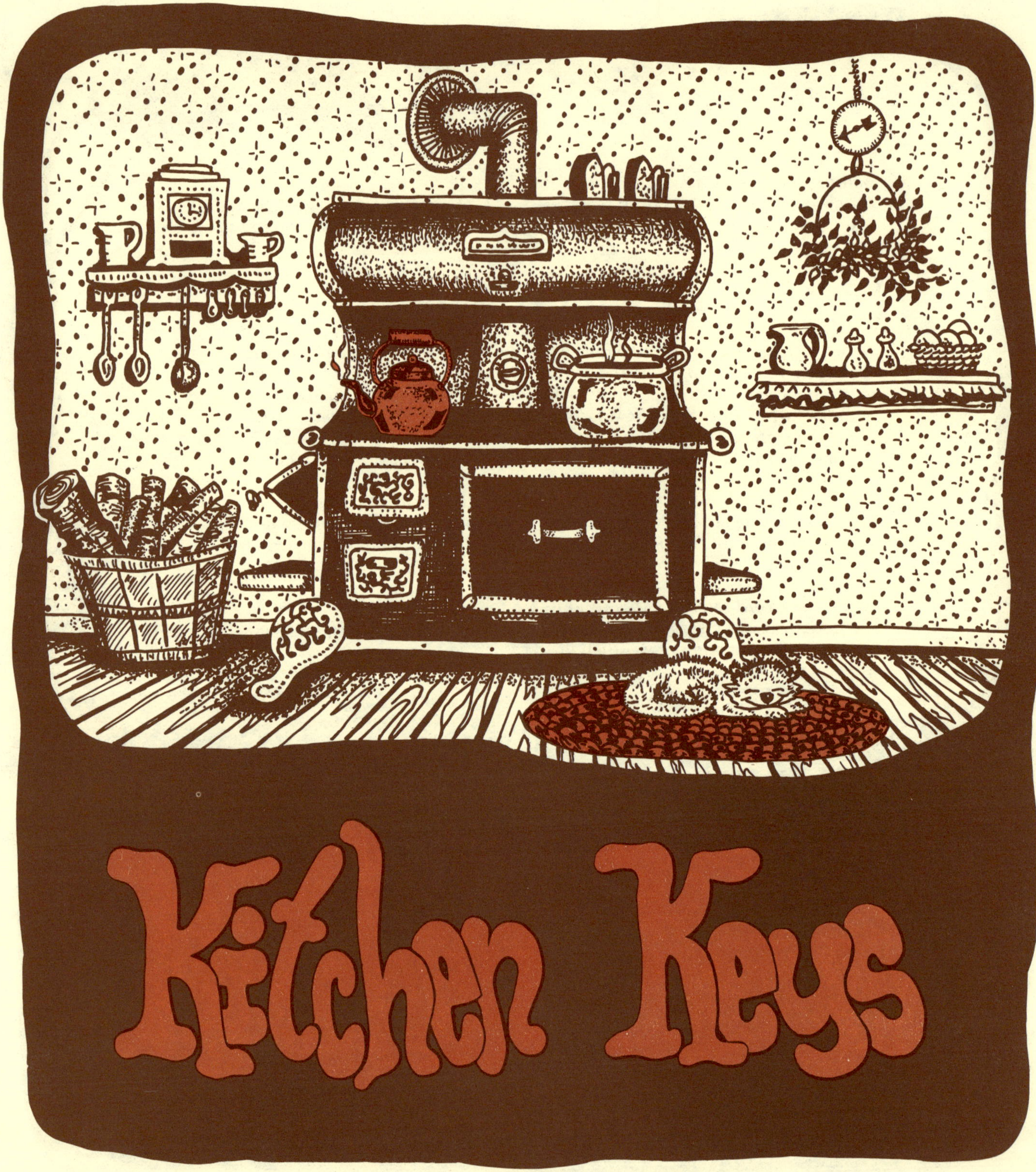
Kitchen Keys

Kitchen Keys

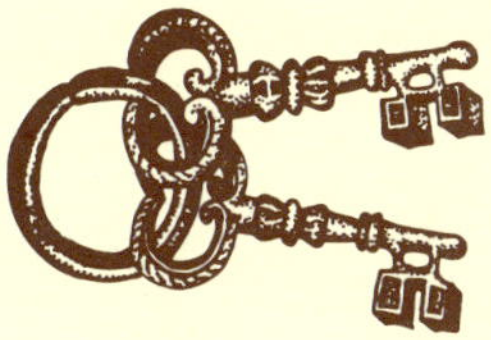

We are learning constantly. With each new book we read, each whole-istic workshop we attend, each friend we meet, a new door is opened and we add to our collection of keys for vibrant living. We have also learned to disperse the drudgery of KP duty by means of a few *kitchen* keys.

The Keys to Efficiency

You can be an avid cook and thoroughly enjoy creating your specialties without being a slave to your kitchen. When you are familiar with terminology, techniques, equipment and methods of preparation, your time in the kitchen is considerably reduced. A systematic recipe file may seem time consuming, but will prove its worth when you're pressed for time later. Overlapping, or doing more than one thing at a time, may just be the ultimate path to maximum productivity in the kitchen (or anywhere).

Double or triple your favorite recipes and freeze the extras; bake tomorrow's squash with today's lentil loaf and potatoes when there is room in the oven. Designate a special space for sprouting so you won't forget about them. Sponsor a "Cook-In" where the whole family devotes one day to quantity preparation of favorite foods (plus clean-up) in exchange for one day of freedom from schedules and obligations. Be sure to record and date recipe revisions and shortcuts. And don't be surprised if, someday, you open your drawer to find that someone has ironed "SUPERWOMAN" on your favorite tee-shirt.

The Keys to Satisfaction

Whatever you remove from your family's diet, you will need to replace with something similar, so that no one feels deprived or punished. But be fair. Don't expect carob to taste just exactly like chocolate or a roasted barley drink to exactly duplicate coffee. Remember that a slice of whole wheat cake will have a coarser texture and stronger flavor than the cottony white stuff. Some honeys are stronger than others while some grains are bland and need artful assistance. That your first soy-burger does not classify as "food for the gods" is no reason to stop trying.

So you may better tune yourself into your own senses, we invite you to perform an Organoleptic test each time you try an unfamiliar food. By definition this means to see, smell, touch, taste and remember. If you truly involve yourself in the experience of enjoying food, then you will be fully satisfied and there will be no need to return to the kitchen between meals to gratify a dangling appetite.

The Keys to Substitutions

So often we read in the news about another food product with questionable ingredients and our thoughts range from, "Why was it ever approved in the first place?" to "If we shouldn't eat *that*, what *can* we eat?" One of the purposes of writing this book is to share with other frustrated parents some of the ways we have found to make healthy food appealing to all ages.

Gurus may live on black beans and rice and dates and nuts and lead you to believe they never tire of mono-diets because of the esoteric beauty of the pure life. Fantastic! We admire them. But we must answer to our seven children three-plus times a day when they are hungry and they should not be expected to maintain rigidly singular diets that may (by the very lack of nutrients) be more harmful to their growth and development than the chemicals and dyes that are added to a variety of processed foods.

Therefore, we must substitute — to achieve that all important variety, to compete with the junk food and snacks industry, and to answer our children when they say, "What's there to eat?" with "How about an Earth-Shaking Shake and a UFO?" They need fun-sounding names of eye-appealing foods that will build their bodies, yet look like and taste better than their commercial counterparts.

So if everyone else is donating a cake for the cake walk, send a date nut cake. If everyone else gets a crunchy candy bar at the movies, send a crunchy Dandy Bar — and make them better with substitutions.

SUBSTITUTIONS

bacon	**TVP bacon-flavored bits without MSG, Bakon yeast**
baking powder with aluminate compounds	**homemade baking powder made from ¼ C. potassium carbonate, ½ C. cream of tartar and ½ C. arrowroot flour; sift, store in tightly covered container.**
black pepper	**cayenne — sparingly.**
buttermilk (for 1 C.)	**yogurt, kefir or milk with 1 T. lemon juice or vinegar.**
cheese, processed or spreads	**undyed, aged, hard cheeses.**
chocolate (1 oz.)	**3 T. carob powder moistened with 1-2 T. water or milk.**
chocolate chips	**carob chips. (Some carob chips have brown sugar. See recipe for homemade chips in** *KID STUFF.)*
coconut, sweetened	**fresh or unsweetened coconut.**
corn starch	**equal parts tapioca, arrowroot flour or twice as much whole wheat pastry flour.**
eggs, mass produced	**farm fresh eggs from exercised hens or ¼ cup nut butter.**
honey, 'pure,' commercial	**raw, unheated, unfiltered, direct from beekeeper.**
ice cream, commercial	**homemade with honey or maple syrup or health store brands made with natural ingredients.**
lettuce (iceberg)	**sprouts — (See P.S.** *Stone-Age Food For Space-Age People* **for nutritional information.) Individual sprout growing directions are in following chapters: alfalfa —** *KID STUFF,* **buckwheat lettuce —** *Labor of Love Lunches,* **mixed sprouts —** *Serendipity Suppers,* **mung bean sprouts —** *Serendipity Suppers,* **sunflower seed sprouts —** *Better Beginnings,* **wheat-grass —** *Better Beginnings,* **wheat sprouts —** *Better Beginnings.*
marshmallows (for salads)	**diced, baked yams or diced banana.**
nuts, roasted, salted	**in shell, raw and unsalted (roast raw peanuts).**
peanut butter, hydrogenated	**unhydrogenated, stir before using; refrigerate.**
salt	**kelp or gomazio (12 parts crushed, roasted sesame seeds to 1 part sea salt), Vege-Sal, Veg-it, Spike.**
shortening	**butter or SunButterBlend (2 parts butter mixed with 1 part cold-pressed oil); refrigerate.**
sugar, white or brown (1 C.)	**½ cup honey, unsulphured molasses, maple syrup, or date sugar (about 2/3 cup to start).**
vanillan (synthetic flavors)	**vanilla extract or other flavor extracts.**
yogurt, sweetened, dyed and flavored	**plain yogurt, preferably homemade.**

The Keys to Measurements and Equivalents

Many recipes in this book do not state exact measurements of ingredients. You may consider us vague and careless not to tell you the exact number of teaspoonfuls or cupfuls, or carrots or onions in a recipe. While it is true that no two people are going to produce the exact same casserole or cookie from a specific recipe, it is also a fact that no two taste buds are alike.

Some families like highly spiced and seasoned foods. We have discovered that the less we depend on salty and sugary condiments to flavor our foods and the more we let the natural flavor of the foods and herbs blend and mingle, the more sensitive our taste buds have become. We are satisfied to savor each vegetable or fruit in the dish. Flavors aren't hidden or smothered by an over-powering sauce or condiment.

Therefore, we sometimes present generalities in measurements. In some cases, you can't go wrong to vary ingredients to suit your family's tastes, such as in soups, loaves, or smoothies. Even young children can combine the ingredients in a recipe to suit their tastes.

In recipes where exact ingredients are important, we so state them. In others, we list approximates or offer suggestions for you to adjust. Just as tacos can be hot or mild, so can our felafels or lentil roasts be strong with chili powder and cayenne, or delicate, using a subtle combination of herbs.

MEASUREMENTS

a handful	**= approximately ½ cup**
a pinch	**= approximately ⅛ teaspoon**
a dash	**= approximately 1 shake from a spice jar or can**
a sprinkling	**= a light sprinkling of cheese or a topping over the surface of a casserole, loaf, pie or cake**
t.	**= teaspoon**
T.	**= Tablespoon**

EQUIVALENTS

1 pound of cheese	**= 5 cups freshly grated cheese**
1 lemon, juiced	**= 2 to 3 Tablespoons of juice**
1 Tablespoon of dried herbs	**= 3 Tablespoons of fresh herbs**
1 cup inst. powdered milk	**= 2/3 cup non-instant powdered milk**

The Keys to Equipment

Though you needn't run out and purchase all new equipment, we have listed articles that are useful and possibly unique to whole foods cooking. You may even have some of these lying dormant. Keep your eye tuned at garage sales or post a "wish list" the week before your birthday. Make sure all of your equipment is operating properly: check oven temperature, sharpen knives, clean and oil wood chopping blocks; keep cast iron and woks seasoned, and freezers defrosted.

A spiral notebook is a most useful tool for keeping track of important information, such as, cost comparisons, list of bulk supplies on hand, freezer contents and dates, menu combinations that were particularly attractive, and individual preferences: "Randy's favorite — make for his birthday," or "Chris can do this one by himself"; "great for a potluck" or "CHEAP, make at the end of the month!"

We encourage you to write in the recipe section of this book, making notations of your own seasonings or ingredient additions or omissions. After each recipe you try, keep a record of its acceptance on the right-hand margin of the page by placing an **!** for "outstanding-make-again," a **Q** for "company quality," an **A** for "entire-family-approved" or "family favorites," and a **K** for "kids-can-make."

EQUIPMENT

BLENDER: Found in nearly every kitchen, indispensible for blending drinks, shakes, smoothies, crumbing bread, grinding nuts and seeds, blending the veggies and soup stock for a thicker soup, or in making mayonnaise.

CAST IRON SKILLET: Properly seasoned and cleaned regularly with salt, will last a lifetime. Because it holds the heat evenly, it can be used for dry toasting of grains and seeds; sauteeing garlic, onions, herbs and veggies, for stir-fry dishes, and for oven baking.

CITRUS JUICER: Much more efficient than hand squeezing for the many uses of fresh lemon juice.

CHOPPING BLOCK AND CHINESE KNIFE: You provide the power and these will do everything a food processor will and more! A variety of sharp cuts will add the gourmet touch to vegetable dishes.

COLANDER: *Always* wash veggies quickly in a colander instead of soaking, as nutrients are lost in the soak water.

CROCK POT: For slow cooking of grains, soups and stews. Works overnight and is a tremendous time-saver.

EGG SEPARATER: No fail way to separate eggs for souffles, waffles, etc.

FOOD PROCESSOR: Time-saver for small or quantity preparation. Grates cheese and coleslaw, whips cream and mayonnaise, crumbles bread and crackers, chops nuts and ice, blends butter and oil, mashes squash, pumpkin or potatoes, and mixes batters, dips and spreads for sandwiches. It reduces veggie preparation to little more than the time it takes to clean them.

FRUIT RIPENER: A large covered container with 2 or 3 holes in the top that helps fruit ripen naturally while it keeps bugs out.

GARLIC PRESS: Handy, but if you don't have one, simply place several cloves of garlic on a cutting board and give them a good whack with the bottom of a cast iron skillet; the peelings slip off and you have instant crushed garlic!

GLASS PANS: Preferable to aluminum for baking.

GRAIN MILL: For grinding hard grains into various textures of flour.

GRINDER: For nuts and seeds too hard to work in the blender. Makes meal or paste.

JUICER: For freshly juiced fruits and vegetables and combinations. Some can also make ice creams, sherbets, crush ice for fruit juice snow cones, and grind nut butters. Hand juicers are also available.

MORTAR AND PESTLE: For grinding small amounts of dried herbs and spices.

NUTCRACKERS AND PICKS: Make quick work of shelling nuts.

PILLOWCASE: To whirl washed greens and sprouts for extra crispness.

PRESSURE COOKER: Saves time and preserves nutrients; watch closely and don't over-cook.

STAINLESS STEEL: Preferable to aluminum for range top cooking.

STEAMER BASKET: Fits inside large pot, water never touches veggies; they steam tender in minutes. Or place fish in cheesecloth, steam until flaky; remove to hot buttered tray for serving and top with herbs or sauce.

STRAINERS: A variety of sizes for a variety of jobs. Tiny strainers for herb teas, fine mesh for separating pulp from juices, medium for rinsing sprouts.

TEA POT: Serve herb teas to guests or just enjoy your solitude, but do keep a tea pot handy.

WOK: Wonderful for short cooking with small amount of oil at high heat to lock nutrients in. Vegetables are stir-fried briefly, then pushed aside while other, shorter cooking time veggies are added in the center. When ready, serve right from wok as the foods are always colorful and the wok makes a centerpiece for dishes of condiments to be served around.

WOODEN SPOONS AND UTENSILS: There's a wooden utensil made for almost every purpose. A rice paddle, tongs, carved ladle, spatulas, noodle spoon, whip, chopsticks and spoons with extra long handles for large pots are all useful and decorative.

WOVEN BASKETS OR TRAYS: Use as hot pot holders, bread servers, or containers for utensils, condiments, etc.

The tragedy of life is not so much what men suffer, but rather what they miss.
Thomas Carlyle

The Keys to Preparation

COOKING GRAINS

1 cup raw grain	Regular Cooking liquid (cups)	time (min.)	Pressure Cooking (15 lb.) liquid (cups)	time (min.)	Yield (cups)
Barley (pearl)	3	45-1 hr.	2	10-12	3½
Brown Rice	2-2½	35-45	1½	15	3
Bulgur (cracked wheat)	2-2½	25-35	2	5-10	2½
Kasha (buckwheat groats)	2-2½	15-25			2½
Millet	3+	30-45	2½-3	15-20	3½
Oats-Rolled	3-4	10-15	2 -3	5	
Whole wheatberries	3	1 hr. +	1½-2	15-20	2¾
Whole oats	3	1 hr. +	1½-2	15-20	2¾
Whole triticale	3	1 hr. +	1½-2	15-20	2¾
Wild Rice	3	1 hr. +			4

Method of Cooking:

(Regular). Rinse grains briefly under cold water using a strainer. Bring water to a boil, add 1 t. oil; then grain, and bring to a boil again. Stir once, cover and turn heat to simmer. Follow above time schedule.

(Pressure). Add 1 t. oil to the water; very important, in order to avoid a clogged vent from the grains foaming.

Alternate Methods:

1. Brown or wild rice may be sauteed in a small amount of oil in a skillet for top-o-stove stir-fry veggie dishes. Then add other veggies like onions, mushrooms, celery, pepper, garlic; saute some more. Finally add two times the water as the grain; bring to boil; cover and steam til tender.
2. Bulgur may also be soaked. Pour 2 c. boiling water over 1 c. bulgar and let set for 15 min. Will be fluffy and ready to use.
3. Millet may be dry roasted in a cast-iron skillet at medium heat until each kernel dances and turns light golden brown. Then slowly add boiling water and cover and simmer for recommended time. This makes the grain nuttier in flavor and less mushy. Bulgur or rice cook this way nicely too.
4. Millet and oatmeal cook well in a crock pot set on low. Add grain and hot water Turn to low and go to bed. In a.m. stir; add milk, honey, butter and raisins and serve.
5. Any whole grain berry can be "cooked" overnight in a thermos. To a 1 quart thermos, add 1 cup berries and 2 cups boiling liquid. Cap, and lay on side overnight. Be sure to leave equal amount of space for expansion.

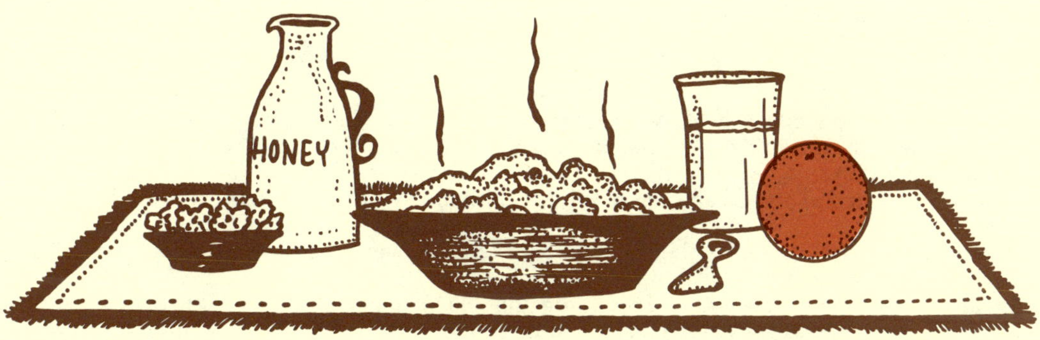

COOKING BEANS

1 cup raw beans	Regular Cooking liquid (cups)	Regular Cooking time (hour)	Pressure Cooking liquid (cups)	Pressure Cooking time (min.)	Yield (cups)
Black beans	4	1½ hrs.	(about	20-25	2
Black-eyed peas	3	1 hr.	same	20-25	2
Garbanzos (chickpeas)	4	3	as	40-45	2
Kidney Beans	3	1½	regular	20-25	2
Lentils	3	45-1 hr.	cooking)	10-15	2¼
Limas	2	1½			1¼
Mung or Adzuki	3	3		30-35	2
Pinto	3	2½			2
Red	3	3		30-35	2
Small white (navy)	3	1½			2
Soy*	4	3+		45-baked 60-mash	
Split peas	3	45-1 hr.		10-15	2¼

*To test a soybean for tenderness, place 1 bean between tongue and roof of mouth. If you can mash bean, it is tender enough to eat.

Method of Cooking:

Wash beans in colander with cold water. Remove pebbles or any bad beans. Place beans in approximately three times the water (see chart above); bring to boil, add 1 T. oil, and simmer (partially covered) until tender.

Alternate Methods:

1. Soak washed beans overnight in water to cover. (Always discard first soak water and add fresh water.) Then bring to a boil; partially cover, and simmer. Cooking time will be shortened by an hour or more. (Lentils and split peas don't need pre-soaking.)
2. Cover washed beans with three times as much water and boil for five minutes. Remove from heat and soak for one to two hours. Change water, then cook until tender. (This is the same as soaking overnight.)

Super Hints for Grains and Beans

1. Although charts are for one cup dried beans or grain, why not cook up two or three cups of dried beans or grain? Use a large pot. Adjust water accordingly; cooking time remains nearly the same. When done, cool slightly, partially drain beans, then spoon grains or beans into plastic baggies using one and two cup proportions. Freeze immediately for future use. When needed, defrost and use as recipe indicates.
2. Save extra bean broth for soup stock. Refrigerate or freeze.
3. Mix leftover beans and rice with mayonnaise, chopped and grated onion, carrot, celery, green pepper for salads or sandwich spreads. Add your own choice of seasonings.
4. Make your own Bean-Grain Patties. Mash beans; mix with rice, millet or barley, sauteed veggies, nuts or seeds (blender ground), hèrbs and spices. If necessary, add an egg for binding. Shape into burgers and dip into crumbs or wheat germ and bake in a buttered pan or lightly saute.

To Roast or Toast Raw Nuts, Seeds or Grains

Cast-Iron Skillet

1. Use a dry skillet and medium heat. Add seeds and stir often until light brown. Remove from pan to cool. Rice and millet will do a little dance and crackle and pop, so be prepared. After toasting, add boiling water and steam until done.
2. Nuts may be roasted in a small amount of oil. Stir until lightly browned. Remove from heat.

Oven

1. Spread nuts or seeds on a cookie sheet and place in a 300° F. oven. Roast until browned. For millet or seeds, it takes only a short time, so check the oven often.
2. Mix half toasted and half raw nuts and seeds together at first to get used to the taste of raw seeds. Gradually decrease toasted; increase raw; even add sprouted sunflower seeds to a raw nut mix. Or toss with green or fruit salads for added crunch and nutrition.

Grains and Beans That Can Be Blender Ground

split peas, rice, whole or cracked corn, lentils, millet, soy beans, pinto beans, red beans.

Use a blender, food processor, wheat grinder, coffee grinder, or nut-seed grinder to grind beans and whole grains to a flour for cereals, pie crusts, cakes, cookies, soup thickeners, casserole additions, or to crack beans and grains for quick soups and stews.

VEGETABLE PREPARATION

You can retain the most nutrients in vegetables by preparing them in the following manner:

1. Wash all leafy-green vegetables quickly and do not soak. A drop or two of a vegetable oil based, non-toxic cleaner can aid in removing pesticide residues. Scrub root vegetables to remove dirt and peel as a matter of choice, but remember that the most nutrients are just under the skin.
2. As a general rule, cut or chop vegetables immediately before preparing or serving. The less you cut veggies the less the loss of nutrients. The enemies of vitamins are air, light, heat and water, so the less exposure to the elements, the better.
3. Some nutrients are more easily utilized by the body when the vegetables are cooked while other nutrients are assimilated better in the raw state. Consequently confusion results as to which vegetables to cook and which to leave raw. To remedy this dilemma, simply serve a vegetable raw one meal and cooked another.

RAW: Sliced, whole, grated — as snacks, with a dip, in salads or sandwiches.

STEAM: Using a steamer basket or colander in a large pot with a small amount of water (not touching basket), vegetables are placed in basket and steamed until just tender (covered). Vegetables look and taste their best while retaining maximum nutrients when steamed. Never add baking soda to veggies for color as it destroys the B-vitamins. Any remaining water can be used in a sauce or gravy or saved for a soup stock. Veggies can be steamed together and still maintain individual flavors.

STIR-FRY: This means to saute in a *small* amount of oil or butter in a heavy skillet at medium-low heat until just tender-crisp, before adding grains. Or saute small amounts of veggies quickly in hot oil in a wok before adding liquids and grains and simmering as in a Chinese dish. Hot oil and quick cooking seals the nutrients in.

BAKE: Fall harvest vegetables such as squashes, yams, potatoes, can be baked whole in a moderate oven. To conserve energy, bake vegetables when you already have the oven heated for loaves, pies, etc. Foil-bake for camp-outs.

SHISH KEBOBS: Use whole or large-chunked veggies, such as mushrooms, green peppers, eggplant, onions, tomatoes, new potatoes. Thread them onto a skewer; then broil or barbeque, basting often and serve beside grains along with a green salad.

Vegetables — Simplified

If you've found yourself hung up on the same old vegetables, four-cans-for-a-dollar, then it's time to step into the incredible world of color, texture, flavor and variety that is vegetables. Vary from day to day your choice of root, stem, leaf and flower veggies, for like people, each has a personality of its own.

ARTICHOKES: Not unlike the human paradox, this aristocrat of vegetables has a spiney surface which must be carefully peeled away to reveal a tender heart. Remove sharp tips with scissors. Steam and serve with individual mini-bowls of hot, herbed butter and/or mayonnaise, for dipping. Be sure to include an extra saucer for discarding leaves.

ASPARAGUS: Take the time to plant them one fall or spring day and asparagus will return, year after year, to grace your table and your tastebuds. Snap stems to separate tender portion from the tough portion, which will be cooked for soup stock. Stand stalks in a clump, tied with string, in one inch of boiling water for five minutes, uncovered, then invert a double boiler pan over top and cook for five more minutes. To serve, drizzle with butter and dust with lemon-pepper seasoning. (The one without MSG)

AVOCADOS: What sheared-velvet does for an evening gown, avocados will do for a salad. Halve, remove seed and place on a chilled, lettuce-leaf-lined plate. Heap centers with any moist vegetable salad mixture and sprinkle with pepitas or use fruit salad and sprinkle with shredded coconut.

BEANS, GREEN: There is no greater pity than for the palate that must endure green beans served in the average cafeteria. To spark renewed interest, steam string or broad beans, just until crisp-tender, then spike with a light touch of Devil Sauce: equal parts SunButter-Blend, honey and prepared mustard with dashes of kelp and cayenne.

BEETS: Only a gardener understands the excitement of the first Spring thinning of baby beets. Scrub whole, with tops (or use mature beets cut into bite-size pieces) and saute in hot butter for two minutes. Cover and steam two more minutes and serve in individual bowls, using juice. Secure a twist of lemon to each bowl for garnish and additional tang.

BROCCOLI: This deep-green flower will embellish your most eloquent tableware. Pile steamed-tender spears estately on a special platter and surround with lemon wedges. Serve homemade mayonnaise in individual goblets, accompanied by dainty hors d'oeuvres forks for dipping.

BRUSSELS SPROUTS: Cut these miniature delicacies in half down the centers to expose the beautiful internal formation of the tender leaves. Steam briefly, serve in a heated dish and drizzle with melted lemon/garlic butter and garnish with sliced, hard-cooked egg.

CABBAGE: If an adverse effect accompanies cabbage consumption, it is probably the result of overcooking. Serve this vegetable raw, chopped fine, but don't hesitate to play a variation on your classic coleslaw medley. Try adding crushed pineapple; chopped nuts, celery or apples, or whole sweet peas, corn or baby beets.

CARROTS: They're like gold; when you wash away the dirt, you find the sweet treasure. Cut carrots on the diagonal, then cut each slice into matchsticks. Steam until tender and toss with basil-butter. Alternate in parfait glasses with garlic croutons, ending with the crunchy croutons. (Warm parfaits with very hot water first, so hot carrots won't break the glass.)

CAULIFLOWER: Remind yourself that this is a delicate flower and must be handled with TLC to prevent overcooking. Break into flowerettes and steam until just tender. Make a Speedy Cheese Sauce in top of double boiler with equal parts mayonnaise, cream and shredded cheese, adding saffron for color if you like. Toss flowerettes with toasted sunflower seeds and cheese sauce and serve in warmed mugs.

CELERY: This pale, sun-deprived vegetable lends crunch to nearly any salad, sauce or main dish, but for sheer pleasure and simplicity, you can take your celery and stuff it! Use cheeses, moist salads, peanut butter, tahini or anything that spreads easily. To send in sack lunches, smack two stalks together (gooey sides) and wrap securely.

CORN: We had so many neat things to tell you about this vegetable, but we changed our minds because they were all too corny. So what you get is a recipe for homestyle creamed corn without the extra starch of a cream sauce. Place half of your corn kernels in a blender with a little cream. Turn blender to low and drizzle a beaten egg slowly into the puree. The heat of the corn will cook and thicken the egg. Add to whole kernels and serve in lightly steamed green pepper halves.

EGGPLANT: The first thing you do to make this vegetable a hit with your family is, use your imagination to change that dull name to one as royal as its shimmering purple exterior. Then you grow some in your own garden, which automatically entices children to be anxious to try even the strangest concoctions. Next, you dice it so fine that it cannot be detected when sauteed with umpteen other veggies. By this time they will be accustomed to the flavor and you can go creative with confidence.

GREENS, LEAFY: Discover and delight in, the pungent flavor and bonus calcium content of the intensely green leafy vegetables, by chopping them very fine and adding to cream sauce or a souffle. Or use the very tiny, tender, center leaves in salads. Either way, you will benefit from the nutrients that are abundant in the sun-drenched leaves.

JERUSALEM ARTICHOKES: Planting these sunflower-like tubers in your garden is a lot like making friends — give them some space and a little loving attention and they'll be with you forever. Low sodium, high iron "sunchokes" will enhance, virtually any recipe in your repertory. They can be diced, sliced or shredded; then steamed, sauteed, broiled, boiled, deep-fried, mashed creamed or simply scrubbed and enjoyed raw for their crunchy texture and mild flavor. For salads, marinate to prevent discoloration.

JICAMA: Pronounce the *j* like an *h* and ask your kids to make up poems about this sweet, juicy, versatile vegetable — you will laugh 'til you cry. But if you are controlling your weight, you won't cry about Crunchy, Color-Wheel Root Salad. In fact it will be a hit at your next exercise luncheon: Individually, shred in food processor, jicama, rutabaga, carrots, broccoli and beets. (Follow that order so you won't have to clean blades between veggies.) Line chilled platter with bronze lettuce leaves. Mound, layer or radiate veggies for color contrast. Serve with breadsticks and a variety of dressings.

LEEKS: Save some space in your garden and time in your day to learn how to grow and harvest leeks. Cut in half lengthwise for easier washing. The whites will impart their unique flavor to everything from cream sauce to souffles while the greens will nicely season soups and stock for cooking grains.

MUSHROOMS: The crown of a good mushroom is much like a baby's bottom after a bath — round, velvety smooth and irresistible. Especially when skewered alternately with pearl onions and dipped in marinade before being quickly broiled for a minute or two and served on a bed of hot, buttered grains.

ONIONS: Don't fret about onion-breath, rejoice in a sweet-heart, for onions have long been associated with keeping the ole' ticker ticking like clockwork. Using a cast-iron skillet, saute rings of sweet onion in SunButterBlend until crisp-tender. Toss with grated Parmesan cheese and turn burner off. The heat of the skillet will continue to soften onions while it melts the cheese. Toss again and serve.

PARSLEY: Use this Jill-of-all-trades fresh, frozen or dried in literally anything. 'Nuff said.

PARSNIPS: When all else seems to have disappeared from the garden, parsnips remain to seal our bond with Mother Earth and entice preparation for yet another Spring. Slice parsnips on the diagonal and saute in butter. Cover and slow-cook until tender. Sprinkle with equal parts herb-buttered bread crumbs and ground, toasted sunflower seeds.

PEAS: Can any Spring scene compare with watching your little ones dance gaily around the pea-patch, stopping only long enough to snap open a crispy green pod and express their fascination with the tiny jewels tucked inside? If you must cook peas at all, steam very briefly and serve with butter and chives.

PEPPERS, BELL RED OR GREEN: "Of course, peppers are stuffed with rice, is there any other way?" Ahem, since you asked: Try millet, bulgur, buckwheat, wild rice (actually a grass), barley, farina, or couscous, in a pilaf. Then there are cornbread, shortbread or savory bread stuffings. How about spaghetti, chile or Sloppy Jose Sauce? You can even fill with leftover casserole and break an egg on top for a quick brunch. And don't forget about the creamed corn! Of course peppers are stuffed with rice, too. But then you already knew that. Use higher-in-vitamin-C red peppers whenever possible.

POTATOES: Although delicious and nutritious plain, we chefs have never been content to leave this staple vegetable unadorned. Since you probably already have 1001 ways to prepare potatoes, promise yourself that, starting today, you will be equally as creative with other veggies. Try your hand at matchmaking; we're sure the single potato will enjoy company: Potatoes and Broccoli Au-Gratin, Creamed Potatoes and Carrots; Sauteed Potatoes and Scallions; Potato and Sunchoke Pancakes; Scalloped Potatoes and Green Beans; Mashed Potatoes and Apples; Potato and Jicama Salad . . . now pair your own.

TOMATOES: If you simply cannot tolerate those hot-house imitations, just plant your own, then next fall, you will have earned the right to relish the regal flavor of your ruby-red gems. For salads that become a light dinner on a hot summer day, remove tops and some pulp of tomatoes and stuff with your favorite salad.

SQUASH, SUMMER: Just how it happens, we're not sure, but the phenomenon repeats itself annually: One day there's a beautiful yellow blossom and the next day there's a zucchini or a crookneck or a patty pan or a strange cross that we don't remember planting! But they're all delicious sliced, sauteed in butter or olive oil and sprinkled with Italian Herb Mix. Now I wonder what kind *this* one is . . .?

SQUASH, WINTER: Some varieties can grow to enormous size. Remember to get a picture of that three-and-a-half foot tall banana squash standing upright next to your three foot tall two-year-old! To further warm a winter kitchen, bake a big squash all day at low heat in the oven. Serve wedges, spread with butter and drizzle with maple syrup for dessert or the next morning for breakfast. Freeze some and share some with a neighbor.

YAMS AND SWEET POTATOES: It doesn't matter which is which, use both yams and sweet spuds often to benefit from their vast store of nutrients and energy. Cooking times vary, but either is delicious baked, buttered and sprinkled with nutmeg. Mash leftovers and use in your favorite holiday pie, reducing honey, as both are sweeter than pumpkin.

Using Herbs, Seeds and Seasonings

ALLSPICE: pies, cookies, puddings, curries.
ANISE SEED: cookies, cakes, tea, fruit salads.
BAY LEAF: soups, stews.
BASIL (SWEET): tomato based casseroles, sauces, soups, stews, vegetables (carrots, green beans), salad dressings, loaves.
CAYENNE: salads, casseroles, grain dishes, egg dishes (use sparingly).
CARAWAY SEED: coleslaw, cottage cheese, cabbage rolls, salads, breads, curry-rice dishes, potatoes, onions, salads.
CARDAMON SEED: cakes, rolls, yogurt dishes, curries.
CELERY SEED: soups, mayonnaise, stews, salads (potato and coleslaw), stuffings, onions.
CHIA SEED: hot cereals, soups, sauces, vegetables, salads, drinks.
CHERVIL: cottage cheese, butter, salads, sauces, soups.
CHILI PEPPERS: refried beans, Mexican dishes, cheese and egg dishes, soups, soybean casseroles.
CHIVES: salads, soups, salad dressings, dips, cheese and egg omelets, potatoes.
CINNAMON: rice and millet puddings, shakes, squash and yam pies, cookies, banana bread, fruit dishes, cereals (oatmeal-millet-4 grain).
CLOVES: squash or yam pies, hot cider, cakes, cookies.
CORIANDER SEED: cakes, cookies, curries.
CUMIN SEED: curries, bean dishes, tomato based casseroles, Mexican dishes, sauces, salads, soybean dishes.
CURRY POWDER: rice and other grain dishes (contains allspice, cardamom, cayenne, cloves, cumin, coriander, dry mustard, fenugreek, ginger, turmeric, nutmeg).
DILL SEED: salad dressings, salads, sandwich spreads, egg and cheese casseroles, soups, vegetables, cucumber-pickles.
FENNEL: cookies, breads, cakes, soups, egg dishes, salads, fruits.
FLAX SEED: cereals, breads, salads, puddings, shakes, teas.
GARLIC: eggplant, soups, stews, sandwich spreads, casseroles, bean and grain dishes, nut and seed patties, salad dressings, Italian dishes, Chinese dishes, etc.
GINGER: breads, cookies, cakes, squash pies, Chinese stir-frys.
MACE: carrot cake, millet pudding, spice cake, banana bread, squash pie, cookies, fruit smoothies.
MARJORAM: spaghetti sauce, green beans, eggplant, potatoes, soups, stews, egg dishes.
MINT LEAVES: tabouleh, carrots, fruit salad, peas, tea.
MUSHROOMS: Chinese dishes, casseroles, egg dishes, vegetable stir-frys, salads, soups, stews, loaves, patties, crepes.
MUSTARD SEED: curries, cabbage dish, spreads, salads.
NUTMEG: spinach, pies, puddings, quiches.
OREGANO: soups, stews, casseroles, bean loaves, pizza, Italian foods, vegetables (broccoli, eggplant).
PAPRIKA: potatoes, eggs, salads, casseroles, fish.
PARSLEY: egg dishes, salads, casseroles, breads, potatoes, fish, stuffings, gravies, sauces, soups.
POPPY SEED: noodle dishes, cakes, breads, salads.
PUMPKIN SEED: salads, loaves, vegetables.
ROSEMARY: soups, vegetables, sauces, peas, potatoes, eggplant, fruit salads, tea.
SAGE: stuffing, rice dishes, lentil loaf, vegetables, casseroles, curries, cottage cheese.
SAVORY: potatoes, beans, grain dishes, salads, sauces, soups, cabbage dishes, corn.
SESAME SEED: tahini, gomazio, fudges, cookies, breads, patties, loaves, casseroles, salads, rice, soups, asparagus, cereals, granola, pie crusts.

SUNFLOWER: nut and seed patties, salads, gravies, casseroles, loaves, vegetables, stir-frys, breads, fruit salads, hot cereals, pie crusts, fudges, granola, desserts (raw, toasted, sprouted).
TARRAGON: egg dishes, tomato based casseroles, salads, vinegar, mayonnaise, broccoli.
THYME: soups, potatoes, cheese dishes, salads, onions, peas, carrots, cheese dishes, green beans, eggplant.
TURMERIC: cream sauces, mayonnaise, curries, corn.

The Keys to Success

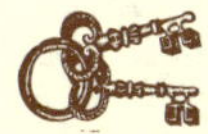

We're not sure if it's really a tradition or just because grandma only had one fancy dish, that dessert always seems to come in the most elaborate receptacle. Since part of the Organoleptic test is visual, try serving herb-buttered carrots in individual parfait glasses with a sprig of parsley and see if the response isn't better than just setting the cook pot on the table and dishing up plain, cooked carrots. Make lentil loaf in a bundt pan and turn out onto a pedestal cake stand, filling the center with a tiny bouquet of freshly picked flowers. Creamed sunchokes are delicious tasting but look plain and simple; zap them up with some sprinkles like chopped chives and toasted sun seeds, and you double the probability of their being enjoyed the very first time.

Literally everything tastes better by candlelight and digestion can be improved with some relaxing background music. Although we're certain no one would notice they were eating stuffed tofu if The Captain and Tenille came to dinner, we haven't yet tried that as a "don't-worry-about-what's-in-it-just-eat-it" technique! We do know that getting as excited about the vegetables or main dish as you do the dessert, will guarantee success.

Send Your Taste Buds Back to School

Although we include honey, maple syrup and other natural sweeteners in our recipes, we hope that you will reserve those treats for occasional use and try to re-educate your taste buds to rely upon fruits and nuts for sweetness and satisfaction. The right combinations can be colorful, crunchy and flavorful enough to tantalize any child or adult.

All of our suggestions and recipes are designed to look, feel and taste great just as they are, but we hope that you will use them only as guidelines and will soon be converting all your favorite recipes to include the best high-energy foods on the market.

Blue Ribbon Criteria

In our years of experiments converting to natural food recipes, we have prepared some dishes that were too unusual, too spicy, too expensive, or too time-consuming to receive our Blue Ribbon status.

Therefore, we have a rule in our kitchens that goes something like this: Everyone in our family has to at least try the new concoction. If someone doesn't like it, s/he is not permitted to influence another family member or guest with such outbursts as: Yuk! Gross! Ghastly!, a grimace, a downward gesture of the thumbs, or feeding Brutus under the table. If they like what they have just eaten, however, they must jump up and down, wave flags, sound horns, yell cheers, release rockets, and carry the cook around on their shoulders to show appreciation.

We pledge on our heretofore Top Secret Recipe Files that every recipe printed in this book has passed the test!

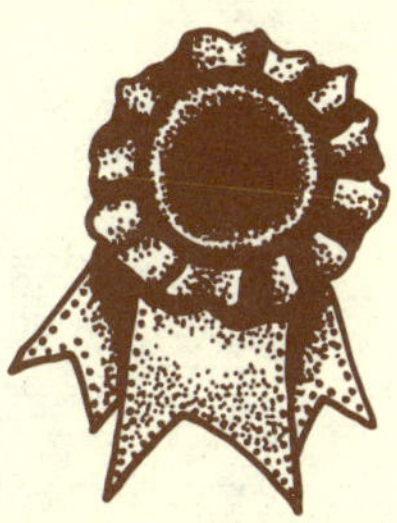

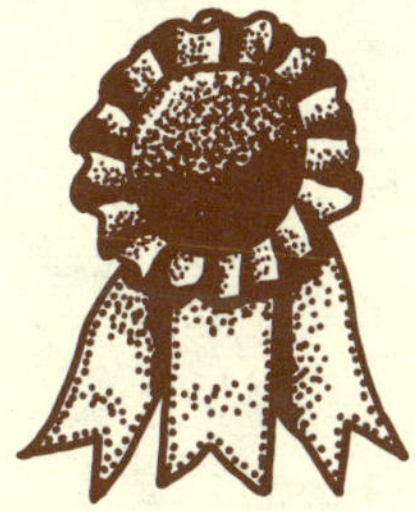

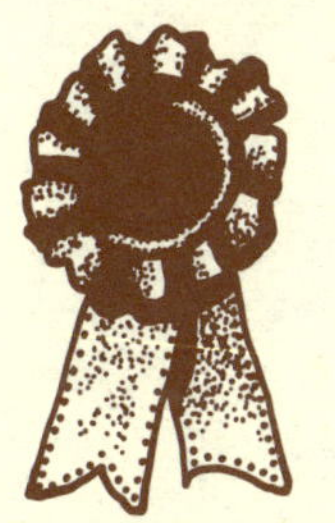

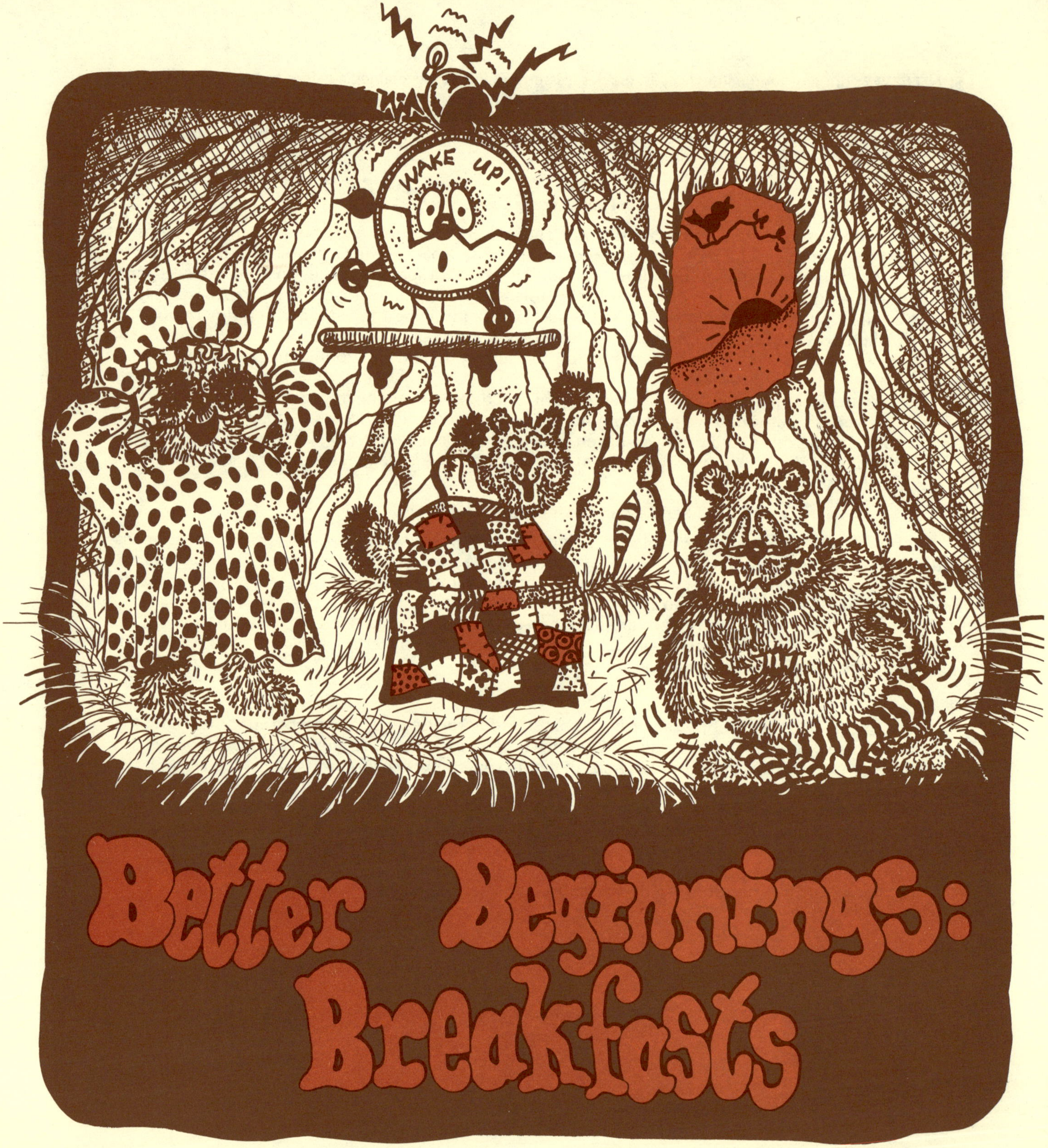

Better Beginnings: Breakfasts

Better Beginnings: Breakfasts

It's really to your behoovement
To undergo muscle improvement.
When you're huffin' and puffin'
Try our Pineapple Bran Muffin.
You're bound to begin a new movement.

High Test Fuel

Many of the recipes in this chapter take a daring detour from standard breakfasts. Whoever said the morning meal had to be cold cereal, or bacon, eggs, toast and juice? Surprise your family some morning with a pot of beans or a tortilla cheese melt. They are high in protein and carbohydrates and will satisfy the adult or child until lunchtime. Besides, the aroma just drifts down the hall into the bedrooms and greets hungry hibernators with a "Hi, wake up and start your day with a hearty breakfast!"

Perhaps mornings are rushed for you and you would rather drink your meal. Try high protein shakes, fruit smoothies, or energy drinks, guaranteed to be delicious while providing enough energy to keep you rolling until noon. Breakfast fruit salads can be crunchy and chewy or smooth and creamy, and are great alternatives to the cold cereal syndrome.

Whether you choose the usual, the unique or the liquid, breakfast shouldn't be skipped. A meal that provides *high test fuel* is necessary to keep you going at an optimum energy level throughout the morning. So challenge your creativity and tantalize your taste buds with any of the Better Beginnings recipes. The variety is here; the choice is yours.

FRUIT SALADS AND PUDDINGS

DESSERT FOR BREAKFAST

papaya or melon
plain yogurt or
strawberry-banana sherbet
sun seed sprouts
cinnamon

Cut papayas in half and scoop out seeds. Fill center with plain yogurt or sherbet, then garnish with sprouts and cinnamon. Sherbet: Blend bananas and strawberries together with a little lemon juice; freeze, then blend again to sherbet consistency just before using.

RICE YOGURT SUPREME

1½ cups cooled, cooked brown rice or millet
1 cup plain yogurt
2 diced bananas
2-4 T. honey
¾ cup crushed pineapple (well-drained)
granola, ground nuts or strawberry

Mix rice with yogurt. Stir in honey, pineapple and bananas. Chill well; top with granola, nuts or berry.

DIANE'S BAKED APPLES SUPREME

apples (winesaps are best)
dates or raisins
walnuts
maple syrup
SunButterBlend
1 to 1½ cups apple juice
cinnamon
honey/vanilla yogurt or honey-sweetened whipped cream

Core enough apples to serve your family or guests. Peel a ring around the top of each and stand upright in an oiled pan. Fill the cavity of each apple with equal parts chopped dates or raisins, and walnuts. Place syrup and a small pat of SunButterBlend on top of each apple. Pour apple juice into the pan around apples and sprinkle the whole thing generously with cinnamon. Cover and bake at 350° for about 40 minutes or until tender. Top with a dollop of yogurt or whipped cream.

PINEAPPLE-ORANGE SALAD

Cut a pineapple in half lengthwise. Remove fruit, core, and slice it into long spears. Peel an orange and remove segments. Arrange pineapple spears and orange segments in reserved pineapple shells. Chill until ready to serve, then top with Sesame Dressing. DRESSING: In a jar, add ½ cup oil, ¼ cup lemon juice, ¼ cup orange juice, 3 T. honey and 2 T. toasted sesame seeds. Cover and shake.

DUTCH APPLE BREAKFAST

Put 4 large apples, cored, through shredding blade of food processor. Add to 1 pint yogurt, ½ cup *each* wheat germ and coarsely chopped walnuts, ¼ cup flaked bran, 2 T. honey and 1 t. *each* cinnamon and vanilla. Stir well and allow flavors to blend in refrigerator.

DELIGHTFULLY DIFFERENT BREAKFASTS

CROCK O' BEANS

¼ cup lima beans
¼ cup red beans
½ cup lentils
½ chopped onion
1 bay leaf
1½ t. crushed basil
1 t. sea salt/kelp
2½ cups boiling water
½ t. cider vinegar
a few teaspoons tomato paste

Begin this the night before. Rinse and drain *dried* beans. Place in crock pot along with onion and seasonings. Pour boiling water over all, place lid on crock and set at low. Just before serving in the morning, add vinegar and tomato paste. Don't be surprised when your family lines up, bowl and spoon in hand, ready to be served. Accompany with whole grain bread.

Variations: Try other combinations of beans — black, Navy, adzuki.

TAMARI RICE CRUNCH

Heat 2 T. oil in a skillet. Stir in 2 cups cooked brown rice and 1 T. tamari-soy sauce. Add fresh chopped vegetables or leftover cooked veggies (broccoli, carrots, onions, celery, mushrooms, sunflower seeds, chopped walnuts, and some mung sprouts). Heat thoroughly (if veggies are raw, saute before adding rice). Grate a little Jack cheese over all and let set until melted.

Variation: Substitute cooked potatoes (cubed, sliced or shredded) for rice and top with toast cubes.

HIGH PROTEIN STRATA

7-8 slices day-old bread
4-5 eggs
1 small can green chili salsa
1-2 T. minced dried onion or
3-4 T. fresh, chopped onion
approximately 1 cup milk
6 oz. cottage cheese
cayenne to taste (a dash goes a long way)
sea salt/kelp to taste
grated Cheddar cheese

Prepare the night before and bake in the morning. Oil an 8"x8" cake pan. Preheat oven to 350°. Tear bread slices into pieces and place in pan. In a bowl, mix eggs, salsa, onions, milk. Add cottage cheese and seasonings. Pour over bread and poke bread with a fork so mixture soaks in. Sprinkle light layer of cheese over top. Bake 45 minutes until firm.

Variation: Substitute corn bread for bread.

CHEESE MELT

Place thin slices of Jack or Cheddar cheese on whole grain bread slices, corn tortillas or whole wheat chapatis. Melt in a 350° oven. Remove and top with tomato slices and alfalfa sprouts. OR spread leftover frijoles on the bread, top with cheese and melt.

WHOLE WHEAT VEGETABLE OR FRUIT PIZZA

See recipes for pizzas in *Serendipity Suppers* and *KID STUFF*. They are quick to make for a hearty breakfast and kids love 'em cold in their sack lunches, too!

GO GOURMET WITH GRAINS

Cold Cereals

"WE LOVE YOUR BODY" MUESLI

3 cups blender-ground oats
¼ cup flaked bran
¼ cup wheat germ
½ cup finely ground nuts
½ cup raisins or dried, chopped dates
½ cup coarsely ground sun seeds
2 T. ground sesame seeds
2-3 t. cinnamon

Mix in a large bowl and store in covered jars in refrigerator. To serve: place portion in bowl and top with 1 T. honey and 1 raw grated apple. Pour milk over all.

Variations: Substitute dates and bananas for honey and apple and pour hot milk over. OR use grated apple with apple juice. OR use dates with orange juice or yogurt. For a creamier texture, soak portion overnight in refrigerator in slightly more liquid than dry cereal. Add fruit, sweeteners and more liquid in the morning.

GRRRRREAT GRRRANOLA BY THE GALLON

5 cups rolled oats
1 cup wheat flakes
1 cup rye flakes
½ cup soy grits
½ cup raw wheat germ
½ cup bran
1 cup coconut
½ to 1 cup honey
½ to 1 cup oil
1 t. vanilla
½ cup sunflower seeds
½ to 1 cup peanuts
1-2 cups chopped, raw nuts (walnuts, cashews, almonds)
1-2 cups dried fruit (dates, raisins, apricots)
½ cup raw sesame seeds or pumpkin seeds
1 T. cinnamon

Mix first 7 ingredients in a large bowl. Heat the liquids and pour over the dry mixture and stir well. (Less honey and oil give a flaky texture; more will make the granola stick together and candy-like.)

Spread on cookie sheets and bake at 325° until dry and crunchy, or toasted to your taste. Stir occasionally and check often.

Remove from oven and add remaining ingredients. Mix well and cool. Place in jars and refrigerate, freeze, or store in a cool, dry place. Makes a gallon.

Variation: Nuts and seeds may be added before toasting, but nutritionally, they're better raw.

Ways to Use Granola

1. Sprinkle on top of other cereals, hot or cold.
2. Top ice cream, puddings, desserts.
3. Use as a trail mix for snacks, hiking, or lunches.
4. Stir into yogurt.
5. Layer granola on peanut butter in sandwiches.
6. Add to cookie dough.
7. Top fruit salads or mix in.
8. Roll bananas in honey or carob sauce and then in granola and freeze.
9. Make a granola pie crust.
10. Use in casseroles where a sweeter, crunchier texture is desired, or as a stuffing for squash or baked apples.

WHEAT BISCUITS

Run cooked, salted whole wheatberries through the meat grinder, using a very fine blade so that wheat comes out in spaghetti-like strands. Place in clumps on cookie sheet and bake at 250°-300° for 1 hour or more. Turn once or twice during baking and drying.

GRAPE NUTTY CEREAL

Run equal parts sprouted wheat and raisins through a meat grinder. Knead the "dough" well; spread on a cookie sheet and dry in an oven, that has been warmed and turned off. When thoroughly dry, crumble and store in a covered container.

MALTED WHEAT CEREAL

Run 1 loaf of 2-3 day old whole wheat bread through a meat grinder. Toss with 1½ T. malt flavoring and 1½ T. date sugar. Bake on a cookie sheet at 250°-300° for 45 minutes to 1 hour.

Hot Cereals

Use any of the wide varieties of whole grain cereals or flaked or cracked multi-grain cereals. They need from 8 to 25 minutes cooking time. Old-fashioned oatmeal is better than instant. Instant hot cereals usually have sugar added and are so refined and processed that nutritional value is low.

BASIC COOKING METHOD: Bring twice as much water to a boil as dry cereal.

When boiling, add cereal, turn heat down, cook desired time (stirring often); then cover and remove from heat for a few minutes longer. Dried fruit may be cooked with cereal or added after cooking. See section on Cooking Grains in *Kitchen Keys* for interesting and time-saving ways to prepare cereals. (Let kids make faces on their own cereal with a variety of toppings.)

MMMMMM MMMMMM MILLET

1 cup raw millet
2 finely chopped apples
2 sliced bananas
¼ cup dried, chopped dates
4 cups boiling water

Simmer above ingredients in water for 30-35 minutes. (Millet needs more water than most grains.)

Variations: Use raisins in place of dates and add cinnamon, honey, and butter after cooking. OR cook millet in milk instead of water over a double boiler and add fruit after cooking.

CORNMEAL MUSH

Boil 2½ cups water. Mix 1 cup cornmeal with 1 cup cold water and add to boiling water. Stir frequently, cooking for 30-40 minutes. Sweeten with maple syrup, cinnamon and butter, OR flavor with cottage cheese and homemade preserves.

MAMA BEAR'S PORRIDGE

2 cups raw brown rice
½ cup millet
½ cup chopped sun seeds
1 T. ground chia or flaxseed
2 T. rice polish

Rinse quickly and drain rice and millet in a colander. Spread on cookie sheets and toast in 300° until very lightly browned (about 10-15 minutes for millet and 15-20 minutes for rice).

Grind grains in blender or grinder to a coarse or fine flour, depending upon how smooth or chewy you like your cereal.

Mix in sun seeds, chia and rice polish and store in covered quart jar in refrigerator. Optional: Rinse grains and dry on *low* in oven; then grind.

Variation: Add chopped raw or toasted almonds, cashews and sesame seeds.

To cook: Add 1½ cups dry mix to 3 cups boiling water. Lower heat and simmer for 5-8 minutes, depending upon texture of ground grains. Serve with dates or raisins, sliced apple or bananas, honey to taste and yogurt or milk.

Cereal Toppings

granola	**fresh fruit**	**chopped dates**	**milk**	**raisins**	**yogurt**
cinnamon	**any seeds or nuts**	**butter**	**homemade jam**	**honey**	**toasted wheat germ**

POWER-PACKED PANCAKES-WAFFLES-MUFFINS

SUNNY BANANA PANCAKES

3 cups whole wheat flour
½ t. salt
1 T. baking powder
2 eggs
2 T. oil
2 T. honey
2½ cups milk
1 cup sprouted or chopped sun seeds
2 diced bananas

Mix dry ingredients. In another bowl, beat eggs, oil, honey and milk. Add to dry ingredients and stir just to blend. Stir in sun seeds and bananas. Makes 25-30 small pancakes.

Variation: For extra nutrition add 1 T. each ground chia, sesame seeds and 1 T. brewer's yeast.

PEPPY POTATO PANCAKES

In large bowl, mix 4 cups shredded, cooked potatoes, 1 cup shredded cheese, ½ cup Snappy-Quick Mix, and ¼ t. *each* vegetable salt, freshly grated pepper, ground celery seed and basil. Beat 2 large or 3 medium eggs with 2 T. SunButterBlend and stir into potato mixture. Shape into patties. Saute in a little sunflower oil until golden on both sides, then finish baking in 375° oven for 15 minutes.

OREGON TOAST A LA CASHEW

1 cup raw, washed cashews
1½ cups water or ½ water and ½ juice
¼ cup chopped dates
½ t. cinnamon

Blend cashews and water in a blender. Add dates and cinnamon and blend again. Pour into a bowl. Dip whole grain bread into mixture and place on well-oiled cookie sheet for approximately 10 minutes per side in a 400° oven until golden brown. Serve with SunButterBlend. Sweet, crusty and delicious!

FRESH FRUIT PUFF

¼ cup SunButterBlend
3 eggs
¾ cup milk
2 T. honey (optional)
¾ cup sifted, whole wheat pastry flour

Put SunButterBlend in a 9" cast iron skillet or other baking dish and melt in a 425° oven until bubbly, about 10 minutes. Beat together eggs, milk, honey and flour. Pour mixture all at once into the hot pan.

Return to oven and bake for 30 minutes, or until edges are puffed and browned. Mix about 3 cups of fresh fruit with a little honey and spoon immediately into center of hot puff. Cut into wedges and dollop with sour cream or yogurt.

YUMMY YAMMY PANCAKES

½ cup dry soybeans
3 cups water
2 cups grated, raw, peeled yams
½ cup finely chopped onion
½ cup finely chopped green pepper
butter
2-3 eggs
sea salt/kelp to taste

Wash beans. Place in blender with water and blend until broken into tiny pieces. Pour mixture into saucepan and bring to a boil. Simmer, covered, for 10 minutes. Add yams and simmer an additional 10 minutes, adding more water if necessary. Cool.

Meanwhile, saute onion and green pepper in butter; then set aside.

Take cooled soybean-yam mixture and place, a little at a time, in the blender along with eggs; blend until smooth, adding more water, if necessary — to make a very thick pancake batter. If batter is too thin, add whole wheat pastry flour to thicken. Stir in sauteed veggies and drop by spoonfuls onto oiled skillet and fry like a pancake. Serve with SunButterBlend. Delicious!

Variation: To make into a pie: add another egg, about 2/3 cup milk, 4 T. honey, 1 T. orange juice, 2 T. butter, and cinnamon, cloves and nutmeg to taste. Omit salt. Pour into a crust of your choice and bake at 375° for 35-40 minutes or until set. (See *Labor of Love Lunches* for pie crust recipes.)

NUTRITIOUS SYRUPS AND TOPPINGS

1. Heat peanut butter and honey until smooth and creamy.
2. 1 or 2 t. frozen orange juice concentrate mixed with yogurt.
3. Fresh fruit, plain or with yogurt.
4. Plain or flavored kefir mixed with strawberries or other fruit.
5. Fresh applesauce with cinnamon.
6. 1 cup softened cream cheese mixed with 1 T. honey, topped with raisins and chopped walnuts.
7. Nutty Butter: In blender, blend ½ cup ground almonds or walnuts, 10 chopped, pitted dates, a pinch of salt, and enough water to make a buttery consistency.
8. Date Orange Syrup: Simmer 2 cups pitted dates in 2 cups boiling water until soft. Add ¼ cup frozen orange juice concentrate. Blend in blender.
9. Heat equal parts SunButterBlend and honey with a little cinnamon and cloves until of syrup consistency.
10. Homemade preserves.

APPLEY MUFFINS

1 cup whole wheat flour
1 cup flaked bran
½ cup wheat germ
1 t. baking soda
1 t. cinnamon
2 T. oil
½ cup honey
1 egg
1 cup apple juice
1 grated, peeled apple
(opt.) 1 small handful each of coconut and chopped sun seeds

In a large bowl mix first 5 ingredients. In another bowl mix egg, oil, honey, apple juice and apple. Stir all together just to blend. Add coconut and sun seeds if desired. Spoon into muffin cups and bake for 20 minutes at 400°. Makes 12 muffins.

PINEAPPLE BRAN MUFFINS

1 cup whole wheat flour
1½ cups flaked bran
½ t. salt
3 t. baking powder
½ cup raisins or chopped dates
1 egg
1 cup yogurt or buttermilk
½ t. baking soda
¼ cup honey or molasses
4 T. oil
½ cup undrained, crushed pineapple

In a large bowl mix first 4 ingredients. In another bowl mix egg, yogurt or buttermilk, soda, honey or molasses, oil, raisins or dates and pineapple. Add liquids all at once to dry mix and stir just to moisten.

Fill muffin cups 2/3's full and bake 20 minutes at 400° until done.

Variation: Omit fruit and place 1 cube of Cheddar cheese in middle of each muffin before baking.

SURPRISE RICE-BUTTERMILK MUFFINS

1¼ cup brown rice flour
½ cup millet flour
2 T. soy flour
2 T. minute tapioca
1 T. baking powder
2 T. arrowroot flour
½ t. baking soda
¼ t. salt
¼ cup melted butter
2 T. honey
2 well-beaten eggs
1 cup buttermilk
Cheddar cheese cubes

In a large bowl, measure the dry ingredients together and mix well. Add liquids all together and stir until moistened.

Fill paper muffin cups with 1 heaping T. of batter. Then place a ½" cube of Cheddar cheese in center of each muffin cup. Fill with remaining batter. Bake at 425° for 12-15 minutes or until browned. Makes 12 muffins.

Variations: Add 2 extra T. of honey to liquids. In place of the cheese cubes, spoon 1 t. of the following mixture in the center of muffin before covering with batter: grated apple, raisins, chopped walnuts and cinnamon. OR fill center with 1 t. homemade jam. Great for school lunches!

DRINK TO YOUR HEALTH

For most of the Fruit Smoothies and Super Milk Shakes, use frozen banana chunks as a sweetener and thickener. This is a healthy replacement for sugar-sweetened ice cream-based shakes. Simply peel ripe bananas, slice into one inch chunks, place in tightly closed glass or plastic containers and freeze. Usually the equivalent of one banana (approximately four to six chunks) will thicken a twelve to fourteen ounce shake or smoothie.

Variation: Freeze peeled bananas whole and cut into one inch chunks with a very sharp knife just before adding to blender.

FRUIT SMOOTHIES

BASIC DIRECTIONS:

1. Fill glass with frozen banana chunks OR use half bananas and half of the following fruit (fresh or frozen): **Apples, Berries, Grapes, Cantaloupe, Pears, Pineapple, Peaches, Cherries, Apricots, Avocados, Papaya, Nectarines, Cranberries, Dates, Strawberries.**
2. Pour fruit juice in space around fruit. Choose from the following: **Orange, Apple, Pineapple, Lime, Grape, Papaya, Apricot, Cherry, Lemon, Berry, Pear, Mixed.**
3. Pour all into a blender. Blend until smooth and thick.
4. For more than one serving, place desired amount of frozen fruit in blender; fill surrounding space with juice and blend.

OPTIONAL: Try adding a pinch or dash of one of the following spices:
cinnamon, nutmeg, mace, anise, cardamon, mint, grated lemon or orange peel.

MELLOW YELLOW

Blend 3 parts apple juice, 3 parts orange juice, 1 part pineapple juice, a few squeezes of fresh lemon juice, and enough frozen banana chunks to make thick.

PINEAPPLE BERRY

Blend pineapple juice with frozen strawberries.

Variation: Use half bananas and half strawberries.

AVOCADO-PAPAYA

Blend 16 to 20 oz. pineapple juice, ½ avocado, ¼ of a papaya, 10 frozen banana chunks and 1/3 cup coconut.

STRAPPLE

Blend apple juice with equal parts frozen bananas and fresh or frozen strawberries.

Variation: 2 heaping T. of plain yogurt per serving blended in.

PINEAPPLE-YOGURT

Blend 1 cup plain yogurt with 1 8 oz. can of undrained, crushed pineapple until smooth. Add enough frozen banana chunks to make desired thickness. Garnish with fresh mint.

PAPAYA

Blend 2 cups mashed ripe papaya, 1 cup plain yogurt, 2 T. honey, ½ t. cinnamon, and 2 to 4 frozen banana chunks.

CAROB-DATE

Blend 4 pitted dates, ½ t. vanilla, 1 T. tahini, 1 T. coconut, 2 t. carob powder, 8 to 10 oz. apple juice, and enough frozen banana chunks to make desired thickness.

PEACH

Blend 6 to 7 frozen banana chunks, 4 frozen peach puree cubes, 4 to 6 oz. apple juice, 5 to 6 heaping T. plain yogurt, 1 small handful raisins. Blend until smooth and icy.

APPLE SPICE

Peel and core 2 large apples. Dice into blender and add 1 cup plain yogurt. Blend until thick and smooth. Add mace, cinnamon, nutmeg, and/or cloves to taste. Optional: 1 t. honey.

NECTARINE

Blend a cup plain yogurt, 1 banana, sliced (fresh or frozen), and 1 sliced nectarine or peach.

GO HAWAIIAN

Blend 1 and ½ cups orange juice, ½ a lemon (juiced), 4 to 6 frozen banana chunks and 1/3 of a papaya. *Mikimiko!* (Very tasty).

LIQUID BREAKFAST

Blend 4 to 6 frozen banana chunks, 1 cup plain yogurt, ¼ cup orange or apple juice, 1 fresh sliced pear, apricot or peach, 2 to 3 T. chopped dates, and ¼ cup pineapple chunks. Add a dash or two of cinnamon, nutmeg, or Almond-Cinnamon Mixture.

SUPER MILK SHAKES

BASIC DIRECTIONS:

1. Fill glass with frozen banana chunks.
2. Pour milk in space around bananas. OR substitute:
   yogurt, soy milk, buttermilk, cottage cheese, nut or seed milk, homemade honey ice cream, powdered milk.
3. Pour into blender and add flavorings or sweeteners:
   1 to 2 T. of: honey, real maple syrup, unsulphured molasses, carob powder, peanut butter, Tahini OR
   ½ to 1 t. of: pure vanilla or almond extract, Almond-Cinnamon mixture, barley malt, or any other spice desired.
4. For more than one serving, place desired amount of frozen bananas in blender; fill surrounding space with milk or substitute, add flavorings to taste and blend.
5. For High Energy Drinks: Add 1 or more T. of your choice of the following Nutritional Fortifiers:
   figs, dates, raisins, sunflower seed sprouts, raw egg, coconut, flaxseed, soy powder, lecithin, peanuts, walnuts, cashews, almonds, sesame seeds, sunflower seeds, rice polish, wheat germ, nutritional yeast, flaked bran, protein powder, safflower oil, nut butters, sprouts (all kinds).
   (May also be added to fruit smoothies.)
6. Blend all ingredients of your choice in blender until smooth and thick.

CAROB-BANANA

Fill a 16 oz. glass ¾ full of frozen banana chunks. Pour milk in space around bananas. Pour into blender. Add 2 raw eggs, 1 t. vanilla, 1 T. carob powder, and 2 T. honey. Blend until smooth.

EARTHSHAKING SHAKE

Blend milk, frozen bananas and 1 t. per glass of Almond-Cinnamon Mixture.

STRAWBERRY

Blend milk, frozen bananas, fresh or frozen strawberries, and 1 T. per glass of vanilla protein powder.

DATE

Blend milk, frozen banana chunks, a few dates, and per glass ½ t. vanilla, 1 T. Tahini, 1 T. coconut, 2 t. carob powder, 1 t. soaked flaxseed.

Variation: Substitute raisins for dates and soy milk for milk.

A SHAKE FOR THE SHAKES

Blend 1½ cups orange juice, 4 to 6 frozen banana chunks, ¼ cup plain yogurt. Add 1 T. each of orange or vanilla flavored protein powder, wheat germ, sun seeds, lecithin, safflower or sunflower oil, nutritional yeast. Blend well and sip slowly.

PEANUT BUTTER

Blend milk, enough banana chunks to make thick, and ½ t. cinnamon and 1 or 2 T. peanut butter per serving.

FRUIT SHAKES

Mix fresh or frozen fruit with milk and frozen bananas for delightful fruit shakes. Add nutritional fortifiers desired for protein.

Pineapple Plus Drinks

Each drink serves four. Juice 1 whole, peeled pineapple for each drink. Remaining ingredients may be blended and strained, juiced, or blended and enjoyed as is.

1. Pineapple juice, 7-10 leaves of spinach (juiced or strained), 1 handful alfalfa sprouts.
2. Pineapple juice, ½ to 1 avocado, ¼ cup ground coconut, 1 banana.
3. Pineapple juice, 1 papaya, 2 bananas, 1 avocado, ½ lemon, juiced.
4. Pineapple juice, 8 oz. apple juice, 1 banana, 6 to 8 oz. carrot juice, 1 T. ground sunflower seed sprouts or mung bean sprouts.

RECIPES FOR DRINK ADDITIONS

ALMOND-CINNAMON MIXTURE

To one cup of finely ground shelled almonds, stir in 1 T. cinnamon. Store in covered glass jar in refrigerator. Keep plenty of this one on hand; many of the *KID STUFF* recipes call for this mixture.

SOY MILK

Blend 6 T. soy milk powder with 2 cups water. Refrigerate. Use within two days.

NUT AND SEED BUTTERS

Finely grind nuts in a blender or nut grinder until a butter is formed. May need to add a teaspoon or so of oil per cup of nuts. Each nut has its own amount of oil. Peanuts are higher in oil than almonds. Choose from: peanuts, almonds, cashews, sesame. Walnuts tend to become bitter after exposure to air. Sesame butter is called Tahini.

NUT AND SEED MILKS

To 1 cup of raw, shelled nuts (blanched, if almonds), slowly add 1 quart of water while blending at high speed. Blend until smooth; then add 1 T. oil, 2 T. honey and a pinch of salt. Blend again, strain, and refrigerate. May be used in any of the shakes, plain or flavored drinks, or in yogurts. When using seeds, use ½ cup of seeds with ½ cup nuts. Almond-Cashew or Almond-Sesame are good combinations.

HOT CAROB COCOA

Heat 1 quart of any kind of milk, but *do not boil.* Mix 3 T. carob powder, 3 T. honey, 1 T. oil and ½ t. vanilla or 1 T. vanilla protein powder. Add to hot milk.

SUNFLOWER SEED SPROUTS

Wash raw, hulled sunflower seeds in a colander. Pick out the dark ones. Place seeds in a glass jar and fill with water. Soak overnight. In morning, drain and rinse. Drain again and cover colander with a paper towel or cloth. Rinse twice more during the day, draining well after each rinse. By evening a tiny sprout will be forming. You may refrigerate at this point or continue to rinse and drain three times a day for one more day until sprout is as long as seed, but no longer. Refrigerate. Use in drinks, salads, puddings, yogurt, soups, and on tostadas. They taste crunchy, nutty, and are high in protein and other nutrients.

WHEAT GRASS

Sprout wheat berries in same manner as sunflower seeds. Then place in an aluminum pie pan which has been pierced with several holes for draining. Cover with damp paper towels and rinse two to three times daily. When stalk grows, remove towels, expose to light and water daily until grass is dark green and about seven inches tall. Cut at base for juicing.

WHEAT SPROUTS

Soak wheat berries overnight. In morning drain, rinse and drain again. Repeat two or three times a day for two days or until sprout is just the length of the grain. Crunchy and surprisingly sweet! Use in salads, sprout candies, cookies.

YOGURT

In a saucepan, mix 1 quart milk (whole, skim, 2%) with ¾ cup instant powdered milk. Blend and stir until milk is warm to touch. If you have a candy thermometer, check to see that milk is not warmer than 114° F. Remove from heat, and when temperature is correct, add 2 T. plain commercial yogurt. Stir gently. Pour into a wide-mouth quart jar or three or four smaller jars. Cover jars and place in a large pot of very warm water and carefully place in a cupboard, near a radiator or in a cooled oven. Leave for 5 to 8 hours, changing water when it becomes cool. When yogurt is yogged, refrigerate. Ideal temperature for yogging is 110-114° F. Other ways to incubate: Wrap well in sleeping bag or blankets and place in a clothes basket overnight. Wrap heating pad turned on medium-low around jar. Place jar on hot pad set on electric food warmer.

USE IN: dips, dressings, salads, soups, popsicles, puddings, shakes and smoothies, refrigerator or frozen desserts, casseroles, and toppings for pancakes and cereal.

FLAVOR WITH: vanilla, maple syrup, honey, dates, raisins, sun sprouts, dried fruit, fresh fruit, ground nuts, granola, cinnamon, nutmeg, and herbs and mayonnaise for dips or dressings.

SOME JUICES FOR FASTING

It is important to use fresh fruit or vegetable juices whenever possible for fasting, but if unavailable, canned or bottled tomato, pineapple, apple, grape, or frozen orange juice is definitely preferable to coffee and colas. Many raw greens, beets, carrots and celery can be washed, chopped, blended in the blender, and strained for a fresh, pure juice.

RAINBOW DRINK

Juice 5 to 6 carrots, 1 beet, and 2 stalks celery. Mix well and sip slowly.

MIXED FRUIT

Blend 3 parts fresh apple juice, 3 parts fresh orange juice, 1 part fresh or canned pineapple juice and a few squeezes of fresh lemon juice.

SUNRISER

Juice 1 lemon. Add water to make a tall glass and stir in 1 scant t. honey.

CARROT COCKTAIL

Juice some carrots for carrot juice. Juice a small handful of alfalfa sprouts, and 1 garlic clove. Sprinkle kelp and cayenne over drink and stir well.

ALOHA NUI

Blend together the following juices: ½ cup pineapple juice, ¼ cup carrot juice, ¼ cup orange juice, juice from ½ papaya. Pour in glasses and squeeze a thin slice of lime into each glass and place slices on rims of glasses.

VITAMIN ENERGIZER

Cut a small handful of wheat grass into 2 inch pieces. Place in blender with a little water and blend. Strain so that only the green liquid drains into a pitcher of fresh pineapple juice. Stir well. This is a lovely, mint green juice that contains a balanced ratio of vitamins and minerals.

POTASSIUM BROTH

2 to 3 quarts bran-oatmeal water
2-3 medium potatoes
1 cup chopped celery
1 chopped onion
¼ cup chopped parsley
1 cup grated carrots
kelp and cayenne to taste
any other herbs for seasonings

This vitamin-mineral broth is essential to drink while fasting.

Soak 1 cup bran and 1 cup oats overnight in water in refrigerator. In morning, beat mixture with egg beater and strain through a fine sieve. Pour liquid in pan and add veggies. Bring to a boil, adding additional water if necessary.

Simmer on low, covered, for approximately 30 minutes. Let cool 30 minutes, then mash veggies with a hand masher and strain through a fine sieve. Drink some warm with kelp and cayenne and herbs, and store the remainder, covered, in the refrigerator.

Reserve the mush for blending into soups or for adding to casseroles.

JUBILATION COCKTAIL

2 cups carrot juice
5 almonds
2 T. sun seed sprouts
1 T. sesame seeds
1 raw egg yolk
4 apple juice ice cubes

Blend all ingredients in blender except ice cubes. Slowly add juice cubes and blend well.

Celebrate with this when in the interval between the end of the fast and getting back to regular solid meals.

If you like a hot drink, there is a wide variety of delightful herbal teas available to suit your tastes. Mint teas are stimulating; chamomile relaxes; comfrey is healing. To better acquaint yourself with these teas and their medicinal value, see *Nothing New; Tried and True.*

PERFECTLY PLEASURABLE PARSNIP For "Coffee Lovers" — Minus the "Caffeine"

Grate 3 washed, unpeeled parsnips. Dry in oven turned to low. (Keep door slightly ajar to let moisture escape.) When dry, turn oven to 300° and roast until light-to-medium brown, about 8-10 minutes. Check oven often as they can easily burn.

To make drink: Pour boiling water over 1 T. of dried parsnips. Let steep for a few minutes. Strain into another cup. It tastes very mellow, sweet and delicious!

Store in covered glass container.

Variation: Add 1 t. honey and 1-2 t. carob powder for a mocha-like drink.

Experiment with grains and beans. Rye berries, wheat berries, garbanzo beans, chicory, barley and dried beetroot can all be roasted, (in 350-375° oven until dark brown), ground and percolated or steeped in boiling water. Amounts will vary from 1 t. per cup to 1 T. per cup, depending upon your taste and strength of the grain.

HEALTHSAVING HINTS

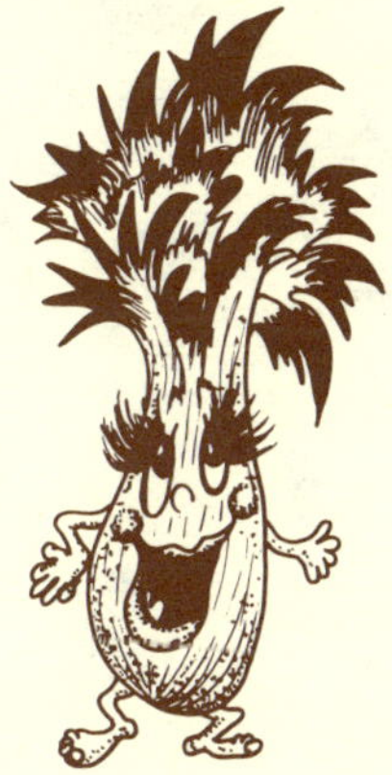

1. Dice cooked, but still firm yams or sweet potatoes and add to salads as a marshmallow substitute.
2. Make sure your children chew nuts and grains slowly and thoroughly for easier digestion and assimilation. Do not serve a chewy breakfast on a rushed morning.
3. When making waffles, sprinkle nuts or seeds over batter before closing lid. Toasty and crunchy!
4. Make lemon ice cubes. Mix 2 cups of water with ½ cup lemon juice. Pour into ice trays. Add a sliver of lemon peel to each cube. Keeps juice cold while adding zing! Can also be used to cool hot teas.
5. Twelve pounds of powdered grass contain more vitamins than 340 pounds of veggies and fruits — more veggies and fruits than the average person can eat in a year. So dry those leftover sprouts and wheat grass, and powder in a blender. Store in a cool cupboard.
6. For supplemental vitamin C, stir powdered ascorbic acid into citrus fruit juice. NEVER give children chewable vitamin C tablets to eat like candy. The highly acid nature may be harmful to teeth.
7. For any chilled party punches, pour some of the punch mixture in a ring mold. Arrange whole cranberries, lemon slices or mint. Freeze. Then unmold and float in punch bowl. OR float fresh orange, lime and lemon slices in punch bowl.
8. Try making your favorite jam or jelly with half as much honey as you used to use sugar. If fruit doesn't jell firmly enough, don't worry, you can still use as fabulous fruit syrup for pancakes and waffles.
9. Rose hips are among the highest natural sources of vitamin C. They are the part of the rose left when all the petals fall off. Make tea from the dried hips and jelly from the fresh or frozen puree. Gather in the fall; remove stalk and flower remnants and stew with water until tender. Then pack in jars and freeze. OR dry in dehydrator until brittle. Use in soups, fruit juices, salads, sauces, jams and teas.
10. To enhance the nutritional value of your favorite waldorf salad, prepare it according to your favorite recipe (omitting the dressing but making sure to include the apples, celery and walnuts); then add 1 cup sprouted sunflower seeds. For the dressing, gently stir one small can of crushed, drained pineapple into one cup plain yogurt. Toss with salad ingredients, top with freshly ground allspice and serve to the family for breakfast.

TIMESAVING HINTS

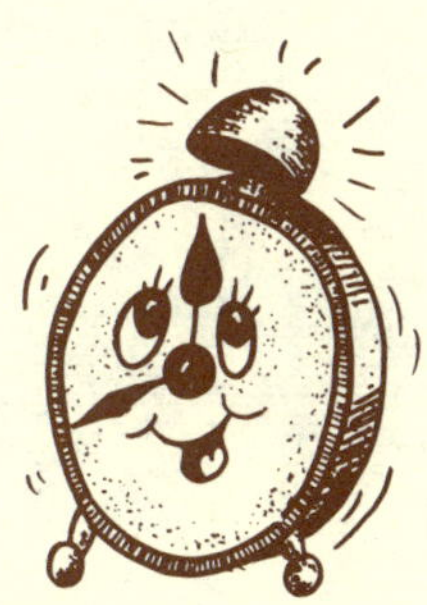

1. When you crack eggs for breakfast, reserve a little egg white in one shell to smooth on your face for a refreshing skin tightener before going out into the polluted atmosphere.
2. When cooking grains for dinner, cook double the required amount and save half for breakfast. For a special treat, press cooked grain into an oiled loaf pan and refrigerate overnight. The next morning slice, dust with flour, saute' and serve with hot maple syrup.
3. Watch for specials on any kind of fresh, ripe fruit and buy in quantity. Wash, peel, core, blend in blender and freeze puree in ice cube trays, OR simply freeze chunks of fruit on freezer trays and then bag when solid. If you think the proverbial hot cakes disappear fast, watch the frozen fruit vanish as your family falls in love with smoothies and shakes!
4. Freeze leftover pancakes or waffles in baggies. Remove from baggies and pop into toaster on a rushed morning for a quick breakfast.
5. Don't forget to make crock pot soups the night before for a hot breakfast on a cold winter morning.

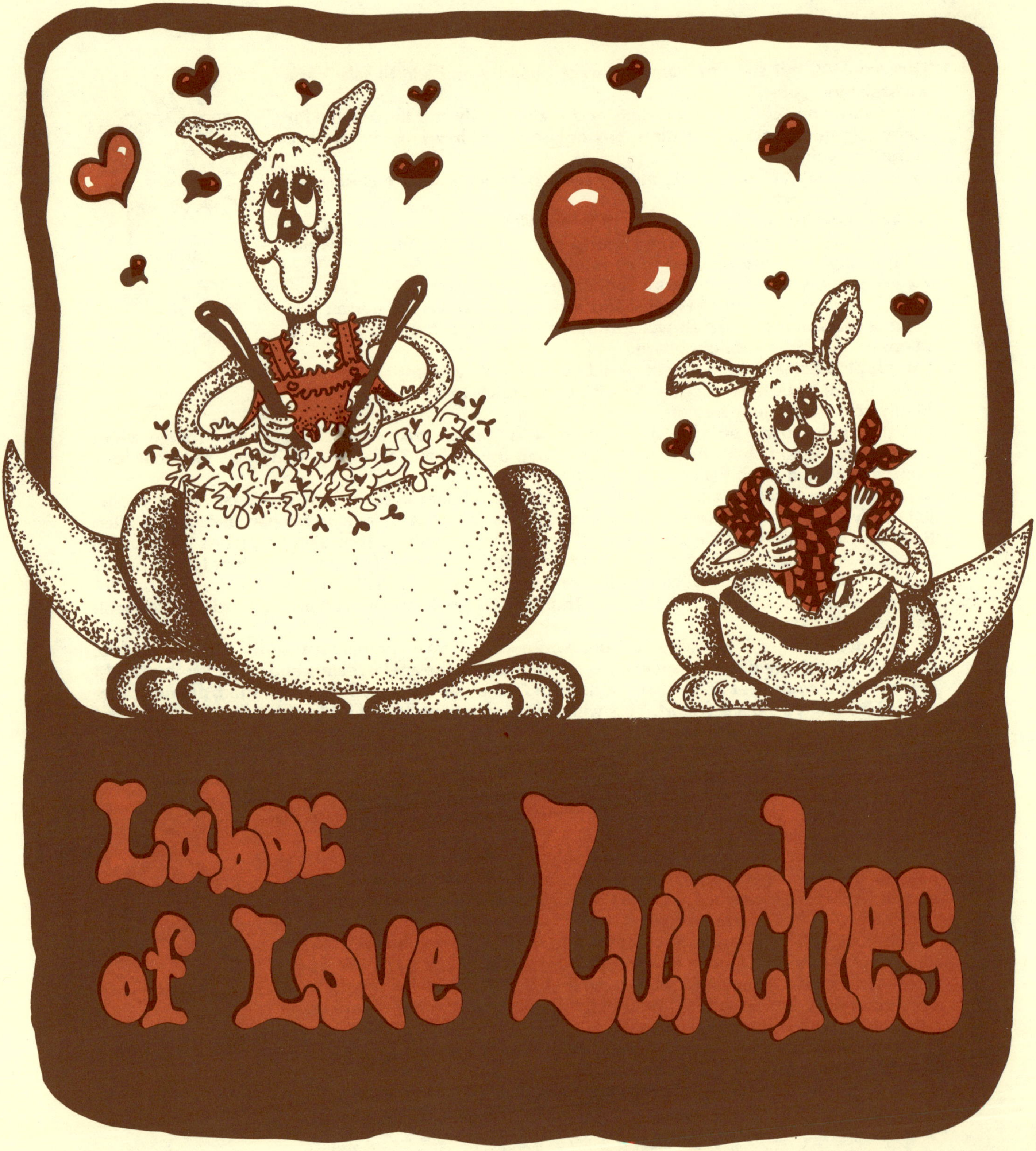

Labor of Love Lunches

Labor of Love Lunches

"We Love Your Body"

After our children exercised at the YMCA
In swimming, racquetball, gymnastics and free play,
There was nothing to eat; for all good intent
A quarter to buy a drink, was not a quarter well-spent.

For the vending machines and concession stand
Dispensed all the junk food that seemed to be in demand.
Kids, hot and thirsty, had no choice of what to eat.
All the things on the menu were either too salty or sweet.

We knew people came to build up muscles and strength.
To have a good shape, they'd go to nearly any length.
But to "reward" their exertions with cola or a candy bar
Just tore down all the good work they'd done so far.

We thought, "Let's provide them the correct building materials
All natural and down-to-earth, nothing ethereal.
We'll increase energy, endurance and prevent over-fatigue
By serving wholesome fast foods with real taste intrigue."

We knew that mixed nuts, fresh juice or a high protein shake
Would "add life" to their living — that's all it would take.
So . . . we bought the snack bar, "We Love Your Body" became its name,
Because we loved all the kids — thin or fat — just the same!

We scrubbed the kitchen, wrote menus; our kids painted signs
In hopes that when school was out we could open in time.
Our recipes were from home; our desire was sincere —
Love and a will to labor hard on this project so dear.

We wanted to offer the best choice for young bodies and minds.
About good nutrition, too many kids grow up blind.
But once they find that fast food can be healthy and fun,
They'll whip up their own delicious snacks — for on-the-run.

We pledged to serve only what is wholesome and best
For "real" nutritious food can pass any test.
If it looks colorful and enticing to the eyes
And tastes fantastic too, they'd have a pleasant surprise!

So when we first opened our little lunch shop
One look at our menu would have made your eyes pop.
Instead of "hot dogs," "gum," "candy" and "coke";
Ours read "felafels," "kefir" and "Please don't smoke."

For sandwiches we offered a variety of spreads,
"Choose your filling, then decide upon one of our breads.
There's whole wheat and rye and sunflower-millet;
Pita has a pocket — just slit it and fill it.

Chapatis; spread the filling and heap on the sprouts,
Then roll it or fold it; don't let anything drop out.
The prices are right, we hope you'll agree.
Our aim is to please — that's our cup of tea."

Aromatic homemade soups were in great demand,
At noon we would stand there with ladle in hand.
We'd say, "Hello, how are you; the soup is on."
And by five after twelve the soup pot was gone.

Fresh salads were prepared with tender loving care.
First, swing the greens in the pillowcase, high as we'd dare;
Then add grated veggies, tomatoes and cheese.
"How 'bout creamy-herb dressing?" "Yes, please."

The drinks were unusual and very nutritious
And all who tried them said, "They're incredulicious!
What did you add to give it such flavor?"
"Take three guesses — now sip and savor."

We'd always take time to tell how to make it,
"Add bananas, cinnamon, milk and then shake it.
Now go home and try your own winning combination.
We guarantee your family will love any variation."

Our juice was delivered fresh-pressed twice a week.
We became the place that health seekers seek.
We offered apple, orange and celery-beet-carrot.
Each passed the taste test on its own merit.

If someone had just come from an athletic event
And looked rather tired, their energy spent;
To their smoothies we'd add wheat germ and nutritional yeast,
Then they'd know they were having an energy feast.

Our new patrons asked them down at the Y
To get rid of all junk foods — give natural snacks a try.
So the candy bars, soda pop and chocolate ice cream
Were removed from the various vending machines.

They were soon filled with yogurt, nuts and sunflower seeds,
All containing vitamins and minerals the human body needs.
Then when "We Love Your Body" was closed for the night,
Kids could still refresh themselves with food, healthy and light.

As word got around, the lines just got longer
And people who waited went away feeling stronger.
In good food our customers had a strong belief.
There were doctors, lawyers, even an Indian chief.

We had a Principal, construction crews and electricians,
Secretaries, city planners and politicians.
From mothers with their toddlers and infants so new,
To bachelors, seniors and counter-culture folk too.

A newcomer might start to walk out the door
But one taste would convince him to come back for more.
And though we often were teased for our strong exclamations,
To each question we'd try to give good explanations.

Sometimes we were surrogate mother or wife
When we'd say, "Now if you want to improve your life,
Stay off the junk food"; "Try our yogurt with dates."
"Chew well"; "Eat slowly"; "Your work can wait."

They came as skeptics and left as believers,
The satisfaction they gave us — left US the receivers.
It felt good to be missionaries of health,
For when ill, to regain it, you'd spend all your wealth.

But our health hints were free; served with the meal,
Just part of our way of making customers feel
That somebody cares about spreading the news
That you CAN feel just as good as you choose!

Through cooking classes and lectures we tried to relate
All our knowledge and experience that helped us feel great.
And people responded; they wanted to know
Our "secret" ingredients and what made us glow!

We truthfully said, "With good diet, positive thinking and exercise,
You too can soon return that sparkle to your eyes.
Love your body; put Labor of Love not only in your lunches,
But in breakfasts, snacks, dinners and mid-morning brunches."

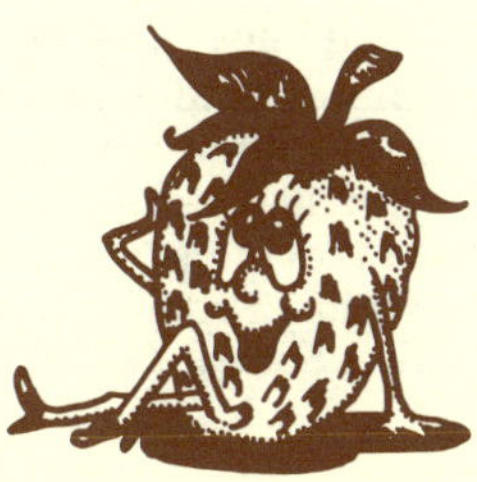

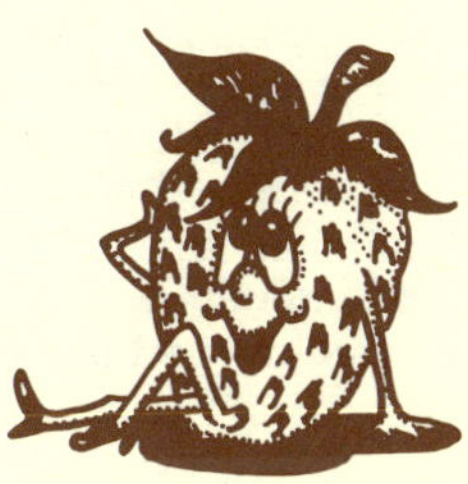

SANDWICH WRAPPERS AND OTHER BREADS

BASIC WHOLE GRAIN BREAD

2 T. dry yeast
2 cups warm water
¼ cup oil
1 scant T. salt
½ cup honey
2 eggs
6-6½ cups whole grain flour. (Use half whole wheat and half unbleached; ¾'s whole wheat and ¼ a mixture of any other whole grain flour, OR 100% whole wheat.)

Dissolve yeast in warm water. Add eggs, honey, oil, salt and 3 cups flour. Beat 3 minutes by mixer. Mix in 3 additional cups flour. Place on a floured board, cover hands with flour, and knead 10 minutes or until smooth and elastic. Place in a greased bowl and cover with a cloth. Let rise in a warm place until doubled. Punch dough down, divide into 2 balls, cover, and let rest for 5 minutes. Grease 2 bread pans. Roll out each ball and form loaves. Tuck under ends and place in loaf pans to double again. Bake in a 375° oven for 35 minutes. Remove from pans and cool. Brush tops with melted butter.

Variation: For sprouted wheat bread; decrease honey to ¼ cup; liquefy 1 cup wheat sprouts with 1½ cups water and ¼ cup oil. Then dissolve yeast in remaining half cup water. All other ingredients are same.

BANANA RICE-MILLET BREAD

5 T. butter
¼ cup honey
1 large egg
1 T. arrowroot
1 T. soy flour
1 T. minute tapioca
2½ t. baking powder
¼ t. salt
½-1 t. cinnamon
1 cup rice flour
1 cup blender-ground millet flour
3-4 mashed bananas
¼ cup buttermilk
5-6 chopped dates
¼ cup plus chopped nuts

Cream butter, honey and egg in large mixing bowl. Measure dry ingredients in a bowl and add to creamed mixture. Mix well. Beat in bananas, buttermilk, dates and nuts. Spoon into 2 greased loaf pans or 6 mini-loaf pans and bake at 350° for 50 minutes or until browned for large loaves and 25-35 minutes for small loaves. Tastes delicious and makes great gifts for teachers, friends, relatives. They freeze well too. When cool, place in plastic bags, squeeze out air, secure end.

CHAPATIS

2½ cups whole grain or whole wheat flour
½ t. salt
2 T. oil
¾ to 1 cup water

In a bowl, mix flour, salt, oil and water. Adjust water, adding a little at a time, to make a stiff dough. Let dough rest for an hour; then divide dough into 8 balls. Flatten each ball on floured surface and roll out until paper thin. Brown on lightly oiled cast iron skillet on both sides until lightly browned or brown spots begin to form. (See recipes for sandwich fillings or *KID STUFF* for Roll-Arounds.)

CREAM PUFFS

½ cup water
¼ cup safflower oil
½ cup whole wheat flour
½ t. salt
2 eggs
1½ T. sesame seeds

Mix water and oil in medium saucepan and bring to a boil. Stir in flour and salt all at once, beating until mixture forms a ball and leaves sides of pan. Remove from heat and cool about 2 minutes. Add eggs, 1 at a time, beating well after each. Continue to beat until no longer glossy. Stir in sesame seeds. Spoon batter in mounds, using about ¼ cup dough for each, set 3" apart on a well-greased cookie sheet. Bake at 400° for 10 minutes; reduce heat to 350° and continue baking for 20-25 minutes, until golden brown and crisp, with no beads of moisture on surface. Remove from oven and cool. Cut off tops and remove any uncooked batter from inside puffs. Spoon in any fruit-yogurt salad or Cucumber-Yogurt Filling. (See recipe this Chapter), and replace lids. Makes 6 cream puffs.

GREEN CRACKERS

1 T. honey
½ cup sunflower oil
1 cup vegetable or potato water
4 cups blender-ground oats
1 t. vegetable salt
1 T. sesame seeds
1 T. fresh parsley or 1 t. dried

Blend liquids, then add dry ingredients. Dough will be stiff. Roll into a log, chill well, then slice off thin rounds. Bake at 300° for 15-20 minutes. Excellent with cheese or a tossed green salad.

GRIDDLE ENGLISH MUFFINS

2 T. active dry yeast
1¾ cups very warm water
2 T. honey or molasses
2 t. vegetable salt
2½ cups whole wheat flour (increase each time you make these muffins)
2½ cups unbleached white flour (decrease until mixture is 100% whole wheat)
¼ cup each: non-instant dry milk powder, blender-ground oats, wheat germ and sunflower seed meal
½ c. cornmeal

Dissolve yeast and honey in water and let stand 5 minutes. Stir together dry ingredients, using only ½ of flours. Add yeast/water and beat for 5 minutes. Gradually add all but ¼ cup remaining flours and stir with a wooden spoon. turn dough onto floured board (use reserved flour) and knead 10 minutes. Form a ball; oil, place in bowl, cover with damp cloth and let rise about 1 and ½ hours in warm place. Punch down and roll out dough to ½" thickness on a board sprinkled with ½ of cornmeal. Using a tuna can, cut dough in rounds. Place muffins, cornmeal side up on baking sheet sprinkled with remaining cornmeal. Cover with damp cloth and allow to rise 1 hour in warm place. Heat electric griddle or cast iron skillet to 300°, oil surface and toast muffins until golden, about 10 minutes. Turn *very* carefully and brown other side. Cut a muffin in center to test for doneness. If more cooking time is required, place in a 300° oven for 10 minutes or until done. Cool, split muffins and refrigerate or freeze. Makes a baker's dozen. Keep plenty in freezer. Use for Eggs Benedict, individual pizzas, etc.

WHOLE WHEAT PRETZELS

1 T. active dry yeast
1 T. honey
1¼ cups very warm water
4 cups whole wheat flour OR 2 cups wh/wheat and 2 cups unbleached white
1 cup sesame seeds

Dissolve yeast and honey in water and set aside for 5 minutes. Combine flour and salt in large bowl and mix in yeast/water. Dough should be stiff. Knead 5 minutes, form into a ball, coat with oil, cover with a damp towel and let rise about 2 hours. Spread sesame seeds evenly on a cookie sheet. Gently pinch off a handful of dough and roll between palms until a rope is formed, 15" long and ½" in diameter. Oil hands and ropes and gently press and roll in sesame seeds until well coated. Shape into pretzel knots and arrange on oiled cookie sheet, with enough space around each to double in size. Let rise in a warm place about 1½ hours. Bake at 350° for 15-20 minutes. Break one to test for doneness. Enjoy warm with butter or cheese or cool and refrigerate and re-crisp in oven for later use. Makes 16-18 pretzels.

MAPLE-NUT ROLLS

1 T. yeast
½ cup warm potato water
1½ cups potato water
½ cup honey
2½ cups whole wheat flour
¾ cup raisins
1½ t. salt
1/3 cup sunflower oil
2½ to 3 cups flour
melted butter
3 T. maple syrup
2 T. cinnamon
½ cup chopped walnuts

In a large mixing bowl, dissolve yeast in ½ cup warm potato water; then add rest of potato water. Dissolve honey in this mixture, then add 2½ cups whole wheat flour and beat with a wooden spoon until smooth. Mix in raisins; cover and set in a warm place to rise for 30-45 minutes until light and foamy. Mix in salt, oil and about 2½-3 cups flour until dough comes away from sides of bowl. Dough will be slightly sticky, but easy to handle. Knead for 15 minutes; then roll out into a 12"x12" square. Brush with melted butter; spread with maple syrup; sprinkle with cinnamon and walnuts. Roll up entire square into long roll. Slice into 1" slices; set on oiled cookie sheet or in square pan to rise until doubled in bulk, about 1 hour. Preheat oven to 350° and bake for 20-25 minutes. Makes about 1 dozen rolls.

NICE TWICE RICE BREAD

2 eggs, separated
1 cup milk, yogurt or buttermilk
2 T. oil
1 T. honey
2 cups Mama Bear's Porridge (dry)
2 t. baking powder
¼ t. salt

Mix egg yolks, milk, oil and honey in a bowl. Sift dry ingredients into bowl. Blend until smooth. Whip egg whites until stiff and fold into mixture. Pour into a well-greased bread pan. Bake at 350° for 40-45 minutes. Makes good toast.

PITA BREAD

1 T. yeast
1 1/3 cups warm water
1 T. oil
1 t. salt
¼ t. honey
1½ cups whole wheat flour
1½ to 2 cups whole wheat flour (or use unbleached flour)
sesame seeds

Dissolve yeast in warm water. Add oil, salt, honey and 1½ cups flour. Beat until smooth. Gradually add additional flour. Knead until firm and smooth, but not stiff (approximately 10 minutes). Return the dough to its bowl, brush top with oil, and let rise for 1 hour. Divide into 6 pieces; shape each in a ball and let rest 10 minutes. On a floured board sprinkled with sesame seeds, roll each ball into a 6½″ circle, about ¼″ thick. Place on ungreased cookie sheet which has been sprinkled lightly with cornmeal. Let rise 30 minutes. Bake in a preheated 450° oven on lowest rack for 5-10 minutes, depending on thickness, until breads puff up and start to brown. The heat of the oven will make the moisture in the pita explode into steam. *As soon as you remove from oven,* slit the bread along one side of the rim and split open, or cut in half and split open. Cover, to keep moist, until stuffed with a filling. To store, place in plastic bags, seal, and freeze or refrigerate for later use. Reheat in oven before using.

LANI'S MUSHROOM HERB HEALTH BREAD

3 T. yeast
¾ cup warm water
7½ cups hot water
10 cups whole wheat flour
4½ t. diastatic malt (see below)
1 cup sunflower oil
2½ T. sea salt
1 cup flaked bran
2 T. brewer's yeast
1 cup soy flour
½ cup powdered milk
½ cup wheat germ
1 T. lecithin granules
½ cup whole millet
5-6 cups whole wheat flour
3 T. mixed, crushed, dried herbs: thyme, basil, rosemary, oregano, sage, savory

Soak yeast in warm water. In a large bowl or bread mixer, place 7½ cups hot water and 10 cups of whole wheat flour. Mix well. Then add malt, oil and salt. Mix again and add yeast/water, flaked bran, soy flour, powdered milk, wheat germ, lecithin, millet, flour and herbs. Mix 10 minutes in dough mixer or as long as necessary to have a smooth, elastic dough. Let rest/rise in bowl for 10 minutes or so. Then divide dough into 6 pieces. Take each piece, flatten into a thick rectangle with a rolling pin, then carefully fold and roll from short end so that you have a fat cylinder. Be sure you don't have any air pockets. Alternate Way: Take each piece and form into a smooth circle. Place each loaf in a well-greased (use shortening) 46 oz. juice can. Loaf will barely reach mid-way to top of can. Cover with towel and let rise in warm place until doubled. Dough will rise to top of can; when baked, will rise above can to form mushroom cap. Bake on lowest rack in preheated oven (upright) at 400° for 10 minutes; then at 375° for 30-35 minutes. Remove from cans immediately and let cool on racks. Brush tops of each mushroom with oil for glossy appearance. Then give to friends, or freeze in plastic bags until needed. Your kids will love this bread as it slices round for a different sandwich shape and there are *no crusts!*

DIASTATIC MALT

This malt can be used in place of honey in many bread recipes. It gets the action of the yeast going and adds sweetness to bread. (1 T. malt = 2/3 cup honey.) Soak 1 cup wheatberries overnight in 1 quart of water. In the morning, drain and rinse and drain again. Rinse 3 times a day for 2-3 days. On the third or fourth day, spread them evenly and thinly on cookie sheets and place in a warm, dry place to dry; room temperature is okay — nothing over 110°. When thoroughly dry (may take 3 days), place a small amount at a time in blender and blend to a fine powder. Store in airtight container in refrigerator or cool place.

SUPER DUPER REFRIGERATOR BISCUITS

This is a most versatile refrigerator biscuit dough. It can be prepared ahead of time, refrigerated, then the children can slice off what they need to prepare their own pizza snacks or Fruit Walk-Aways. It can also be frozen until needed. Keep some always on hand.

2¼ cups whole wheat pastry flour
1 T. baking powder
½ t. baking soda
1 scant t. salt
4 T. instant powdered milk
½ cup sunflower oil
2 T. honey
2/3 cup milk

In a large bowl, mix together dry ingredients. In a smaller bowl, mix together liquids, then add all at once to dry ingredients and stir well with a fork and/or wooden spoon. With oiled hands, form dough into a long roll, about 2"-2½" in diameter. Wrap well in wax paper and foil and refrigerate. When ready to bake, using a sharp knife, slice into ¾"-1" slices and place a few inches apart on oiled cookie sheet. Brush tops with oil and bake in a preheated 400° oven for 10-15 minutes or until browned. These biscuits are very light and taste delicious hot with butter and honey or homemade jam.

PIZZA

Prepare Super Duper Refrigerator Biscuit dough. Roll out in an oiled pizza pan. Add toppings and bake at 400°-425° for 12-18 minutes. (See *Serendipity Suppers.)*

INDIVIDUAL PIZZAS

Prepare dough as stated above. Slice with a sharp knife into ½"-¾" slices. (Size depends on whether you like a thinner or thicker crust.) Place up to 6 rounds of dough on a *large* oiled cookie sheet. Using an oiled glass, roll out each round to a 4"-6" flat circle. Spoon Easy Pizza Sauce onto each pizza. Top with chopped onions, green pepper, mushrooms and black olives. Sprinkle grated Swiss, Cheddar, Jack or Parmesan cheese over all and bake at 400° for 8-10 minutes.

VEGETABLE POT PIES

Prepare dough as stated above, omitting baking powder if you don't want the crust to expand. Use for bottom and top crusts of large or small pies.

FRUIT WALK-AWAYS

Prepare dough as for individual pizzas, rolling out rounds into 6" circles. Add 1 T. fruit mixture; fold over dough like a turn-over and pinch ends. Bake at 400° until browned. (See *KID STUFF* for filling ideas.)

SNAPPY — QUICK MIX

Measure first 5 ingredients in a large bowl, then sift to distribute baking powder evenly:

5½ cups whole wheat pastry flour
1½ cups soy flour
2/3 cup non-instant powdered milk
(¾ cup instant)
4 T. baking powder
1 T. sea salt
1 cup wheat germ

Add and stir in wheat germ. Store in covered jars in refrigerator or freezer. To use in your favorite recipes, substitute mix for flour, omitting the salt and baking powder or soda. Mix spices into dry mix before adding liquids.

COBBLER TOPPING

Measure 2 cups Snappy-Quick Mix into large bowl. Make a well in center and add ½ cup milk, buttermilk or yogurt, 1 egg, ¼ cup honey and 1 T. oil. Stir just until batter is moistened, batter should be lumpy. Drop like dumplings onto very hot fruit mixture and continue baking 15-20 minutes or until golden brown.

SHORTCAKE

Prepare just as for cobbler topping except use 2 2/3 cups Snappy-Quick Mix and stir thoroughly. Roll out on floured board ½" thick and cut rounds with a tuna can. Bake on an oiled cookie sheet at 350° for 25 minutes or until done. Serve with fresh berries and whipped cream or yogurt or kefir. Or shape like Ladyfingers before cooking and use to accompany a fruit compote.

PANCAKES

Measure 1½ cups Snappy-Quick Mix in large bowl. Make a well in center and add 1 cup milk, buttermilk or yogurt, 1 or 2 eggs and 2 T. *each* honey and oil. Pour on hot oiled griddle.

WAFFLES

Measure 2 cups Snappy-Quick Mix. Make a well in center and add 1 cup milk, buttermilk or yogurt, 3 T. oil and 3 egg yolks. Whip egg whites until stiff and carefully fold into batter. Pour in center of hot, oiled waffle iron and cook until steam ceases to escape.

DATE-NUT BREAD

Measure 3 cups Snappy-Quick Mix in large bowl with 1 cup chopped walnuts and ½ cup chopped dates. Mix 1 cup milk or kefir, 1 egg and ½ cup *each* honey and oil. Bake at 350° for 1 hour in a greased loaf pan.

CURRY CUPS

1. Crumble 6 large, shredded wheat biscuits into a large bowl with 1 cup shredded coconut, ½ cup finely chopped peanuts and ¼ cup blender-ground sunflower seeds.

2. Melt ½ cup butter, then stir in 2 T. honey and ½ t. curry powder. Drizzle over dry ingredients and mix well. Then press into well-buttered muffin cups to form nests and bake in a 275° oven for 10-12 minutes or until lightly browned. Cool slightly, then remove carefully.

3. Spoon steamed rice into cups. Spoon gravy over rice and proceed with the garnishes indicated in Make-Ahead Curry *(Serendipity Suppers).* Makes 12 muffin cups or 6 large custard cups.

COMPLEMENTARY PROTEIN CUPS

These wheat-seed-egg-cheese cups will complement any bean-grain dish with high quality protein to form a complete protein dish. They taste delicious and are as versatile in a meal as your imagination.

1. In a large bowl, crumble 6 large, shredded wheat biscuits. Add ½ cup blender-ground sesame seeds and 1 cup blender-ground sunflower seeds. Stir in ¼ cup grated Parmesan cheese.

2. In a saucepan, melt ½ cup butter. Stir in 1 T. plus 1 t. tamari-soy sauce and ½ t. garlic powder. Drizzle over dry mixture and stir well. Beat 2 eggs in a small dish and stir into dry mixture. Press into well-oiled muffin cups or large custard cups to form nests. Bake at 300° for 15 minutes or until browned. Makes 12 muffin-sized nests or 6 large nests.

3. Spoon any of the following prepared fillings into baked nests, then heat in 350° oven until hot: Stan's Stuffed Zucchini, Millet Stuffed Green Peppers, Sunflower Cabbage Rolls, Summertime Squash, Frijoles Refritos, Mexican Beans and Rice (all from *Serendipity Suppers),* Split Pea Soup, Chili Bean Soup *(Labor of Love Lunches),* Sloppy Joses or Heidi's Mashed Po-Lentil Pie *(KID STUFF).*

4. OR fill baked nests with mashed potatoes and sprinkle with grated Cheddar cheese and a pat of butter. Heat in oven until melted, then dollop with sour cream and garnish with chopped chives and TVP bacon bits.

5. OR melt 2-3 T. grated cheese in baked cups in oven. When cheese is melty, serve nests as a cracker accompaniment with soup or add any of above fillings to grated cheese nests and heat.

6. Prepare a souffle and spoon into pre-baked cups and bake at 350° until set.

SANDWICH FILLINGS AND SPREADS

Bean

CRUNCHY TOASTY SPREAD

Mix 1 cup cooked, green split peas, 2 T. mayonnaise, ¾ to 1 cup toasted sunflower seeds, and salt and cayenne to taste. Spread on your choice of sandwich wrapper; add sprouts and tomato slices OR grated carrots and chopped cucumbers.

Variation: For a dip, add additional mayonnaise and a little yogurt.

YELLOW SPLIT PEA SPREAD

Cook 1 cup yellow split peas in 2½ to 3 cups water about 35 minutes. Drain any excess water and save for soups. Refrigerate overnight. In morning, place in large bowl. Mash with fork; add mayonnaise, ½ chopped dill pickle, 1 T. dried, minced onion, 1 dash garlic powder, sea salt/kelp to taste, 2 T. toasted sun seeds, and 2 T. each grated carrot and finely chopped celery.

Variation: Add 2 T. chopped olives.

MOCK TUNA SPREAD

Grind 2 to 3 cups of cooked soybeans through a meat grinder. Add mayonnaise, grated carrot, chopped celery, minced onion, chopped pickle to taste, finely ground cashews or almonds (about ¼ cup), and 1 T. of tamari-soy sauce. Delicious! Looks like tuna or crab.

BEAN-NUT BUTTER

Mash some cooked soybeans with a fork. Add a little peanut butter, mayonnaise and cottage cheese until like tuna consistency. Then add finely chopped celery, dill pickles, minced onion, and chopped sun sprouts. Spread on bread, place thin cucumber slices on spread; then thin slices of Jack cheese. Top with thin tomato slices and alfalfa sprouts. Season all with sea salt/kelp.

Cheese and Egg

JACK OR CHEDDAR

Grate and mix with mayonnaise. For variety add chopped nuts, chopped onion, chopped olives, OR crushed pineapple.

SWISS

Mix ½ pound grated Swiss cheese, 2 hard-cooked eggs, diced, ½ cup chopped almonds, and 1/3 cup mayonnaise.

COTTAGE

Mix cottage cheese with diced cucumber, tomatoes, green pepper, green onion, and/or avocado.

CREAM

Add dates and walnut pieces to cream or Neufchatel cheese and a dash or two of cinnamon.
Variation: Substitute raisins and chopped almonds.

EGG SALAD

Chop hard-cooked eggs and mix with mayonnaise. Add one or a combination of: onion, celery, raisins, green pepper, bean sprouts, grated carrot, chopped raw spinach, grated cheese, black olives, sun seed sprouts, mashed lentil loaf.

EGG LENTIL

Dice 3 hard-cooked eggs; add to 1 cup mashed, cooked lentils, ¼ cup cottage cheese and 1 T. minced onion. Add seasonings to taste.

Peanut Butter

PEACH LOVER'S DELIGHT

Spread peanut butter on bread of your choice. Slice fresh peaches on top.
Variation: Sliced nectarines, green grapes or fresh strawberries.

MONKEY MASH

Mash ½ cup peanut butter, 1 large ripe banana, ½ t. cinnamon, a handful of raisins OR dates, and 1 to 2 t. shredded coconut.

SUN SPROUTS WITH PB

Mix peanut butter, a little cottage cheese and some sunflower seed sprouts.
Variation: Layer above ingredients.

PB AND OJ

Spread crunchy peanut butter mixed with raisins and a little frozen orange juice concentrate on whole grain bread.

CARROT AND RAISIN

Mix peanut butter with a little mayonnaise and some grated carrot and raisins.

ALFEE PB

Heap alfalfa sprouts on a peanut butter sandwich. It's a great way to introduce sprouts to kids. If you start with just a few, they will add crunch, and taste delicious with the peanut butter!

NUT BUTTER SUPREME

1. Spread Tahini (sesame seed butter), almond, peanut OR cashew butter on your choice of bread.
2. Add apple chunks, banana rounds, peach slices, grapes, OR chopped dates.
3. Sprinkle with cinnamon OR nutmeg.
4. Cover with ricotta, cottage cheese OR grated Jack.
5. Drizzle with honey OR maple syrup.
6. Top with sunflower seeds, pumpkin seeds, OR chopped raw nuts.

PEANUT BUTTER-CARROT LOAF SPREAD

Mix 2½ to 3 cups finely grated carrots, ¾ cup peanut butter, 1 12 oz. can tomato paste, 1 T. honey, 1 to 2 T. tamari-soy sauce, 1 scant cup water, 1 to 2 t. sea salt/kelp, 1 t. basil, 1 t. garlic powder, 1 t. onion powder, 3 pieces of blender-ground toast. Place into an oiled loaf pan and bake, covered, at 350° F. for 40 minutes. Let cool. Slice thin and use in sandwiches. Tastes great hot too.

Tofu

TOFU PEANUT BUTTER

In a blender, puree 12 oz. tofu, ½ cup peanut butter, 1 and ½ bananas, 2 T. lemon juice and 2 to 3 T. honey. Serve as is on whole grain bread or top with nuts, raisins and thinly sliced bananas.

Variation: Freeze until firm; blend again, refreeze and serve as a sherbet.

SPROUTS AND TOFU

In blender, blend ½ cup hulled mixed sprouts, 1 t. lemon juice, ½ t. vegetable salt and 3 to 4 T. tofu. Puree and spread on bread. top with avocado slices, alfalfa sprouts and 2 dashes or cayenne.

Other

Nearly any lentil, bean, rice and/or nut loaf, when cold, can be sliced or mashed and spread on any bread with a little mayonnaise, catsup, and salad garnishes.

ROLL-AROUNDS

Spread a chapati with either mayonnaise or cream cheese. Spoon on any bean, vegetable, or fruit "salad" filling and roll up like a burrito.

FOR THE LOVE OF YOUR LIFE

Spread a whole grain chapati with Herb-Yogurt Dressing. Then spread Guacamole all over it. Now heap one side with alfalfa sprouts. Sprinkle a grated carrot-radish-zucchini mixture over sprouts. Lay 3 thin tomato slices on top. Dollop with more dressing and fold the chapati in half.

MOROCCO TACO (or FELAFELS)

Felafel Mixture: In a blender, mash 6 cups cooked garbanzo beans, the juice from 2 lemons, 1 cut-up onion, 3 to 4 garlic cloves, 1 bunch chopped parsley. Mash a little at a time. Use some bean liquid if necessary and blend until mushy. Transfer to a large bowl. Add dashes of garlic powder, about 1 or 2 t. salt, 1 to 2 T. cumin and 1 to 2 T. chili powder. Mix well, shape into patties; dip in bread crumbs and saute lightly in a buttered skillet. Spread one-half a pita bread with Herb-Yogurt Dressing on both sides of the pocket. Insert 3 or 4 felafel patties. Add finely chopped tomatoes and cucumbers, sprouts, and dollop with a Thousand Island Dressing.

OPEN-FACED ZUCCHINI

Slice zucchinis in half lengthwise. Spread mayonnaise on top of each slice, then Guacamole. Sprinkle with grated Cheddar cheese. Top with small tomato chunks and alfalfa sprouts.

Variation: Slightly hollow zucchini boats to accommodate more filling. Use pulp for a salad, or casserole.

CUCUMBER-YOGURT FILLING

Sprinkle 1 cup chopped cucumbers with salt and leave standing for 5 minutes. Drain well. Mix cucumbers with 2 cups plain yogurt, ½ cup broken walnuts, 2 thinly sliced green onions, and a dash of cayenne. *Chill.* Add some fresh, chopped mung bean sprouts. Spoon into Cream Puffs. (See recipe this Chapter), allowing about 1/3 cup filling per puff. Replace lid of puff.

Sandwich Garnishes

VEGETABLE

Anything that goes in a salad can be heaped on an open-faced sandwich or arranged on the plate to add color to Roll-Arounds and regular sandwiches.

FRUIT

Nut, spices, honey or syrup, sun sprouts, yogurt or cream cheese, toasted seeds.

HEARTY HOMEMADE SOUPS

VEGETABLE SOUP STOCK

Save everything but the kitchen sink for savory stock: potato peelings, carrot tops, celery leaves, wilted celery stalks, leaves of cauliflower and hard green stems from broccoli, wilted greens of any kind. Keep covered in containers or plastic bags and use weekly. Place in a large pot of water, add 1 or 2 onions, a parsnip or turnip, and 1 or 2 carrots. Simmer, covered, about 1 hour.

After cooking, strain and reserve liquid. The nutrients and flavor are in the water. Optional: Blend the onions and carrots in a blender and put back into the stock for a thicker consistency.

Add herbs. A good herb mixture for tasty stock is: 2 parts each of basil, celery seed (ground), chervil, marjoram, and parsley to 1 part each dried lemon balm, rosemary, summer savory, and thyme.

Once the soup base is prepared to your taste and texture, it can be served the following ways: a. as a clear broth (everything is strained out). b. as a stock to which you add cooked noodles, rice, beans, barley, etc. c. as a base for a thicker soup to which sauteed veggies, thickeners and other seasonings will be added. d. freeze and save for a leftover vegetable or bean soup.

BASIC METHOD OF SOUP FROM SCRATCH

1. Saute herbs in a wok or cast iron skillet in SunButterBlend with minced garlic and chopped onion. See below for tasty herb combinations.
2. Saute cubed veggies: carrots, celery, potatoes, turnips, squash, yams, parsnips, Jerasalem artichokes, green pepper, etc.
3. If adding a grain such as rice, bulgur, millet or barley, prepare in 1 of 2 ways: 1. Stir-fry in butter and tamari-soy sauce until it pops or lightly browns; then add liquid, cover, and steam until done, and add to soup pot. OR 2. Add steamed grains to soup pot.
4. Add the sauteed veggies to the soup stock in 1 of 2 ways: 1. Blend ½ of the sauteed veggies (mostly potatoes) in a blender until fairly smooth; add with remainder of veggies to soup stock for a creamy, thick and chunky soup. OR 2. Add all of the sauteed veggies to the soup stock for a thinner broth.
5. **Variation:** Disregard all of the above instructions and cook everything together in 1 large soup pot of water or stock: herbs, seasonings, vegetables, grains, beans.

Tasty Herb Mixtures For Soups

FOR A MEATY-TASTING SOUP: In a skillet with SunButterBlend, saute these herbs: 2 parts oregano, 1 part cumin, ½ part mustard powder, ½ part caraway, and some chopped onion, or dried, minced onion.

FOR TOMATO-BASED SOUP: Saute in SunButterBlend, dashes of crushed basil, bay leaf, marjoram, oregano, and thyme.

FOR BEAN AND VEGETABLE SOUP: Saute in SunButterBlend, dashes of basil, bay leaf, curry, rosemary, sage, tarragon, thyme, cumin, chili powder.

Flavor Enhancers For Vegetarian Soups

Miso (soybean paste), tamari-soy sauce, Bakon Yeast (a hickory-smoked yeast), AminoTone (similar to Kitchen Bouquet), vegetarian boullion cubes OR vegetable stock, lemon juice, wine OR vinegar, added during the last few minutes of cooking.

Garnishes

1. Fresh, ground black pepper — added just before serving.
2. A dollop of yogurt or sour cream — stirred into soup at the last minute.
3. Whole grain, herb-buttered croutons, or popcorn — mixed with garlic butter and Parmesan cheese.
4. Chopped fresh parsley or other fresh herbs — added just before serving.

5. A couple Tablespoons of butter — stirred into soup just before serving for richness and flavor.
6. Whole toasted sesame seeds, chopped nuts, or Gomazio — sprinkled lightly.
7. Sunflower seed sprouts, mixed sprouts or alfalfa sprouts — added for nutrition.
8. A thin slice of cheese placed in bottom of bowl, or grated cheese sprinkled on top — for flavor and protein.

CREAMY MUSHROOM SOUP

3 T. SunButterBlend
½ pound coarsely chopped mushrooms
1 large, coarsely chopped onion
2 T. whole wheat pastry flour
1 T. Bakon yeast (opt.)
4 cups milk

In a 3 quart saucepan, melt SunButterBlend over medium heat. Add mushrooms and onion and saute, stirring until onions are limp and juices evaporated. Stir in flour and yeast. Remove from heat. Stir in milk. Whirl soup, a little at a time, in a blender until smooth. Season to taste. Heat, but *do not boil.*

Variation: Replace 2 cups milk with 2 cups vegetable water.

OLD-FASHIONED HARVEST TOMATO SOUP

1 large, chopped onion
2 T. SunButterBlend
3 T. whole wheat pastry flour
1 t. sea salt/kelp
3-4 cups chopped tomatoes (skin if desired)
3 cups milk
1 t. honey

Saute onion in SunButterBlend until transparent. Sprinkle with whole wheat pastry flour and stir until a smooth paste forms on onions. Add salt and tomatoes. Mash down with a potato masher and cook, stirring constantly, until thickened. In a separate pan, heat milk and stir in honey. Then, gradually add tomato mixture to the hot milk, stirring constantly to prevent curdling. Keep hot, but *do not boil.* Serve with herb and cheese breadsticks or Parmesan-coated popcorn.

Variation: Add 1 cup cooked brown rice, millet, barley or bulgur and 1 t. tamari-soy sauce. Make a double batch and freeze half.

BEST VEGETABLE SOUP EVER

8 cups water or stock
1-1½ cups dried lentils
½ cup dried pearl barley
SunButterBlend
1½ t. celery seed
2 t. Italian Herb Mix
(See *Serendipity Suppers*)
½ large, chopped onion
3 crushed garlic cloves
3 chopped carrots
4 chopped potatoes
1 chopped celery stalk
1 small can tomato sauce or paste
1-3 t. sea salt/kelp
½-1 t. chili powder
dashes cayenne

Bring water or stock to boil in a large pot. Add lentils and barley, cover and simmer. Meanwhile, saute celery seed, Italian Herb Mix, onion and garlic in SunButterBlend and add to soup pot. Then, in same pan, saute carrots, potatoes and celery, adding more butter if necessary. When lentils and barley are tender, add veggie mix to soup pot. In a blender, place tomato sauce or paste and 1/3 blender full of vegetables and broth (mostly carrots and potatoes), and blend until smooth. Repeat: 1/3 blender full of some veggies and liquid and blend. Return to pot. Rinse blender in a little liquid and add to pot. Add salt, chili powder and cayenne. Very flavorful and spicy.

CREAM OF LENTIL SOUP

1½ cups dried, rinsed lentils
4 cups water
1 medium, chopped onion
1 chopped celery stalk
½-¾ cup instant powdered milk
1 t. sea salt/kelp
1 T. olive oil

Simmer lentils, onions and celery in water for 30-40 minutes. Place in blender and liquefy. Add some water if necessary and powdered milk, and blend again. Season, heat and serve in bowls topped with grated Jack cheese and alfalfa sprouts. Serve with Green Crackers. (See recipe this Chapter)

Variation: Add 1-2 minced garlic cloves.

THICK ROOT SOUP

8 cups boiling water
4 potatoes
2 turnips
1 rutabaga
3 celery stalks
4 carrots
1 onion
1-2 garlic cloves
¼ cup fresh, chopped parsley
large pinch marjoram and basil
1 T. tamari-soy sauce
1 t. Bakon yeast (opt.)
3 t. vegetable salt
up to ½ cup powdered milk

To 8 cups boiling water, add first 5 ingredients, all coarsely chopped. Simmer, 1 hour or more until tender. Chop onion, and garlic and saute in butter, along with herbs and seasonings. Add to soup pot. When veggies are tender, blend, little by little, in blender until liquefied, adding soup broth if necessary. Add ½ cup total of powdered milk. Reheat until hot and smooth. Serve. Soup should be thick and creamy and a mellow yellow-orange. Goes well with whole grain crackers and cheese and a fresh green salad.

"WE LOVE YOUR BODY" CREAM OF SPLIT PEA SOUP

2½-3 cups dried split peas
1 chopped onion
1 chopped carrot
1 chopped celery stalk
1 minced garlic clove
6-7 cups boiling water
¼ c. melted butter with 2 t. Bakon yeast (opt.)
2 t. sea salt/kelp
1½ t. basil
1 t. sage
cayenne, pepper or garlic powder to taste
1 finely grated, raw potato
2 T. fresh, chopped parsley
½ cup instant powdered milk

Simmer first 5 ingredients in water. When tender, add seasonings and butter. Place half of mixture in blender and add potato and powdered milk. Blend until smooth. Do the same with remaining mixture.

Variation: Substitute 2-3 cups whole milk for powdered milk and use less water when cooking split peas. Serve hot with croutons and shredded cheese, hot, herb-buttered bread, OR make soup with less liquid and spoon over buttered rice or toast.

BEST CHILI BEAN SOUP

1 cup dried lentils
2 cups dried red beans and pintos (mixed)
6 cups boiling water
1½ t. crushed basil
1½ t. crushed celery seed
1 chopped carrot
1 chopped garlic clove
1 chopped onion
SunButterBlend
1 can V-8 juice (6 oz.)
1 small can diced green chiles
2 small cans tomato paste
½ t. each of garlic powder and onion powder
2 t. cumin
2½ t. chili powder
1-2 t. sea salt/kelp
dash cayenne

Set crockpot at low and add legumes, boiling water, basil and celery seed. After 8-10 hours, or when nearly tender, add carrot, garlic, onion (all of which have been sauteed in SunButterBlend). Stir in V-8 juice, chiles, tomato paste, and seasonings, adding more water if necessary. Heat until beans are tender and seasonings are blended. Before serving, add 1½ T. butter. Serve with cornbread.

SENSATIONAL SALADS

Vegetable Salads

SUPER SPROUT SALAD

In any amounts, mix chopped buckwheat lettuce, sunflower greens, sunflower seed sprouts, alfalfa sprouts, a handful of mixed sprouts (garbanzo, adzuki, lentil, mung, soy), chopped green onion, grated carrot, diced celery, diced cucumber, chopped avocado and mushrooms. Toss with your favorite dressing or a lemon juice and oil dressing and garnish with tomato wedges. Sprinkle kelp and cayenne over all.

UNFORGETTABLE FRESH SPINACH SALAD

1 lb. fresh spinach
¼ lb. fresh mushrooms
4 hard-cooked eggs
Bleu Cheese Dressing
soy bacon bits (without MSG)
Bakon yeast (opt.)
green onions or chives
toasted sunflower seeds

Wash spinach, whirl in pillowcase and tear. Clean mushrooms and slice. Finely chop eggs. Divide spinach into 6 individual salad bowls. Top with mushrooms, then chopped egg. Drizzle each with about 2 T. Bleu Cheese Dressing and sprinkle with bacon bits, sun seeds and sliced green onions or chives.

BUCKWHEAT LETTUCE

To grow pesticide-free buckwheat lettuce indoors, year-round: Soak 1½ cups unhulled buckwheat overnight in a large jar with 3 cups water. In morning, pour off water into a bowl and save. Spread seeds on a tray of soil (3 parts organic soil to 1 part peat moss) and pour soak water over all until soil is nice and moist. Cover with a sheet of plastic until light and air-tight and put away for 3 days. Then uncover and place in light. Water as needed until leaves appear and hulls begin to fall off, about 10-15 days total. With scissors, clip lettuce near base just before using in a salad; rinse in colander and remove any hulls. (Buckwheat is high in rutin — a member of the vitamin C family).

Stuffed Salads

LENTIL STUFFED TOMATOES

2 cups cooked lentils
1 cup mung bean sprouts
1 small, chopped onion
1 cup chopped celery
4 T. oil
3 T. tamari-soy sauce
1 T. molasses (opt.)
¼ cup cider vinegar
¼ t. sea salt/kelp
a few dashes cayenne
6 large, ripe tomatoes
grated carrots

Combine all ingredients except tomatoes and carrots and refrigerate. Cut core from tomatoes and drain. Cut each tomato, not quite all the way through, to form a 6-wedge star. Spoon lentil mixture into tomatoes. Arrange on serving plates surrounded with red lettuce, alfalfa sprouts and parsley. Grate a little carrot on top of each tomato.

OTHER STUFFINGS FOR TOMATOES

1. Mock Tuna mixed with chopped celery, cucumbers and Herb-Yogurt Dressing.
2. Mock Crab Salad.
3. Any bean or vegetable sandwich filling.
4. Cottage cheese mixed with diced avocado, tomato and green onion.

GARDEN STUFFED CUCUMBERS

Cut cucumbers in half lengthwise and scoop out a hollow. Mix pulp with chopped celery and tomatoes, chopped walnuts and mayonnaise. Stuff the boats with this mixture and garnish with grated Jack cheese and fresh basil and oregano. Place boats on a bed of alfee sprouts.

SALAD IN A CREPE

Grind ½ cup sunflower seed sprouts and ½ cup raw almonds. Mix with an oil and vinegar or lemon juice dressing. Now mix with finely chopped tomatoes and form a stiff roll. Form in hot dog shapes and roll up like a burrito in a Romaine leaf with alfee sprouts inside.

ROLL-AROUNDS

Any of our Roll-Around bean or vegetable fillings can be rolled up with a Romaine, Spinach or Red Leaf lettuce leaf instead of a whole grain chapati, for a delicious salad in the hand. (See *KID STUFF* and sandwich fillings in this Chapter for additional ideas.)

Variation: Before rolling, drizzle with Herb-Yogurt Dressing and alfee sprouts.

MARINATED CHICKPEAS

Marinate sprouted or cooked garbanzo beans in oil, lemon juice or vinegar, parsley, minced garlic clove, dash of nutmeg, salt and cayenne. Great as is or in salads.

MOCK CRAB SALAD

4 cups cooked, drained soybeans
2 sweet or dill pickles
1 onion
1 carrot
1/3 cup almonds or cashew nuts
dash garlic powder
¼ cup chopped, green onions
2 T. chopped parsley
½ t. sea salt/kelp
dash cayenne
½ t. freshly ground pepper
dash ground dill seed
2 t. prepared mustard
½ cup mayonnaise
1-2 T. tamari-soy sauce
Herb-Yogurt Dressing

In a meat grinder, grind soybeans, pickles, onion, carrot and nuts. Place mixture in a large bowl. Add remaining ingredients and mix well. Consistency should be like tuna salad. Serve on individual lettuce cups, ringed with tomato wedges, topped with Herb-Yogurt Dressing and alfalfa sprouts.

BUFFET PARTY SALAD

mixed greens — (iceberg lettuce, Romaine, butter, red leaf) rinsed and whirled dry
alfalfa sprouts
grated carrots
grated purple cabbage
mixed sprouts (lentil-mung-adzuki)
olive oil and fresh garlic
Garnishes: chopped tomatoes, grated beets, sliced green onions, thinly sliced raw zucchini or crookneck squash, herb-garlic-buttered croutons, fresh, thinly sliced mushrooms, sliced celery, sliced green peppers, sliced cucumbers, sliced radishes, roasted tamari nuts and sun seeds (mix nuts with tamari-soy sauce and sea salt and roast)

In a large wooden salad bowl that has been seasoned and rubbed with olive oil and fresh garlic, place greens; toss in a quantity of fluffed, rinsed alfalfa sprouts. In another seasoned salad bowl, place grated carrots, purple cabbage and a smaller proportion of mixed sprouts. Place each of the garnishes in small, separate salad bowls. To serve: Let your guests begin with the two larger bowls, dishing out the proportions they want in their own salad bowls. Then, using spoons from each bowl of garnish, they can top salad with their favorite toppings. Have a choice of two dressings: Herb-Yogurt and an oil-vinegar dressing.

BEAUTIFUL 10 STEP HIGH PROTEIN LUNCHEON SALAD

1. On each plate arrange torn lettuce and Romaine.
2. Sprinkle as many alfalfa sprouts over the greens as desired.
3. Sprinkle 2-3 T. mixed sprouts over alfalfa sprouts.
4. Make a circle of cucumber slices in center of salad.
5. On top of this, place a scoop of cottage cheese.
6. Arrange avocado slices and tomato wedges around cottage cheese.
7. Spoon 2-3 T. of Bean-Nut Butter sandwich spread over cottage cheese.
8. Sprinkle kelp and a little cayenne over veggies and grate pepper over all.
9. Drizzle lemon juice over greens and veggies.
10. Grate a little Jack cheese over bean-nut mixture for added flavor and protein.

WE LOVE YOU TRULY TABOULEH

This is a colorful red and green salad from the Middle East. It is very nutritious and different tasting. Three-day old Tabouleh, refrigerated, is better than one; six-day is better than three.

4 cups boiling water
2 cups bulgur
1 cup olive oil
1-2 finely chopped onions or several sliced green onions
3-4 minced garlic cloves
1 small bunch of finely chopped, fresh parsley
½ t. sea salt/kelp
juice from 2 lemons
¼ to 1/3 cup finely chopped fresh peppermint (optional)
5-6 finely chopped fresh tomatoes.

Pour boiling water over bulgur and let set for 30 minutes to an hour or until all water is absorbed and bulgur is fluffy. Transfer to a large bowl. Add olive oil, onions, garlic, parsley, salt, lemon juice and mint. Allow flavors to blend at least 4-8 hours in the refrigerator. Just before serving, add finely chopped tomatoes. Serve on lettuce cups with crisp whole grain crackers. This is a meal in itself.

Variations: For extra protein add ½ cup diced tofu and/or ½ cup cooked garbanzo beans.

Fresh Fruit Salads

The best way to serve fruit is to pick it ripe from the tree. Second best is to select it from the fruit bowl, wash and/or peel, and eat *a la natural.* (See *KID STUFF* and *Better Beginnings: Breakfasts,* for additional fruit salad recipes.)

PDQ (PRETTY DARN QUICK)

Chop an apple or 2, slice 2 peeled bananas, cut up 1-2 peeled oranges and mix all together in a bowl. Add up to 1 cup plain yogurt, a Tablespoon of Almond-Cinnamon Mixture. (See *Better Beginnings: Breakfasts),* a handful of chopped dates and 1 T. frozen orange juice concentrate. Mix gently and serve.

AVOCADO-ORANGE SALAD

Cube 1 peeled orange and 1 peeled avocado. Toss with 1 Tablespoon honey and ¼ cup shredded coconut. Scoop this mixture onto 2 round slices of pineapple; sprinkle lightly with cinnamon and serve.

PINEAPPLE BOWL

Cut a fresh pineapple in half lengthwise through the crown. Remove fruit, leaving shells intact. Core and dice the fruit. Toss pineapple with 2 cups fresh strawberries, 1 cup sliced celery, ½ cup chopped walnuts, ½ cup green grapes, ½ cup cantaloupe or other melon balls and ½ cup sun seed sprouts. Spoon back into pineapple halves and serve with your favorite fruit dressing. Orange-Yogurt Dressing is good.

MAIN COURSE OR DESSERT FRUIT SALAD

Any combination of fruits and nuts is good in this simple, natural salad. Toss 4 cups diced, fresh fruit (several kinds), 1 cup thinly sliced celery, 1 cup chopped nuts, 1 cup real whipped cream, and ½ t. crushed anise. The anise gives it a distinctive flavor. Another time try mace or cardamom or allspice. Experiment, but always strive to give your foods *flavor* instead of just sweetness.

PASTEL PARTY SALAD

Alternate peeled slices of cantaloupe, honeydew melon and avocados on a bed of lettuce leaves. Drizzle with Orange-Cashew Cream. Sprinkle with fresh raspberries and shredded coconut. ORANGE-CASHEW CREAM: Blend 1 cup *each* orange juice and washed cashew nuts with 1 T. frozen orange juice concentrate until smooth. Optional: Add a dash nutmeg or mace.

FRUIT AND FIBER

Line a bowl with torn lettuce. In the center, place a Pineapple Bran Muffin. Lay banana slices around the muffin. Then place slices of peaches or nectarines, whole grapes, apple wedges, pineapple chunks, or any mix of fruit in season. Slice a thin round of an orange; cut it to center, twist and stand up on the side of the salad. Drizzle with Orange-Yogurt Dressing and sprinkle nutmeg over all.

Variations: Drizzle with crushed pineapple and sprinkle with caraway or anise seeds. OR substitute a scoop of cottage cheese in center of salad for the muffin, then drizzle with crushed pineapple and sprinkle with nutmeg and ground walnuts or nutmeg and poppy seeds.

DRESSING UP THE SALAD

NEVER FAILS HOMEMADE MAYONNAISE

2 eggs plus 1 egg yolk
2 T. lemon juice
2 t. apple-cider vinegar
or 2 T. vinegar and no lemon juice
¼ t. paprika
1 scant t. sea salt
1 t. honey (opt.)
½ t. dry mustard
2 cups chilled Safflower or Sunflower oil

Place eggs and lemon juice and/or vinegar in blender. Blend on low, then high until creamy. Add paprika, salt, honey and mustard and blend briefly. *Slowly,* very slowly, pour in oil, blending continuously on high, with oil being poured at a very fine trickle. Blend until desired consistency. The longer you blend, the thicker it gets. You may need a spatula to help coax it to blend in the last few Tablespoons of oil.

Variations: Substitute an equal amount of sesame oil for the oil. OR add 1 or more of the following ingredients after preparing: chopped pickles, basil, chives, 2 t. dill, 2 t. curry, parsley, 2 T. caraway seeds, 2 T. scallions, ¼ cup green pepper, ¼ cup diced celery, 3 T. chopped mushrooms, 1 clove minced garlic, chervil, tarragon, 3-4 T. health-store or homemade catsup. Makes 2½ cups plus.

SIMPLE OIL AND . . . In a shaker or blender mix: ¼ cup fresh lemon juice, ¼ cup water, 2/3 cup Sunflower oil and your choice of herbs: basil, carawav seeds, dill, marjoram, oregano, rosemary, sage.

Variations: Mash 1 garlic clove and add to mixture; after a day, remove clove, flavor remains. Substitute ¼ cup apple-cider vinegar for the lemon juice.

FRENCH DRESSING: Blend in a blender: 1/3 cup apple-cider vinegar, 1 t. honey, ⅛ t. dry mustard, ½ t. garlic powder, ¼ t. salt, 2 grinds fresh pepper, 2 dashes cayenne, 1 cup Sunflower or Safflower Oil. A little V-8 juice is optional.

MOCK SOUR CREAM: Mix ½ cup mayonnaise plus ½ cup yogurt, 1 t. dill and a few drops of lemon juice.

Variation: Add bleu cheese to mixture for a bleu cheese dressing.

COTTAGE CHEESE SOUR CREAM: In blender, blend: 1 cup creamed cottage cheese with 1 T. lemon juice and 5 T. milk until smooth. Use as a base for dips, or on baked potatoes, or as a salad dressing. Season with own choice of herbs.

HOMEMADE BLEU CHEESE DRESSING: Stir together until well-blended: ¼ cup crumbled bleu cheese, ½ cup mayonnaise, ¾ cup plain yogurt.

CREAMY TOMATO DRESSING: In a blender, blend: 1 6 oz. can tomato or V-8 juice, 3 T. cider vinegar, 1 T. honey, 1 egg yolk, 1 T. chopped parsley, 1 T. sliced green onions, and 1 T. nutritional yeast (opt.). When smooth, gradually add ½ cup oil. Blend continuously until smooth and thickened.

GREAT GREEN GOO: In a blender liquefy: 1 cup yogurt, 3-4 T. mayonnaise, 1-2 minced garlic cloves, 1 t. lemon juice, 1 T. chopped chives, 2 T. or more of chopped, fresh parsley, dash cayenne, dash kelp powder.

HERB-YOGURT: In a bowl, mix: 2 cups plain yogurt, 2-3 T. mayonnaise. Now comes the creative part. Experiment by adding crushed herbs and seasonings such as basil, garlic, kelp, sea salt, oregano, celery seed, thyme, marjoram, fresh parsley, etc. If you don't feel adventurous, go to your local health food store and you will find natural, old-fashioned herb dressing mixes, as well as other favorite dressing mixes (no additives or preservatives) to which yogurt, mayonnaise, buttermilk, or vinegar and oil may be added.

DESIDERATUM DIP: Stir together in a bowl: 2 cups yogurt, or 1 cup yogurt plus ½ cup sour cream and ½ cup cottage cheese, 2 t. minced onion and/or 2 t. chopped chives, ½ t. crushed basil, tarragon, parsley, and dash sage, dill or thyme. Stir all ingredients and allow herbs to permeate dip in covered container in refrigerator. Serve with crisp, raw vegetables.

TOFU DRESSING: In a blender, blend: ½ cup oil, 1 T. tamari-soy sauce, 2 cups tofu, ½ cup lemon juice and 1 t. kelp powder. Tastes great with hot or cold potato salad in place of mayonnaise.

CREAMY TOFU DIP OR DRESSING: In blender, blend: 6 oz. tofu, 1½ T. lemon juice, 2-3 T. oil, ¼ t. sea salt/kelp. Add 1/3 cup chopped onion, 1 T. dried parsley, 4 T. catsup and blend. Stir in 2 T. chopped dill pickle.

GUACAMOLE: Mash 2 ripe avocadoes in a bowl with a fork. Add about 2 parts mayonnaise to 1 part yogurt until dip consistency. Squeeze a little lemon juice over mixture and stir in chopped onions, garlic powder, vegetable seasoning and chili powder to taste. Add finely chopped tomatoes (opt.).

ORANGE-YOGURT DRESSING: In a bowl, mix: 1 cup of plain yogurt, 2 T.frozen orange juice concentrate.

Variation: Add ½ t. dried mint and 1 t. grated orange peel. OR add 1 small can crushed pineapple.

PLAIN DRESSING: Sweeten 1 cup plain yogurt with 1 t. honey. Add cinnamon, nutmeg, mace or other spice.

Variation: Substitute 1-2 T. of any frozen fruit juice concentrate for honey. OR flavor with vanilla, almond or maple extract.

SESAME DRESSING: In a blender or shaker: ½ cup oil, ¼ cup lemon juice, ¼ cup orange juice, 3 T. honey and 2 T. toasted sesame seeds.

OIL-LESS-AVOCADO DRESSING: In a blender, blend: 1 small-medium avocado, juice of 1 lemon, 2 minced garlic cloves, 2 dashes of ginger, 3 T. tamari-soy sauce, 1½ cups apple juice, 2 sliced green onions and ½ t. dried, minced onion. This freezes well. Tastes best with mixed greens and sprout salads.

SUNFLOWER SEED YOGURT

1 cup sun seeds
1 T. plain yogurt (use only if using plain water)
1 cup water OR ½ cup water and ½ cup Rejuvelac (2-day, fermented soak water from wheat berries)

Blender grind the sun seeds. Add water and yogurt or water and Rejuvelac. Blend on high until smooth and creamy and the consistency of heavy cream. Pour into a container; loosely cover and let set in a warm place until set up. It will have a black cap, which can be discarded.

DIP: Mix yogurt with chopped tomatoes, onions and celery. Add herbs, crushed garlic and sea salt/kelp. OR mix yogurt with grated carrots and beets and add favorite herbs.

DRESSING: Mix yogurt with mashed avocado, chopped green onion, a little lemon juice, garlic powder, and 1 t. tamari-soy sauce. Great spooned over a sprout salad!

FRUIT TOPPING: Mix yogurt with grated apple, mashed banana, a few squirts of lemon juice and honey to taste.
Variation: Substitute almonds, brazil nuts or ½-¾ cup sesame seeds for the sun seeds. Add apple, banana, lemon juice, honey and poppy seeds and cinnamon.

PRAISEWORTHY PIES

Pies are delicious to eat and fun to make, but they can be difficult for a beginning cook, especially the crust. Practice does make perfect, so prepare the pies with your young cook the first few times. Then after some first-hand experience s/he will be ready to try alone.

Perfectly Delicious and Different Pie Crusts

GRAHAM CRACKER: Mix 2 cups crushed graham crackers, ½ cup melted butter, 4 T. honey, a dash of nutmeg and ¼ cup Almond-Cinnamon Mixture. (See *Better Beginnings: Breakfasts* or *KID STUFF* for recipe). Press firmly into sides and bottom of pie pan. Chill or bake to brown.

WHEAT SPROUT: Spread 1 cup 2-day wheat sprouts on bottom of 10" pie pan. Pour filling in and bake with the pie. Works best with an egg-milk custard-type pie.

WHEAT GERM: Sprinkle wheat germ all over an oiled pie plate. Fill with a custard-type pie and bake.

GRANOLA: Blend 2 cups granola in blender with ¼ cup whole wheat flour and approximately ¼ cup melted butter. Mix and press into pie pan. Bake.

OATMEAL: Mix 1 cup blender-ground oats, ½ cup whole wheat pastry flour, ¼ cup shredded coconut, ½ cup wheat germ, 1 T. sesame seeds, ¼ cup honey, ¼ cup oil, 1 t. cinnamon and just enough orange juice or apple juice to make a dough. Press into pie pan and bake at 375° for 12 minutes.

NUT CRUST: Mix together 2/3 cup of blender-ground oats, 1/3 cup rice-millet flour (equal parts rice flour and millet flour) OR 1/3 cup whole wheat pastry flour, 1/3 cup mixed ground walnuts and almonds, and ½ t. cinnamon. Stir in 2 T. honey and 1/3 cup oil until like a dough. Knead; then press into a 9" or 10" pie pan and bake at 350° for 12-15 minutes or bake with the filling.

FLAKY PASTRY: Mix 3 cups whole wheat pastry flour and ½ t. sea salt. Then add mixture of ½ cup oil, 1 egg, 1 T. vinegar, 5 T. ice water. Knead lightly. Roll between wax paper. Transfer to pie pan and bake at 425° for 8 minutes.

TENDER RICE FLOUR PIE CRUST

1½ cups brown rice flour
4 T. arrowroot flour
¼ cup soy flour
½ t. salt
1 T. baking powder
¾ cup plus of butter
2 medium eggs
(opt.) ¼ cup sesame seeds and 1 t. nutmeg or cinnamon for pumpkin or fruit pies

Measure dry ingredients together. Using pastry blender, cut in butter. Beat eggs well and stir in. Add seeds and spice if desired. Divide dough in 2 and form 2 balls. Roll gently onto a pastry cloth using flour as necessary on rolling pin or cloth. Transfer to 9" pie pan very carefully. Chill before baking. Makes 2 9" crusts. Bake at 425° for 10 minutes.

PERFECT PAT-IN WHOLE WHEAT PIE CRUST

1 cup whole wheat pastry flour
¼ t. salt
¼ cup oil
3 T. ice water

Add flour and salt to a 9" pie pan. Measure oil and water into a cup and stir with a fork; then slowly add to flour mixture in pan, mixing well with fork. Add more water if necessary. Then press into shape with fingers, making sure crust covers entire surface evenly. Prick bottom with fork and bake 20-25 minutes at 375° for a prebaked crust.

Toppings for Pies, Fruit Desserts or Cakes

GRANOLA TOPPING: Mix 1 cup granola, ½ cup melted butter, ¼ cup honey and ½ t. cinnamon or nutmeg. Spread on top of a fruit cobbler.

NUTTY TOPPING: Mix 1 cup oats, 1 cup shredded coconut, ¾ cup chopped nuts, ½ cup butter, 1 t. vanilla and ¼ cup honey. Spread on fruit cobbler or cake before baking.
Variation: Spread on baked cake and broil for a couple of minutes.

CRISPY: Mix ½ cup wheat germ, 1½ cups whole wheat flour, 1 cup blender-ground oats, ½ cup regular oats, ¼ cup oil, ½ cup honey, ½ cup finely chopped walnuts, 1 t. cinnamon, and 1 t. vanilla. Spread over fruit, dot with butter and bake.

COMPLETELY, THOROUGHLY, ABSOLUTELY IMPOSSIBLE PIE

4 eggs
2 cups milk (not raw)
½ cup honey
¼ cup butter
1 t. vanilla
½ cup whole wheat pastry flour
1 T. non-alum baking powder
1 cup shredded coconut
dash nutmeg

In a blender, blend eggs, milk, honey, butter, vanilla, flour and baking powder. Pour into unbaked crust of your choice. Wheat Sprout crust works very good. Sprinkle with 1 cup shredded coconut and a little nutmeg. Bake at 325° for 30 minutes or until set. Makes a large pie.

HEAP BIG CRUSTY

5 cups apples, cherries or peaches
1-2 T. cinnamon
¼-½ cup maple syrup
Crispy Topping

Wash and core apples. Slice into very thin slices. Add cinnamon and mix. Spread into a buttered 9"x13" pan until full. Drizzle with syrup and top with Crispy Topping. Bake at 350° for 30-40 minutes.

GOOF-PROOF TOFU BANANA CREAM PIE

3 bananas
1 T. lemon juice
2 t. vanilla
1/3 cup oil
½ cup honey
dash salt
2½ cups tofu

In a blender, blend bananas, lemon juice, vanilla. Add oil, honey, salt and blend again. Add tofu and blend until smooth and creamy. Pour into a prebaked pie shell (Graham Cracker is good) and refrigerate for a couple hours. Just before serving, slice 1 banana on top.
Variation: Add 3 T. carob powder for a creamy carob-banana pie.

SMOOTH AS SILK FROZEN STRAWBERRY PIE

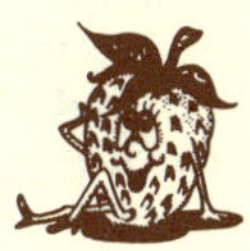

4 oz. softened cream cheese
2 large bananas
1-1½ cups fresh or frozen whole strawberries
1/3 cup instant powdered milk
1 t. vanilla
½ cup honey
1½-2 cups plain yogurt

In a blender, blend cream cheese, bananas and strawberries, milk, vanilla and honey. Remove from blender and stir in yogurt. Pour filling into a baked pie crust (Granola is great) and freeze until hard. Serve as soon as you remove it from freezer. Tastes like ice cream!

DELICIOUS FRUIT PIE

1 cup fresh strawberries, sliced
½ cup fresh rhubarb, sliced
2 cups fresh pineapple, sliced
2 cups fresh bananas, sliced
¼ cup honey or as needed
double recipe Perfect Pat-in Whole Wheat Pie Crust

Mix together sliced fruit with honey. Place into unbaked 9" pie crust. Roll out top crust and place over pie and seal edges. Slit with a knife in 2-3 places. Bake at 400° for 30-40 minutes or until fruit is cooked and juices run out of top crust and sides.

CREAMY PRUNE PIE

1 8 oz. package softened cream cheese
2 T. honey
½ t. vanilla
1 t. cinnamon
1 cup plain yogurt
2 cups dried, pitted, chopped prunes

Beat cream cheese, honey, vanilla and cinnamon until smooth and light. Fold in yogurt. Pour half of this mixture in bottom of a crust. (Nut Crust is good). Add prunes and top with remaining cream cheese-yogurt mixture. Refrigerate before serving.

HEALTHSAVING HINTS

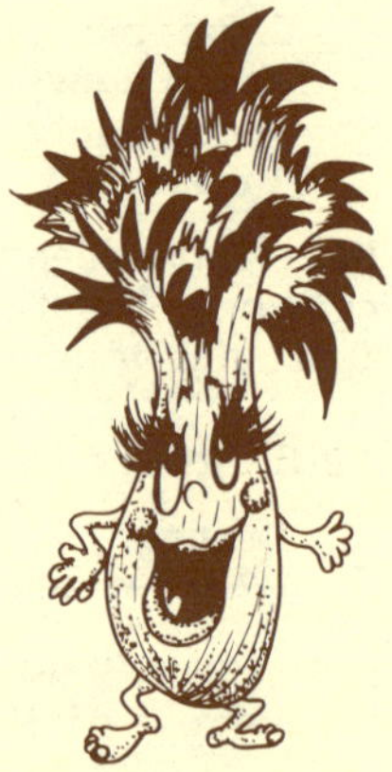

1. **There are no such things as failures when baking bread. If bread doesn't turn out as planned, slice and dice and make into croutons or spicy stuffing. Slice, dry and crumb for extra body in loaves and patties. Slice very thin and bake in moderate oven until it resembles melba toast. Tear in bite-sized pieces and make old-fashioned bread pudding, adding plenty of nuts and dried fruits. Use your imagination to utilize the bread wherever it doesn't have to be perfect. Breadmaking gets better with practice!**
2. **Here is a nutritious butter spread for breads, potatoes, rice and rolls. In a mixer or blender, mix together 1 cup fresh butter, ½ cup sesame seed oil and 4 T. powdered lecithin. When smooth, place in covered container and refrigerate.**
3. **Soybeans are high in protein and low in carbohydrates. They are rich in calcium, phosphorous and iron, and contain vitamins A,B,C,D,E,F, and K. They are also rich in lecithin — nature's cholesterol emulsifier. Include them sprouted or cooked in salads, sandwich spreads, burgers and casseroles. Use tofu in place of meat or cheese or as an added protein ingredient in salads.**
4. **To make any nut butter, grind nuts fine in blender or nut grinder, adding only as much oil as necessary to hold together like a butter. Usually 1 or 2 t. oil per cup of ground nuts will suffice.**
5. **Restaurants often use parsley to increase eye-appeal and appetites for an otherwise bland-looking plate. It may be the most nutritious item on your plate, so don't neglect it.**
6. **A favorite for kids and the young at heart: Place a thin slice of cheese in the bottom of each bowl of soup. Ladle soup into bowls. Cheese will melt and taste delicious with soup. It motivates children to eat all of the soup to get to the cheese at the bottom. Especially good with split pea soup or chili.**
7. **Be sure to rinse all grains and beans before cooking; drain in a colander or strainer and remove bad beans or pebbles. Soak or cook for one hour, then discard first water (contains phytic acid) and start with fresh water. Continue as directed in recipes.**
8. **When using whole spices in soups and stews, place them in a tea ball. Then remove when soup is done. Works well with hot spiced cider too.**
9. **Never wash mushrooms; they absorb water like a sponge. Carefully wipe with a soft, damp cloth. Special mushroom brushes are available.**
10. **Use chopstix to eat salads, vegetables and other dishes. This will prolong your meal, force you to eat one bite at a time, and remind you to chew each bite thoroughly.**

11. To fluff alfalfa sprouts and remove hulls, place alfalfa (or any other) sprouts in a large bowl. Fill with cold water and swish them around with your hand. Hulls will float to the top where you can skim them off with your hand or a spoon. Then place sprouts into a colander; transfer to pillowcase, and go outside and whirl. They'll be crisp and fluffy for salads or sandwiches.
12. Add a handful of cabbage or radish sprouts to green salads for an extra zing. Be sure to sprout with seeds meant for sprouting. Seeds for planting are often chemically treated with fungicides and mercury.
13. Use leftover fruit juices and sweet spices to transform plain yogurt into tangy fruit salad dressings.
14. In selection of salad ingredients consider: texture combinations (some soft, some crunchy), variety in color and taste, protein quality, produce in season, whether a main dish or side, family's tastes, and type of dressing used.
15. For dips or salad dressings calling for yogurt, *gently* stir yogurt into the other ingredients. Blender blades kill the friendly bacteria that are the main reason for using yogurt in the first place. High speed mixing also makes yogurt thin as milk.
16. If small children pick certain vegetables — like onion, celery or green pepper — out of their salads, simply mince those veggies super-fine, and add to the salad dressing.
17. The average American diet is low in fiber. Our teeth and digestive systems were meant to chew and digest foods in their natural state, so the more salads, nuts and seeds you can incorporate into your meals, the better. You will benefit from a high amount of vitamins, minerals and enzymes not so abundant in cooked foods. Not only your palate, but your plumbing will thank you!
18. Dry thin slices of zucchini. Season with kelp and use in place of potato chips for dipping.

TIMESAVING HINTS

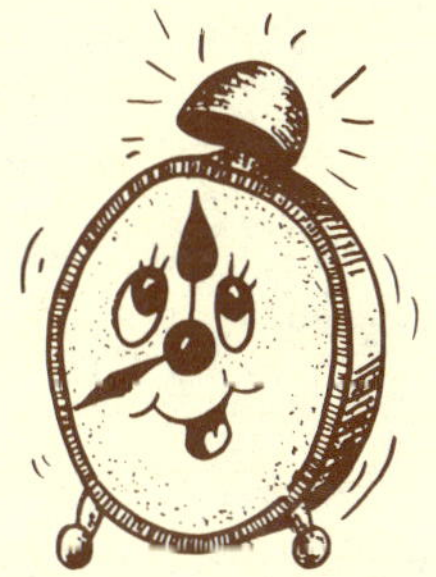

1. Make sandwiches in bulk, wrap in plastic, then foil and freeze. Those that freeze well are bean spreads, leftover loaf spreads, peanut butter, nut butters, and cream cheese.
2. Store whole grain bread in paper bags in cupboard. Freeze what you cannot use within five days of baking.
3. Always keep a variety of fruits and cheeses on hand. When company drops in unexpectedly with a jug of freshly-pressed apple juice, just arrange fruits and cheeses on a cutting board and provide each person with a knife and saucer. Crackers, popcorn, or variety breads accompany nicely.
4. Purchase natural, undyed cheeses and fresh, creamery butter in bulk, cut in portions and freeze. Butter, when thawed, remains the same. Jack and Cheddar will be a bit more crumbly.
5. For a full-bodied soup: During the last few minutes of cooking, finely grate one small potato into soup. Thickens and flavors while adding nutrition.
6. Any of these soups and stews can be started the night before in a crock pot and served in the morning for breakfast.
7. A pillowcase is more effective than a colander and more economical than paper towels for drying greens and sprouts. Simply place washed greens in a clean pillowcase and go outside. With your strong arm, swing the pillowcase as though you were winding up for a pitch. Centrifugal force will force all the water out of the greens. Your plants will love you if you swing near them, but be careful about doing it in front of strangers or windows. Neither takes to unexpected showers!

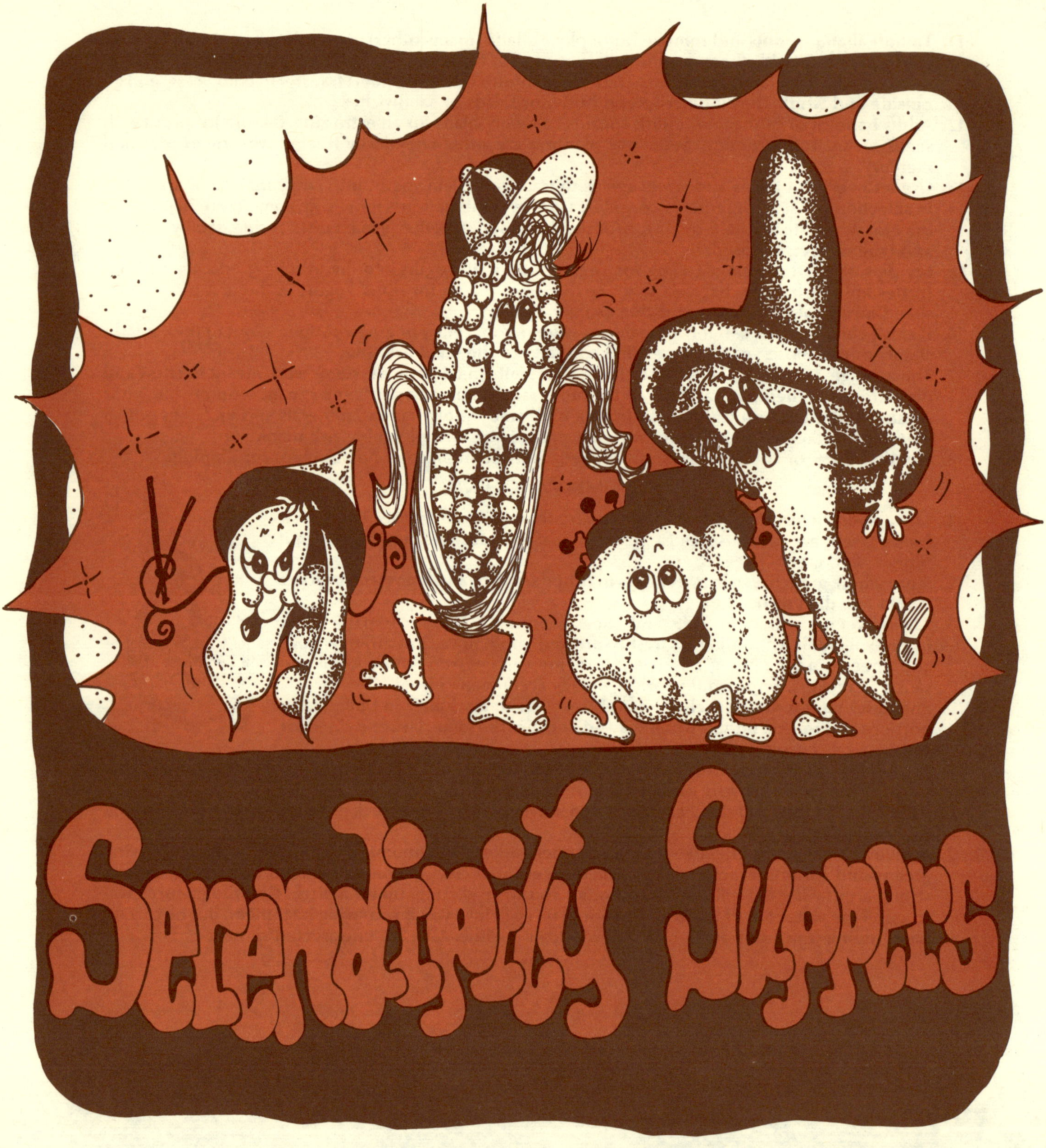
Serendipity Suppers

Serendipity Suppers

Serendipity

Serendipity is the happening upon fortunate discoveries, though not necessarily searching for them. That's how we developed some of our main dishes that taste so scrumptious that you'll forget there's no meat on the table. Menu planning, protein combining, quantity preparation, high-energy additions and leftover suggestions abound. From lazy-day-quick-pot-luck to elegant-ethnic-entertaining-extravaganzas, we share our most delectable discoveries.

Muddle-Free Menu Planning

One of the most interesting aspects of vegetarian cookery is learning what to prepare for variety, protein complementarity, good nutrition and taste. The key to successful vegetarian meal preparation is in the planning.

Whether you work out of the home, have hobbies or children, or just plain don't care to spend all of your time in the kitchen, it pays to be thrifty and organized. The following guide will help you organize shopping, menu planning and food preparation to produce maximum nutrition with minimum time and expense.

A Resourceful Recipe File

As we became more selective about food purchases, and more aware that not just the quality of the food, but the method of preparation is important to maintain optimum nutrients, we found it quite a challenge to organize a new, natural foods recipe file.

We put our *"instant meals"* recipe box in a dark closet and saved only those family favorites we wanted to convert to healthy ingredients, such as substituting honey for sugar, whole wheat flour for white, SunButterBlend for shortening, brown rice for white rice, or home-cooked potatoes for instant. Using a 4"x6" card file we included the converted family favorites plus other recipes which used unprocessed foods only.

The recipes within this book are the result of our trial and error experiences and careful selection of health saving, time saving and money saving meals. As your family develops favorite taste sensations from this book or your own creative experiences, you may wish to record them on cards for easy access and durability. Recipes have a way of becoming wet or oily during food preparation; a card can be replaced much easier than your special cookbook.

Our convenient headings for filing your converted recipes work well, and all the recipes in this book can be filed under the various subject headings according to your choice. You might wish to file a Chinese wok dish under Ethnic Foods or under Vegetable Dishes; a yogurt-rice pudding under *KIDSTUFF* or Yogurt-Kefir. This is a flexible file; add new tabs to fit your family's needs.

Who is wise? He who can learn from every man. — *Hebrew Proverb*

RESOURCEFUL RECIPE FILE

From front to back, tab headings read as follows:

1. **Anxious to Try; Not Yet Tested**
2. **Appetizers, Dips**
3. **Better Beginnings: Breakfasts: cereals, pancakes, toppings**
4. **Breads, Muffins, Rolls: include pita, chapati, pie crusts**
5. **Camp-Outs-Back Packing: menus using dried, easy to pack and prepare foods**
6. **Creative Cosmetics: recipes for facials, shampoos**
7. **Desserts: fruit, nuts, seeds packed into cakes, pies, tortes**
8. **Drinks: yummy fruit smoothies, super shakes, juices, teas**
9. **Egg-Dairy-Cheese Dishes: quiches, souffles, puffs**
10. **Ethnic Dishes: extravaganzas, Chinese, Mexican, Italian, gourmet**
11. **Fish Dishes**
12. **Household Herbs for Healing: simple remedies for sore throats, colds**
13. **KIDSTUFFKIDSTUFF: snacks, cookies, puddings, candies**
14. **Menus for Company and Holidays: buffet, entertaining, using color, texture, seasonal foods**
15. **Patties-Burgers-Loaves: grain, nut, seed and veggie combinations**
16. **Rice and Bean Casseroles: protein complementarity**
17. **Salads, Fruit**
18. **Salads, Vegetable**
19. **Sandwiches and Spreads: home and brown bagging lunch ideas, sandwich fillings**
20. **Sauces-Gravies-Salad Dressings-Seasonings-Nut Butters**
21. **Soups and Stews: includes seasonings and accompaniments**
22. **Sprouts: how to grow, how to use, recipes using them**
23. **Vegetable Dishes: stir-frys, main dishes, side dishes**
24. **Yogurt-Kefir: frozen or refrigerator desserts, drinks, ice creams**

A Rotating Menu Plan

For conservation of time and energy, you can develop a weekly rotating menu plan for the evening meal for four weeks and a corresponding shopping list for the ingredients in the recipes. Though this will *take* time in the initial planning stages, it will *save* you a tremendous amount of time later on. For instance, when you have plans that will take you away from home at mealtime, *any* member of your family will know by reviewing the rotating menu cards, what to prepare for that particular day, and how to prepare it, using ingredients that are already in the cupboards, because the shopping was taken care of earlier in the week.

Notice that all of the dinners for Monday are EGG-DAIRY-CHEESE dishes; all of Tuesday's dinners are PATTIES OR LOAVES; Wednesday's are SOUPS OR STEWS WITH BREAD, ROLL OR MUFFIN; Thursday's are always a CASSEROLE OR SANDWICH WITH A STOVE-TOP VEGGIE; and each Friday, serve an ETHNIC dish. By dividing the dinners into five basic types, the planning is easier and more systematic, yet still provides a great variety with little repetition. The Menu Plans can be accumulated for a year rather than repeated every four weeks, using the five basic meal types but without using the same recipe twice. It's up to you.

To further clarify the plan for other members of the family, color-code each of the meal plans listed on the cards for Monday red, along with their corresponding recipe cards, Tuesday's meal plans and recipe cards can be color-coded orange, Wednesday's, yellow, Thursday's, green, and Friday's, blue. Shopping lists are titled *Week 1, Week 2*, etc., to correspond with each weekly menu card.

In our homes, we have listed Saturday as "Parent's Night Out" and while we go out with our husbands, our children plan and prepare their meal. Even if we don't leave the home, it is still fun for the children and great experience for them to prepare the dinner. Sunday evenings are reserved for trying a new recipe. Be creative! Go Gourmet! Involve other family members and take the time to create something really spectacular! Don't forget to plan ahead to include the ingredients for these nights in your weekly shopping list.

Each of the recipes listed in the sample cards are the main dish. In vegetarian cooking, most of the nutrients are packed into one main dish, rather than the traditional meat-potatoes-vegetable plate. Of course, every main dish should be accompanied by a seasonal raw vegetable salad, raw vegetables for dipping, sprouts for a garnish, or a fresh, steamed vegetable. Drink a minimum of liquids with a meal. Your digestive juices work better when not diluted. Wait at least an hour after the meal to have dessert and try to meet the balance of the day's nutrient needs in your desserts; i.e., fruit, rice or bread pudding.

If you have children, a roommate or a friend, involve them in shopping and preparing the meals. Then in an emergency, by following the cards and recipes, they can be assured the ingredients will be available and will be able to prepare the meal with ease and enjoyment, while you'll be able to relax.

Be flexible. If you've planned apple cake for dessert, but when you shop, ripe bananas are 10¢ a pound, then opt for banana cake this time. Follow ads for specials and plan your menus around in-season produce.

Why do we recommend that you become so organized? First of all, by following these guidelines, you will have variety due to pre-planning. Consequently you won't have to search your mind or cookbook or file each night for something "different." Second, by relieving your mind from the daily hassle of meal *planning*, the actual preparation of the meal can be fun and headache-free.

So read on; try our recipes; experiment! Alter your old favorite recipes or concoct your own. RELAX and enjoy the freedom you'll feel from knowing that you need not *live* in your kitchen in order to serve naturally nutritious food. You *can* start from scratch and still have it ready in half-a-jiffy if you just implement the Resourceful Recipe File and Rotating Menu Plan.

SAMPLE WEEKLY MENU CARDS

	Week 1
Monday	San Francisco Quiche
Tuesday	Mama's Veggie Burgers
Wednesday	Chili Bean Soup Corn Bread
Thursday	Stuffed Cabbage Rolls
Friday	Eggplant Egg Rolls

	Week 2
Monday	Zucchini Souffle
Tuesday	Lentil-Nut Loaf
Wednesday	Split Pea Soup Appley Bran Muffins
Thursday	(Leftover) Lentil-Loaf-French Toast Basil-Buttered Carrots
Friday	Whole Wheat Pizza

	Week 3
Monday	Cauliflower-Broccoli Pie
Tuesday	Sun Burgers Potato Strips with Cheese
Wednesday	Harvest Tomato Soup Herb-Buttered Bread
Thursday	Busy Day Buckwheat Dinner
Friday	South India Upma

	Week 4
Monday	Mushroom-Spinach Crepes
Tuesday	Simple Simon Says
Wednesday	Best Veggie Soup Ever Yogurt Bran Muffins
Thursday	Millet-Stuffed Green Peppers
Friday	Eggplant Enchiladas

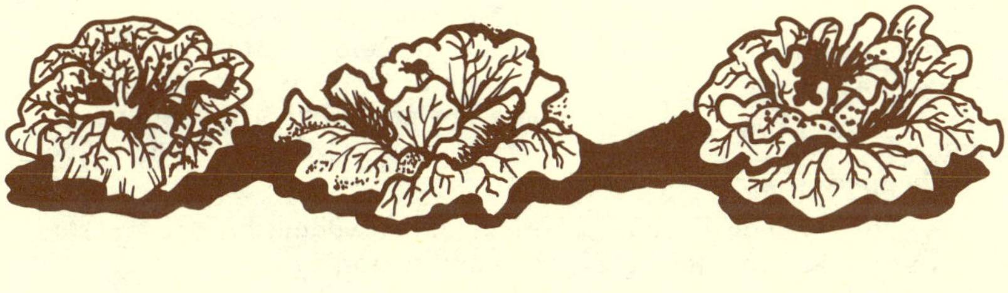

PROTEIN ADDITIONS

The following additions, when included in casseroles, loaves, salads or soups, ensure complete, top-quality protein:

1. **Milk: Yogurt, powdered, low-fat, raw, kefir or buttermilk can be added to grain and bean casseroles or desserts for increased protein and B vitamins.**
2. **Cheese: Cottage, ricotta, Jack, raw, undyed Cheddar, or soybean curd (tofu) can be grated, diced, cubed or sliced into hot dishes, salads or desserts for increased nutritional value.**
3. **Eggs: This complete protein food can be added to anything for nutrition, flavor or as a binder in patties and loaves.**
4. **Raw Nuts or Seeds: Almonds, walnuts, pecans, cashews, filberts, sunflower or sesame seeds will increase important vitamins, oils and minerals as well as protein.**
5. **Sprouts: Alfalfa, mung, lentil, sunflower, adzuki, soy, garbanzo, rye or wheat can be garnished on salads, sandwiches, soups, stir-frys, casseroles. They contribute enzymes, protein, vitamins and fiber.**
6. **Others: Adding wheat germ, peanuts or peanut butter, flaked bran, rice polish, soy flour or grits, brewer's or nutritional yeast, Bakon yeast or carob powder will increase nutrients and ensure the protein quality.**

CASSEROLE AND VEGETABLE PIE TOPPINGS

CRUMBLY TOPPING

½ cup wheat germ
¼ cup flaked bran
¼ cup dry Parmesan cheese
1 T. butter
2 minced garlic cloves

Mix wheat germ, bran and cheese. Cut in butter and garlic cloves. Top any nearly baked casserole or quiche and return to oven to toast about 10 minutes more at 300° F. or under broiler for 2 minutes.

CRUSTY TOPPING

1 cup plain yogurt
1 egg yolk
¼ cup wheat germ or ⅛ cup flour
1-2 T. melted butter
Parmesan cheese

Mix yogurt, egg yolk and wheat germ or flour. Stir in melted butter, pour over casserole, sprinkle with Parmesan and bake with casserole.

OTHER TOPPINGS

wheat germ
any grated cheese
mixed, chopped or ground nuts
croutons
bread crumbs
sprouts

GARNISHES

olives
parsley
tomato slices
sprouts
toasted sesame seeds
sprouted sunflower seeds

SAUCES AND GRAVIES

MUSHROOM GRAVY

3 T. butter
2 cups chopped mushrooms
2 T. whole wheat flour
1½ cups milk
½ t. dried, minced onion or 1 T. fresh chopped
1 t. tamari-soy sauce
sea salt/kelp to taste
dash of cayenne
a few grates of black pepper
optional: ½ t. Bakon yeast

Saute mushrooms in butter until nearly tender. Sprinkle flour over mushrooms and stir until brown. Gradually add milk and tamari-soy sauce. Stir until thickened, then add seasonings.

CASHEW GRAVY

2 cups water or stock
½ cup raw cashew nuts
1½ T. arrowroot flour or
3 T. whole wheat flour
2 T. oil
1 t. dried, minced onion
1 t. tamari-soy sauce
2 T. fresh, chopped parsley

In blender, blend liquid, nuts, flour, oil, onion, tamari sauce and parsley. Pour in saucepan and heat, stirring continuously until thickened. Alternate Method: Saute ¼ cup chopped onion in 2 T. oil until translucent. Add ½ cup ground cashews and arrowroot or whole wheat flour. Stir until light brown. Add liquids and tamari and stir until thick.

SALSA

2-3 fresh, diced tomatoes
1 diced, medium onion
¼ cup fresh, chopped parsley
2 minced garlic cloves
½ t. sea salt/kelp
⅛ t. fresh ground pepper or dash cayenne
⅛ t. ground cumin
⅛ t. chili powder
1 t. olive oil

Combine ingredients. Refrigerate until well-chilled.

BASIC WHITE SAUCE

2 T. butter
2-3 T. whole wheat flour
1 cup milk
your choice herbs: thyme, parsley, rosemary, basil
sea salt/kelp and cayenne to taste

Melt butter in skillet along with herbs. Stir in flour until it browns. Gradually add milk, stirring until thickened. **Variation:** Toast flour in dry skillet before adding butter for a brown sauce.

CHEESE SAUCE

1 recipe Basic White Sauce
½ cup grated cheese
¼ t. paprika
¼ t. dry mustard

Prepare above white sauce; then stir in cheese and spices until just melted.

CREAMY TOMATO SAUCE

½ chopped, green pepper
2 T. butter
2 T. flour
2 8 oz. cans tomato sauce
½ cup water
⅛ t. sea salt/kelp
½ cup plain yogurt

Saute green pepper in butter until tender. Stir in flour, then add sauce, water, and seasonings. Bring to a boil, remove from heat and stir in yogurt very gently.

HEARTY SPAGHETTI SAUCE

olive oil or butter
1 chopped onion
1 chopped green pepper
3 chopped garlic cloves
4 chopped mushrooms
1 stalk chopped celery
2 t. Italian Herb Mix
2 8 oz. cans tomato sauce
1 6 oz. can tomato paste, equal amount water
dash each sea salt/kelp and cayenne

Saute onion, green pepper, garlic, mushrooms, celery, and herbs in butter or oil. In saucepan, heat tomato sauce, paste, water and salt and cayenne. Add saute mixture and simmer, covered for about 30 minutes, stirring often.

EASY PIZZA SAUCE: Mix 1 8 oz. can tomato sauce with 1 t. Italian Herb Mix.

ENCHILADA SAUCE

2 T. SunButterBlend
1 finely chopped onion
3½ cups tomato sauce
2 minced garlic cloves
2 T. chili powder (more or less)
½ t. cumin
¼ t. oregano
1 t. sea salt

Saute onion and herbs in SunButterBlend. Add tomato sauce, cover and simmer about 10 minutes, stirring often. Makes 3 cups for 20 enchiladas.

Seasonings for Sauces, Soups, Stews

ITALIAN HERB MIX: Mix 4 parts marjoram, 4 parts oregano, 4 parts basil to 2 parts rosemary and 2 parts thyme. Store, covered, in a cool, dry place. Use 1-3 t. mix per 2 quarts of soup or sauce.

MEXICAN HERB MIX: Mix 5 parts basil, 4 parts oregano, 4 parts cumin, 3 parts chili powder, ½ part ground coriander. Store, covered, in a cool, dry place. Use 1-2 T. mix per quart of sauce.

GOMAZIO: Stir ¾ cup sesame seeds in dry cast iron skillet over medium heat until just turning brown. Stir constantly as they burn easily. Combine with 1 T. sea salt in a mortar and grind until powdery. Store in covered container and use in place of salt or as a seasoning for a casserole, salad or vegetable pie topping.

SEA SALT/KELP: Start with 1 part kelp powder or granules to 3 parts sea salt and mix in a shaker. As your family adjusts to this, work your way up to a 3 part kelp-1 part sea salt mixture.

SALAD SEASONING: Combine ¾ cup grated Parmesan cheese, ¼ cup dried parsley flakes, 1 t. garlic powder, ¼ t. cayenne, ¼ t. freshly ground pepper, 1 t. dried, minced onion, 1 t. bell pepper flakes, 1 t. crushed basil, 1 T. toasted sesame seeds, 1 T. toasted sunflower seeds, 1 T. toasted oats and ½ t. vegetable salt. Store in air-tight bottle in refrigerator. Sprinkle on vegetable salads.

(See *Kitchen Keys* for other suggestions for using herbs.)

Crusts for Vegetable Pies and Pot Pies

RICE CRUST

2 cups cooked, brown rice
2 T. butter
1 beaten egg
¼ cup Parmesan cheese plus 2 T. chopped onion
1 t. dried parsley or 2 T. fresh, chopped parsley
¼ cup toasted sesame seeds

Mix everything well and pat into oiled pie plate. Bake for 10 minutes at 350° or until browned and crisp.

CHEESE CRUST

1 cup whole wheat flour
¼ t. salt
¼ t. dry mustard
1 cup grated Cheddar cheese
1/3 cup plus of water

Mix ingredients, roll out, place in oiled pie pan and bake 5 minutes at 375° before adding vegetables.

POTATO CRUST

2½ cups packed, grated, raw potato
½ t. salt
1 beaten egg
¼ cup grated onion or 1 T. dried, minced onion
½ t. paprika

Place potato in a colander, sprinkle with salt and let sit for 10 minutes. Drain and squeeze out excess juice. Important! Then mix with remaining ingredients and pat into a well-oiled pie pan, building up sides of crust. Bake 35 minutes at 375°. Brush with oil and bake for 5-10 minutes longer, before adding veggies.

SUPER DUPER REFRIGERATOR BISCUITS' CRUST: Follow recipe for Super Duper Refrigerator Biscuits in *Labor of Love Lunches* under breads. Roll out as for any crust and use for both upper and lower crusts.

ZUCCHINI CRUST

3½ cups grated zucchini
(squeezed and drained)
3 beaten eggs
½ cup flour
1 cup grated Jack or half Jack and half Cheddar
1 t. crushed basil
sea salt/kelp to taste

Mix all ingredients and spread into long baking pan. Bake 20-25 minutes at 350°, brush with oil, and bake for 5 minutes more at 400°.

PERFECT PAT-IN WHOLE WHEAT PIE CRUST

1 cup whole wheat pastry flour
¼ t. salt
¼ cup oil
3 T. ice water

Measure flour and salt into a 9" pie pan. Measure oil and water into a cup and stir with a fork; then slowly add to flour mixture in pan, mixing well with fork. Add more water if necessary. Then press into shape with fingers, making sure crust covers entire surface evenly. Prick bottom with fork and bake 20-25 minutes at 375° for a pre-baked crust.

AMERICAN POT-LUCK

VEGETABLE PIES OR POT PIES

For delicious vegetarian pies follow these step-by-step directions:

1. Saute or steam 4 cups of vegetables: any combination of carrots, celery, cauliflower, broccoli, cabbage, cubed potatoes, green beans, peas, corn, onions, eggplant, mushrooms, green pepper, etc. Cook until crisp, not mushy.
2. Place veggies in an unbaked or baked pie crust or in individual pot pie pans lined with a crust.
3. Pour Basic White Sauce or Cheese Sauce over vegetables.
4. Top with pie crust, cheese cubes, toasted sesame seeds, bread crumbs or your choice of any of the vegetable pie toppings.
5. Bake at 350° for 20-25 minutes or until sauce bubbles.

CAULIFLOWER-BROCCOLI PIE

cauliflower
broccoli flowers and stalks
1 minced garlic clove
1 cup chopped onion
basil
sea salt
pepper
1 cup grated Cheddar cheese
3 T. butter
2 eggs
¼ cup milk
paprika

Steam cauliflower and broccoli and sliced stalks. Saute garlic, onion, basil in butter. Beat eggs and milk; mix all together and place in a potato crust.

Variation: Use mushrooms and spinach in place of cauliflower and broccoli and season with ¼ t. nutmeg in place of basil.

ELEGANT VEGGIE PIE

cooked broccoli
cooked green pepper
cooked cauliflower
cooked onion
Perfect Whole Wheat pie crust
or Super Duper Biscuit Crust
cooked potatoes
cooked, slivered carrots
sauteed eggplant cubes
Mushroom Gravy
grated cheese

Place first 4 veggies in a baked pie crust. Add 1 layer each of potatoes, carrots and eggplant. Pour Mushroom Gravy over all; top with cheese and bake for 20 minutes at 375°.

EGGPLANT-SOYBEAN PIE

½ chopped onion
2 minced garlic cloves
1½ cups cooked, ground soybeans
1 8 oz. can tomato sauce
1 T. tamari-soy sauce
½ of an eggplant, cubed
4 T. oil
½ cup whole wheat flour
¼ cup wheat germ
thinly sliced tomatoes
Crusty Topping

Saute onion and garlic in butter; then add soybeans and stir gently to brown. Add tomato sauce and tamari and simmer for 7-10 minutes. In another skillet in oil, saute eggplant which has been shaken in a paper bag with the flour. Shake and coat a few at a time. Drain. Oil a 10" pie plate and evenly sprinkle wheat germ over bottom and sides. Then alternate layers of eggplant and soybean mixture. Top with tomatoes and Crusty Topping. Bake for 35-40 minutes at 350° or until browned and bubbly.

CASSEROLES AND VEGETABLE DISHES

LANI'S COMPANY CHEESE-CASHEW 3 LAYER CASSEROLE

¾ cup raw brown rice
¾ cup raw pearl barley
4 cups water
2 T. butter
1 thinly sliced onion
2 minced garlic cloves
5-6 chopped mushrooms
1/3 chopped green pepper
2-3 T. butter
1 T. tamari-soy sauce
½ cup raw cashews
5 oz. cubed tofu
double recipe Basic White Sauce
1 cup fresh corn or 1 10 oz. package of frozen corn
2-3 dashes cayenne
½ t. basil
1 T. Aminotone (opt.)
grated Jack cheese

Steam grains in water for 35 minutes; remove from heat and add butter. In a skillet saute onions, garlic, mushrooms and pepper in butter. After a few minutes add tamari sauce, cashews and tofu, stirring until tofu and nuts brown. Spread barley-rice mixture in an oiled 9"x13" pan. Spread the saute mixture on top. In same pan as saute, prepare the white sauce and set aside half of it. Add corn, cayenne, basil and pour mixture over barley-rice mixture and spread. Pour reserved white sauce over entire casserole. Prick with a fork so sauce goes into rice. Bake covered for 20 minutes at 350°, uncover, top with grated cheese, return to oven for 10 minutes more or until cheese melts.

NITA'S ZUCCHINI SOUFFLE

1 cup milk
1 t. crushed basil
¼ t. garlic powder
1 cup diced mushrooms
6 well beaten eggs
3 cups thinly sliced or chopped zucchini
4 sliced green onions
½ chopped green pepper
1¾ cups grated Jack cheese

In a large bowl, beat eggs and milk. Add remaining ingredients except cheese. Pour into an oiled 8"x8" pan. Bake at 325° for 35-45 minutes or until set. Then add cheese and bake 10 minutes longer or until cheese is melted. May use an oblong pan and shorten baking time.

Variation: For a fluffier souffle, separate whites from yolks, whip until stiff and gently fold into the beaten yolks-zucchini mixture.

MILLET SOUFFLE

1 cup milk
4 egg yolks
1½ cups cooked millet
(steam 1 cup millet in 4 cups milk over double boiler until tender)
1 T. minced, dried onion
a few dashes of sea salt/kelp
½ cup grated cheese
4 egg whites, stiffly whipped
2 T. melted butter

In a large bowl, beat together milk and egg yolks. Add 1½ cups millet (there will be plenty leftover in double boiler), onion, salt, cheese and butter. Carefully fold in whipped egg whites. Bake in a buttered casserole or souffle dish for about 20 minutes at 350° or until golden. Use leftover millet to mix with yogurt, honey and fruit for a dessert pudding.

SUZANNE'S SAN FRANCISCO QUICHE

1 Perfect Whole Wheat Pie Crust
butter
1 cup grated Swiss cheese
1 T. whole wheat flour
1 cup steamed 1" asparagus pieces
1½ cups steamed artichoke hearts
4 beaten eggs
1 t. salt
¼ t. grated black pepper
1½ cups half and half
wheat germ or sesame seeds

Prepare pie crust but do not bake. Brush crust with a thin layer of soft butter. Mix together cheese and flour and spread evenly in pie pan. Add veggies. Mix eggs with half and half and spices and pour evenly over the veggies. Sprinkle with wheat germ or sesame seeds and bake at 375° for 40-45 minutes or until set.

Variation: Substitute zucchini and broccoli for asparagus and artichokes.

WONDERFUL WINTER SQUASH

3 acorn or 2 butternut squash
1 small can drained, crushed pineapple
1 large, chopped apple
¼ cup chopped walnuts
1 T. honey or maple syrup
SunButterBlend

Wash, halve, seed and place squashes cut side down in baking pan or cookie sheet with a little water (for steam). Bake at 350° for 45 minutes or until almost tender. Turn cut side up and fill cavities with this mixture: mix pineapple, apples, walnuts and honey or syrup. Spoon into cavities and dot with SunButterBlend. Bake at 350° for 20-30 minutes more until tender. Sprinkle with nutmeg or cinnamon. (Opt.)

Variation: Substitute ½ cup chopped cranberries for pineapple.

DENNY'S DINNER OMELET

3 eggs
2 T. water or milk
dash sea salt/kelp
dash freshly grated pepper
2 T. SunButterBlend
Filling: alfalfa sprouts, green onion slices, avocado slices, shredded Jack cheese, slices of tomatoes, dollop of sour cream

Beat eggs, water or milk and seasonings together. Heat SunButterBlend in large cast iron skillet until it sizzles. Pour in egg mixture, which should start setting up immediately. Lift edges with fork or spatula and tilt pan so uncooked egg mixture will run under to bottom of pan and cook. Turn burner to low. Place filling on half of the omelet. Slip spatula under other half and fold over. Warmth from omelet will melt cheese; keep warm by tipping omelet onto heated plate for table service. Serve with thick slices of beefsteak tomatoes and a dollop of sour cream.

Variations: other fillings: 1. sauteed onions and mushrooms topped with crumbled bleu cheese. 2. steamed broccoli and cauliflower topped with Cheddar cheese. 3. steamed tender asparagus tips topped with Swiss cheese. Another time, try making individual omelets using 1 egg, 1 t. water and 1 t. butter per serving. Cook in a small skillet.

ELEGANT OMELET TORTE: Triple recipe for Denny's Dinner Omelet. Make 3 individual omelets, but do not fold over. Keep warm. Place 1 omelet on a heated serving platter and spread evenly with filling of your choice (see variations). Cover with second omelet and add another layer of filling. Top with third omelet and remaining filling. Sprinkle fresh, chopped parsley over all. Garnish platter with colorful, complimentary vegetables and cut torte in wedges to serve.

MAKE AHEAD CURRY

brown rice, steamed with basil, sage and butter
2-3 cups Mushroom or Cashew Gravy, adding 1-3 t. curry powder
tofu cubes sauteed in butter, tamari-soy sauce, poultry seasoning and garlic powder
Garnishes: chopped tomatoes, green onion bits, chopped peanuts, toasted coconut, crumbled, hard-cooked egg yolks, diced, hard-cooked egg whites, sun sprouts

Steam rice — amount depending on the number of people being served. Prepare gravy. Saute tofu in seasonings and butter. To assemble: spoon some rice in individual bowls. Spoon a little gravy over rice. Spoon some tofu cubes over gravy. Then garnish with your choice of curry condiments. This is a quick and easy dish to prepare for company that should earn you many compliments. Makes a beautiful party buffet. Serve with fresh pineapple strips.

THE ULTIMATE BAKED POTATO

Scrub desired number of large, #1, smooth, good quality baked potatoes. (#2's are often split and discolored in centers, which normally doesn't hurt anything, but for this recipe it would be a disaster!) Oil each potato and wrap in aluminum foil. Bake in a 350° oven for 1 hour or until done in center; remove foil. Slit an X in top of potato and gently press edges with towel-covered fingers, to fluff insides of spud. Have a variety of garments ready to dress your naked potato:

	Sauteed:	**Toasted:**	**Colorful:**
Butter			
Garlic Butter	**Mushrooms**	**Sun Seeds**	**Chopped Egg**
Sour Cream	**Onion Rings**	**Sesame Seeds**	**Green Onions**
Cream Cheese	**Celery Slices**	**Peanuts**	**Chives**
Cottage Cheese	**Broccoli Tips**	**Tamari Almonds**	**Sliced Olives**
Shredded Cheddar	**Tofu Chunks**	**Pepitas**	**TVP Bacon-Bits**
Grated Parmesan	**Asparagus Tips**	**Pine Nuts**	**Nutritional Yeast**

MOUTHWATERING MUFFIN MELT

English Muffins, halved and toasted, become delicious conveyers of vegetables in this easy-going version of the patty melt: Spread warm, toasted, English Muffin halves with soft cream cheese. Top with a slice of tomato and your choice of steamed green veggies — broccoli spears, asparagus spears, French-sliced green beans, baby sweet peas in pods, drained spinach, etc. Mix ¼ to ½ cup *each:* mayonnaise, cream and crumbled bleu OR shredded Cheddar cheese. Dollop on veggies and return to moderate oven until cheese sauce is melted. Add your choice of herbs and seasonings, according to vegetable selection.

VARIATION ON "LA MELODY FRENCH TOAST"

For each serving, you will need: 2 slices whole grain bread, enough cheese of your choice to cover one slice, 4 or 5 thin slices of apple and a few thin slices of onion (rings are nice). Spread bread with mayonnaise, add cheese, apple and onions. Cover with other slice of bread and dip both sides into egg mixture consisting of 1 egg to 1 cup milk and 1 t. prepared mustard. Grill as for French toast, placing in oven for 15 minutes to continue cooking, after browned.

Variation on a variation: Disregard egg/milk mixture. Spread both outsides of sandwich with SunButterBlend and place in a waffle iron. Grill until golden brown and enjoy a very interesting sandwich.

STAN'S STUFFED ZUCCHINI

¾ cup raw millet
2¾ cups hot vegetable stock
4 medium zucchini (cut in half lengthwise)
olive oil
4 chopped mushrooms
3 chopped green onions
2 crushed garlic cloves
3 T. sunflower seeds
1 cup grated Jack cheese
1 cup cottage cheese
2 T. tamari-soy sauce
1 t. crushed basil
dash cayenne
paprika

Stir raw millet in a dry skillet over medium high heat until it begins to brown. Add water, cover, and simmer until moisture is absorbed (about 35-40 minutes). Hollow out each zucchini half, leaving a ¼" border of zucchini to hold shape. Place halves in an oiled 9"x13" pan. Chop unused zucchini pulp into small cubes and saute in olive oil along with mushrooms, green onions, garlic and sun seeds, until barely tender. In a large bowl, mix zucchini-veggie mixture with 1 cup of the cooked millet, grated cheese, cottage cheese, tamari sauce, basil and cayenne. Mix well and spoon generously into zucchini boats. (Leftover mixture can be baked in small, oiled pie tins or custard cups.) Sprinkle everything with paprika and bake at 350° for 35-40 minutes OR make in the morning and refrigerate all day and bake in preheated oven. Freeze remaining millet or save for the next morning's breakfast.

Variations: Substitute cooked brown rice, mashed, cooked soybeans, or cooked lentils for the millet. Substitute cubed, cooked eggplant for the zucchini and spoon into green pepper halves.

MEDITERRANEAN MELT

- **2 chopped, medium onions**
- **6 minced garlic cloves**
- **3-4 thinly sliced celery stalks**
- **12-14 large, chopped mushrooms**
- **½ to ¾ cup sun seed sprouts**
- **1/3 to ½ chopped green pepper**
- **¾ to 1 cup mixed sprouts**
- **oil or butter**
- **3½ to 4 T. tamari-soy sauce**
- **5-6 beaten eggs**
- **3 cups grated Jack cheese**
- **1 scant cup Parmesan cheese**
- **1½ cups cottage cheese**
- **Batter: 3-4 eggs, ¼ cup whole wheat flour, 1½ to 2 cups milk**
- **2 plus eggplants**
- **tomato sauce**

In a wok or skillet saute first 7 ingredients in oil or butter. Add tamari sauce. In a large bowl place eggs, cheeses and mix well. Add saute mixture to cheese mixture in bowl and mix well. Make batter: Mix eggs, flour and milk. Should be fairly thin. Peel and slice at least 2 eggplants into long slices, lengthwise. Each slice should be 1/16" thick. Use a sharp knife. Some slices will be wide and tall and others shorter and not as wide, as you slice through the eggplant. As long as they are very thin, it's okay. Dip each eggplant slice into batter and saute on both sides in hot oil for 3-5 minutes or until slightly browned and soft enough to fold. Drain on paper towels.

To assemble: Spoon 1 heaping T. of saute-cheese mixture onto an eggplant slice. Roll up eggplant from wide to narrow end. Proceed with others. Place seam side down in well-oiled baking dishes (side by side). Sprinkle grated cheese over the tops. Drizzle tomato sauce over rolls. If you don't plan to bake right away, omit the tomato sauce until baking time. Bake at 375° for 20-25 minutes or until melty. If coming from refrigerator, bake at 375°, covered, for 20-25 minutes, and 5-10 minutes, uncovered.

This is an excellent dish for entertaining as it can be prepared the day before. Though it takes time to prepare, the result is an unusual and tasty dish that will be a real conversation piece. Makes enough to serve 15 people.

SUMMERTIME SQUASH

- **1½ cups raw brown rice**
- **3 plus cups water**
- **1 thinly sliced yellow crookneck squash**
- **4 thinly sliced medium zucchini**
- **4 chopped mushrooms**
- **1 large, chopped onion**
- **½ chopped green pepper**
- **butter**
- **1-2 T. hot sauce**
- **½ t. garlic powder**
- **1 T. Worchestershire sauce**
- **3 T. tamari-soy sauce**
- **1 t. crushed basil**
- **2 8 oz. cans tomato sauce**
- **3 cups grated Jack cheese**
- **fresh, chopped tomatoes**
- **1 recipe Crusty Topping**
- **Parmesan cheese**

Steam rice in water until absorbed. Saute veggies in butter until barely tender. Mix rice in a large bowl with seasonings, then spoon mixture in bottom of 2 oiled casseroles. Add the squash mixture and spread evenly. Pour tomato sauce over casseroles. Top with cheese, tomatoes and Crusty Topping. Sprinkle Parmesan over all and bake for 25 minutes at 350°. Cover loosely with foil while baking.

SOUTH INDIA UPMA

- **¼ cup oil**
- **1 t. mustard seed**
- **½ cup chopped almonds or cashews**
- **1 chopped onion**
- **½ chopped green pepper**
- **1½ cups bulgur or 4 grain cereal**
- **3 cups boiling water**
- **1 t. sea salt**
- **1 T. curry powder**
- **¼ t. chili powder**
- **1 t. cumin**
- **1 t. coriander**
- **1 t. caraway seeds**
- **2 cups mixed veggies (fresh steamed or leftover)**
- **plain yogurt**
- **applesauce**

Saute mustard seed and nuts in oil. Then add onion and green pepper and stir until barely tender. Add bulgur or cereal and stir until slightly browned. Slowly pour in water and stir well. Add seasonings and veggies. Simmer, covered, until bulgur or cereal is soft and fluffy. Serve with plain yogurt or applesauce. Very delicious and spicy!

Variations: Use ¾ cup raw millet in place of bulgur or 3 cups of cooked millet and omit water OR use about 3 cups of cooked mixture of lentils and rice. Omit water or use just enough to help cook veggies and soften grains.

MILLET-STUFFED GREEN PEPPERS

4-5 chopped mushrooms
2-3 chopped green onions or
¼ cup chopped onion
2 mashed garlic cloves
½ cup chopped celery
thyme to taste
sage to taste
parsley to taste
1-2 T. tamari-soy sauce
3 to 3½ cups cooked millet
½ small can tomato paste
2 eggs
½ cup cottage cheese
4 green peppers, cut in half lengthwise
tomato slices
sliced Jack or Cheddar cheese
Gomazio

In a large skillet, saute first 8 ingredients in butter or oil until tender. Stir in millet, tomato paste, eggs and cottage cheese. Remove seeds from peppers. Parboil in boiling water until they begin to turn color, but are still crisp. Place drained pepper halves in oiled oblong pan and spoon millet-veggie mixture into each half. Lay tomato slices on top of each along with a slice of cheese on top of tomato slices. Sprinkle with Gomazio and bake at 350° for 20-30 minutes. Very tasty and colorful. Can be prepared in morning and baked in evening.

Variation: If you like, omit parboiling of peppers. Substitute Hearty Spaghetti Sauce for tomato paste and rice for millet.

SUNFLOWER CABBAGE ROLLS

3 T. oil
1 medium, cubed zucchini
3 mashed garlic cloves
1 small, chopped onion
3 T. toasted sun seeds
2 T. tamari-soy sauce
3 cups cooked, brown rice
1 cup cottage cheese
¾ cup grated Jack cheese
½ t. crushed basil
sea salt/kelp to taste
cayenne to taste
parboiled cabbage leaves
1 8 oz. can tomato sauce

Saute veggies in oil; then add sun seeds, tamari sauce and rice. Stir in cottage cheese, Jack cheese, basil, salt and cayenne. Spoon into cabbage leaves and roll, placing each face down in an oiled 9"x13" pan. Pour tomato sauce over all and bake at 350° for 20-30 minutes or until bubbly.

Variation: Use mashed soybeans or cooked millet in place of rice.

BUSY DAY BUCKWHEAT DINNER

2 cups boiling vegetable water
1 cup hulled, raw buckwheat
3 T. SunButterBlend
2 T. tamari-soy sauce
1 chopped onion
2 stalks finely sliced celery
2 minced garlic cloves
½ cup sunflower seeds

In cast iron skillet, dry-toast buckwheat, and while still hot, pour buckwheat into veggie water; bring to a boil, cover, turn burner off and let sit. Saute onion, celery, garlic and sun seeds in butter and tamari sauce. When buckwheat has absorbed liquid (15-20 minutes), add sauteed veggie mixture and toss lightly. Serve immediately with a mound of herbed whipped potatoes and steamed broccoli or brussel sprouts.

Variation: Add 1 egg to buckwheat mixture and pack firmly into an oiled pie plate that has been dusted with wheat germ. Top with the herbed potatoes like a shepherd's pie. Shred a little cheese on top and put under broiler to lightly brown. OR stuff into partially steamed green peppers.

Dine like royalty at breakfast time,
At lunch, enjoy full measure.
But serve the evening meal on a smaller plate;
Eat simply, happily and at your leisure.

LOAVES

CREATE YOUR OWN LOAF

In a large bowl, measure one choice of ingredients from each group, mix well and pack into an oiled loaf pan. Bake 1 hour at 350° F. Melt cheese on top the last few minutes or slice and serve with a gravy.

1. 2 cups cooked, mashed beans: kidney, lentils, pinto, soy, lima, etc.
2. 1 cup grain: steamed brown rice, bulgur, barley or millet OR rolled oats, whole grain bread crumbs, wheat germ, flaked bran or corn meal.
3. ½-1 cup nuts or seeds (chopped or ground): almonds, brazil, cashews, walnuts, sunflower seeds, peanuts, etc.
4. Binding: 1 or 2 eggs, 1 small grated raw potato, 3 T. arrowroot, ¼ cup grated raw yam, ½ cup cooked oatmeal or rice, ¼ cup tapioca, OR ½ cup mashed tofu.
5. Liquid (1-1½ cups as needed to make a meat loaf-consistency): tomato paste with water, V-8 juice, nut milks, gravy, vegetable stock, etc.
6. ½-1 cup vegetables: In a small skillet, saute 1 small, chopped onion in 3-4 T. butter, along with your choice of the following herbs and seasonings. Optional: Saute 1 grated carrot, 1 thinly sliced celery stalk, 3-4 sliced mushrooms, and/or 3 T. chopped green pepper, along with the onions.
7. Herbs and Seasonings (½-1 t. of 1 or more): Italian Herb Mix, sweet basil, cumin, chili powder, sage, tamari-soy sauce, vegetable seasoning, Bakon yeast, parsley, etc. (See Kitchen Keys for use of seasonings.)

SIMPLE SIMON SAYS

3 T. SunButterBlend
1½ cups chopped celery
1½ cups chopped onions
½ cup chopped walnuts
1 cup cashew pieces
¼ t. crushed basil
¼ t. sage
¼ cup rolled oats
1 cup cottage cheese
1 cup grated Jack cheese
3 eggs
½ cup ground almonds
½ cup ground sunflower seeds
½ cup cooked, brown rice

In butter, saute celery, onions, walnuts, cashews, basil and sage. In a large bowl, mix oats, cottage cheese, Jack, eggs, almonds, sun seeds and rice. Add saute to oat-nut mixture and pack in well-oiled 8"x8" pan. If desired, top with tomato sauce and more grated cheese. Bake 45 minutes to 1 hour at 350°. Great served with Mushroom Gravy.

LENTIL-NUT LOAF

2 cups dried, rinsed lentils
2 cups dried, rinsed split peas
8 cups boiling stock
1 t. oil
1 cup dry Mama Bear's Porridge
(See Better Beginnings) **cooked in**
2 cups water for 5-8 minutes
4 medium grated carrots
2 large grated onions
3 grated garlic cloves
3 stalks grated celery
½ grated green pepper
1¼ cups grated walnuts
1¼ cups grated sunflower seeds
1¼ cups grated cashews
1 12 oz. can tomato sauce
4 t. sage
3 t. crushed basil
3 t. sea salt/kelp
¼ t. cayenne
½ t. thyme
½ t. oregano
¼ t. garlic powder
3 t. chili powder
1½ t. cumin
grated Jack cheese

Simmer lentils and split peas, covered, in water and oil for 35-40 minutes. Cook porridge in water for 5-8 minutes. In the largest bowl you can find, mix veggies, nuts and seeds. Mash lentils-split peas with a hand potato masher and add to the bowl along with the porridge. Mixture will be mushy. Add tomato paste and herbs and seasonings. Mix well with a wooden spoon or hands. Spoon into 4-5 oiled loaf pans. Pans should be ½ to 2/3's full. If baking for a large crowd, bake, uncovered, at 350° for 1 hour. Then sprinkle on grated Jack and bake 10-15 minutes more. If freezing loaves, bake at 350° for 35-40 minutes. Cool slightly; cover with foil and freeze. To reheat: defrost halfway and bake at 350° for 40-50 minutes, sprinkling with grated cheese the last 10 minutes.

Variation: Use 2 small grated raw potatoes and 2-3 bread slices, blender ground in place of the porridge.

WHAT YOU CAN DO WITH LEFTOVER LENTIL LOAF

1. Use as a sandwich spread with mayonnaise, catsup and grated cheese.
2. Use with rice in stuffed cabbage rolls or stuffed peppers.
3. Spread on oven-crisped tortilla shells; add grated cheese and heat in oven.
4. Use in pocket bread with sprouts or in a Roll-Around.
5. **Lentil "Sausage":** Mix 1 t. honey, 1 t. tamari-soy sauce, 1 t. minced garlic, ½ t. prepared mustard, 2 dashes oregano, 1 dash allspice, 1 dash cayenne. Start with 1 t. of seasoning mixture. Thoroughly mash into 2 cups leftover lentil loaf. Taste and continue to add seasoning until it tastes like you want your "sausage" to taste. Shape into links or patties and brown in oil in heavy skillet. Serve with breakfast or as a dinner with potatoes, onions and spiced apples. Make less spicy for children.
6. **Egg-in-a-loaf:** Add some sage and mix well. Press mixture thinly to line the bottoms and sides of well-oiled muffin tins, individual pottery bowls or heat-proof custard cups. Break an egg into center of each cup and heat in 350° oven for 10-15 minutes. Last few minutes top with a Jack cheese strip and paprika OR sprinkle with basil and insert a sprig of fresh parsley just before serving.
   Variation: Line bottoms and sides as above with lentil loaf mixture. Spoon in 1 T. of chile salsa; then break egg.
7. **Lentil Loaf French Toast:** Spread 1 slice of bread with SunButterBlend, the other slice with good catsup; spread lentil loaf on one slice and cover with other. Dip sandwich in egg mixture and grill as you would French toast. Egg Mixture: 3 eggs beaten with 3 cups milk.
8. **Lentil-Cottage Enchiladas:** Mix equal parts lentil loaf and cottage cheese. Add some chopped green chiles, shredded Cheddar cheese and a little Enchilada Sauce. Fill prepared corn tortillas, roll up and place seam-side down in baking dish. Pour more sauce over all and top with more cheese. Heat through and serve with a dollop of sour cream.

BETTER BOLOGNA-HEALTHIER HOT DOGS

¼ cup almonds
1 cup sunflower seeds
½ cup rolled oats
½ t. coriander seeds
1 t. celery flakes
2 t. minced, dried onion
1 t. parsley flakes
3 T. potato flour
OR 1 T. tapioca
2 T. powdered milk
½ cup whole wheat flour
1 t. Bakon yeast
½-1 t. cumin powder
½-1 t. chili powder
½ t. Italian Herb Mix
½ t. sage
½ t. mace
1-1½ t. garlic powder
1 t. sea salt/kelp
dash cayenne
1 t. paprika
½ t. curry powder
½ t. oregano
1 t. dry mustard
1 T. vinegar
1 T. honey
1½ cups hot water
½ cup peanut butter
¼ cup tomato paste
1 t. Liquid Smoke
1 T. tamari-soy sauce

Blender-grind the almonds, sun seeds, oats, coriander, celery flakes, minced onion, parsley flakes, potato flour or tapioca and powdered milk. Place in a large bowl and add the remaining dry ingredients and spices. Stir well. Mix liquids and pour over all and mix very well. Pour into 3 well-oiled pint canning jars and pack well. Place lid on and seal loosely with canning ring. Place jars on rack in large pan and add water to ¾'s level of jars. Cover and boil gently for 2 hours. Cool. When ready to eat, remove carefully from jar. Slice in thin round slices for Better Bologna. Cut lengthwise into long wedges or sticks for Healthier Hot Dogs and heat in oven. Cube or dice for macaroni or vegetable dishes.

BURGERS OR PATTIES

Most of these patties are mixed in a large bowl to burger consistency. They may be sauteed quickly in a small amount of oil or butter, or oven baked at 350° on a cookie sheet, turning once, until browned. They may be served on whole wheat burger buns or open-faced on ½ a bun or toast, topped with slices of tomatoes and onions and a Thousand Island dressing. They may be served on the plate plain, or accompanied with a gravy or sauce and steamed veggies. A thin slice of cheese and a heap of alfalfa sprouts are great between the buns or atop the stately open-faced sandwich.

CHEESY NUT BURGERS

- 2 cups chopped nuts
- 1 mashed garlic clove
- ½ cup wheat germ
- ¼ cup ground sesame seeds
- ¼ cup ground sun seeds
- 1 small, chopped onion
- ½ cup cottage cheese
- ½ cup grated cheese
- 2 beaten eggs
- 1 t. salt
- 1 t. chili powder
- ⅛ t. curry powder or cumin
- a few chopped mushrooms

Mix all ingredients together and form into patties. Cook as suggested above.

OAT NUT BURGERS

- 3 T. butter
- ¼ cup finely chopped onion
- 1 cup whole wheat bread crumbs
- 1 cup cooked oatmeal
- 1 egg
- 1 cup chopped walnuts
- 1½ t. tamari-soy sauce
- ½ t. thyme
- ¼ t. sage
- 2-4 T. ground, roasted sun seeds
- tomato sauce

Saute onion in butter until tender. Remove and put in a bowl. Add remaining ingredients, using enough tomato sauce to make a good consistency. Shape into 6 patties, cook, and serve with flower vegetable: broccoli, cauliflower, asparagus.

MAMA'S VEGGIE BURGERS

- ½ to ¾ cup cooked, brown rice
- 1 to 1½ cups cooked, mashed beans
- ¼ cup chopped sun seeds
- 1 T. soy flour
- 1 T. flaked bran
- 2-4 finely chopped mushrooms
- ¼ to ½ cup grated Cheddar cheese
- 1-2 T. dried, minced onion
- ⅛ t. garlic powder
- ½ to ¾ t. chili powder
- 1 T. catsup
- ½ to 1 t. sea salt/kelp
- 1 T. chopped cashews
- 1 egg
- 1 T. sesame seeds

Mix together, shape into patties and sprinkle sesame seeds on one side. Saute in safflower oil, turning once when golden brown.

MILLER'S MUTTLETS

- 1 cup finely chopped mushrooms
- 2 minced green onions
- 2 slices whole grain bread, blender ground
- ¾ cup grated Cheddar cheese
- 1 T. tamari-soy sauce
- 2 eggs

Mix together, form into silver dollar-sized patties and saute in butter at medium heat. Makes 8 small patties. Even people who aren't overly enthusiastic about mushrooms will like these.

SUNBURGERS

- ½ cup grated carrots
- ½ cup finely chopped celery
- 2 chopped green onions
- 1 T. chopped parsley
- 2 T. chopped green pepper
- 1 beaten egg
- 1 T. oil
- ¼ cup V-8 juice
- 1 cup ground sun seeds
- 2 T. wheat germ
- ½ t. salt
- ⅛ t. basil

Mix well and bake in oiled pan for 15 minutes each side at 350°. Makes 4 large patties.

Variation: Substitute grated, raw yam for carrot and add 1½ cups cooked millet and an extra egg to above mixture.

LENTIL PATTIES

- 1 to 1½ cups cooked lentils
- 1 grated carrot
- 2 stalks finely chopped celery
- ½ to 1 cup finely grated green cabbage
- ½ to 1 cup whole grain bread crumbs
- 2 beaten eggs
- 1 t. sea salt/kelp
- dash cayenne

Mix well, form into patties and bake at 350° in oiled baking pan for 10 minutes per side or until cabbage is cooked and patties are firm. Tastes great with cheese and Creamy Tomato Sauce.

TASTY SOYBURGERS

- 2½ to 3 cups cooked, ground soybeans (use meat grinder)
- 2 T. fresh, chopped parsley
- 1 carrot
- 1 small onion
- 1 small handful raw sunflower seeds
- 1 small handful cashews
- 1-2 T. sesame seeds
- 2-3 T. oil
- 1-2 eggs
- 2 T. whole wheat flour
- 2 T. corn meal
- ½ t. garlic powder
- 1 T. minced onion if omitting fresh onion
- 4 finely chopped mushrooms
- 1-2 T. tamari-soy sauce
- 3 dashes cayenne
- ½ t. sea salt/kelp
- Jack cheese

Grind soybeans, parsley, carrot, onion, walnuts and cashews in meat grinder. Mix well with remaining ingredients, except cheese. Bake or saute. At last minute place a thin slice of cheese on each pattie. These patties may be pre-formed and frozen for camping trips. Then slightly defrost and saute.

Variation: Pat mixture into oiled loaf pan and bake at 350° for 1 hour and 10 minutes. Let cool 10 minutes and slice.

CHEESEBURGERS

- 1½ cups dried lentils
- 1 cup raw, brown rice
- 1 chopped onion
- 3 minced garlic cloves
- 1 t. sea salt/kelp
- ½ t. oil
- 5¼ cups boiling vegetable stock
- 2 t. sage
- 1 cup ground sun seeds
- flour
- butter
- Cheddar cheese

Simmer, covered, the oil, lentils, rice, onion, garlic and salt, for 35 minutes or until tender and still soupy. Add sage. Take *2 cups* of this mixture and add sun seeds. Mix well. Add a little flour if necessary, to make mixture the consistency of ground beef. Shape into patties and saute in buttered skillet. Serve on open-faced buns with a thin slice of cheese, mayonnaise, catsup and sprouts. Delicious!

Variation: With remaining lentil-rice mixture, add 1 small can of tomato sauce and a handful of finely ground walnuts. If thicker consistency is needed, add some ground sun seeds. Pack into small loaf pans and bake at 350° for 45 minutes. Freeze or use as a sandwich spread OR prepare Cheeseburgers as indicated and bake in an oiled pan with Creamy Tomato Sauce poured over. Bake 20-25 minutes at 350°.

FROM THE SEA

BAKED RED SNAPPER

- 1 lb. red snapper
- 1 beaten egg
- a little milk
- 1 cup dry Mama Bear's porridge or flour or wheat germ
- 2-3 T. sesame seeds
- several dashes paprika
- several dashes garlic powder
- several dashes vegetable salt
- melted SunButterBlend

Cut snapper into 1½" chunks. Dip into a mixture of egg and milk. Place chunks in a paper bag (a few at a time) that contains porridge, wheat germ or flour, and seasonings. Shake, remove and place, separated, in a buttered casserole dish. Bake at 425° for about 15 minutes or until browned and flaky.

Variation: Drizzle SunButterBlend over each chunk before baking and broil the last 2 minutes of baking time for a crispy, browned top.

COAST-TO-COAST QUICHE

2 large, thinly sliced onions
¾ cup finely chopped celery
3 T. SunButterBlend
1 cup fresh mung bean sprouts
½ t. crushed thyme
1 baked 9" pastry shell
2 cups shredded Cheddar cheese
1 cup cooked crab, salmon or shrimp
Sauce:
4 eggs
½ cup milk
2 T. flour
1 t. vegetable salt
pinch cayenne

Saute onions and celery in SunButterBlend. Remove from heat and stir in bean sprouts and thyme. Sprinkle half the cheese over pie crust; layer half the onion-sprout mixture over cheese; then all of your choice of fish; then cover with remaining onion-sprout mixture and cheese. For sauce: beat eggs with milk, flour and seasonings. Pour over all ingredients in pie. Bake at 350° until custard appears firm in center or about 40-45 minutes. Let stand 10 minutes before serving.

SEAFOOD SOUFFLE

2 cups cooked, flaked fish (sole, halibut, haddock, perch)
2 T. lemon juice
1 t. vegetable salt
½ t. dried, minced onion
½ t. dill
dash cayenne
4 beaten egg yolks
double recipe Basic White Sauce
4 whipped egg whites (stiff)
2-4 T. wheat germ or bread crumbs
Yogurt Dill Sauce

Combine fish with next 5 ingredients. Stir in beaten egg yolks and Basic White Sauce; then fold whipped egg whites carefully into mixture. Line a 1½ quart, buttered casserole or souffle dish with wheat germ or bread crumbs. Spoon in souffle mixture. Bake at 375° for 30 minutes or until knife inserted comes out clean. Serve in wedges with **Yogurt Dill Sauce:** Combine 1 cup plain yogurt with 1 T. finely chopped green onions and ½ t. dill.

DILLED SALMON LOAF

16 oz. cooked salmon, with juice
1 cup dry bread crumbs
1 medium onion, minced
½ cup chopped, fresh parsley
½ cup ground sunflower seeds
½ cup flaked bran
1 egg
1 T. fresh lemon juice
2 dashes each vegetable salt and fresh grated pepper
½ t. crushed dill weed
1 T. Bakon yeast (opt.)

Thoroughly mix all ingredients. If necessary, add more bread crumbs to make a firm loaf. Shape into oiled loaf pan and bake at 350° for 40 minutes.

SCRAMBLED SALMON

2 T. SunButterBlend
¼ cup *each* finely minced onion and celery
8 oz. salmon, drained and flaked
2 T. mayonnaise
dash cayenne
6 eggs, well beaten

Saute onion and celery in SunButterBlend until soft. Add salmon and while it heats beat eggs with mayonnaise and cayenne. Pour in eggs and scramble until eggs are set. Serve on heated platter surrounded by steamed broccoli spears and raw carrot curls.

SMOKEY SALMON SPREAD

8 oz. softened cream cheese
8 oz. salmon, drained and flaked
2 t. Bakon yeast
½ t. crushed dill weed
½ t. prepared horseradish (opt.)
2 T. minced onion (opt.)

Mash all ingredients together until well blended. Spread on warm whole wheat bagel for "mock" lox. Or thin with juice reserved from salmon and use as a dip for veggies.

SUNNY CHEDDAR-SALMON LOAF

2 cups cooked salmon
1 T. minced onion
½ cup finely diced celery
1 egg
½ cup grated Cheddar cheese
½ cup milk
2 T. powdered milk
2 cups soft crumbs OR ½ cup flour plus ½ cup ground sunflower seeds
1 T. melted butter
sea salt/kelp to taste
OR 1-2 t. tamari-soy sauce

In a large bowl, mix together all ingredients. Pack into an oiled loaf pan or shape into a fish on an oiled cookie sheet. Bake at 350° for 45-55 minutes. Garnish with additional cheese 10 minutes before removing from oven. Serve with mushroom or onion gravy, steamed rice and green peas.

THE CREPERY — USA

BASIC CREPES

6 eggs
1 1/3 cups whole wheat pastry flour
2 cups milk
butter

In a blender, blend eggs with flour until smooth. Gradually blend in milk. In a 7″ or 8″ skillet on medium-low heat, swirl ¼ t. butter. When melted, pour in about 1½ to 2 T. crepe batter, tilting pan until it flows quickly over entire flat surface. Crepe should set at once, forming tiny bubbles. Cook until edge is lightly browned; then loosen edges with spatula and flip over to brown other side. Repeat for each crepe, stirring batter *often.* Stack crepes atop each other. Allow to come to room temperature before separating. Makes about 3 dozen crepes. Keep covered in refrigerator until used or wrap carefully and freeze.

EGGPLANT CREPES

2 cups steamed cubed eggplant
1 T. dried, minced onion
1 T. fresh, chopped parsley
grated Parmesan or Jack cheese
Cheese Sauce or Creamy Tomato Sauce
Basic Crepes

Mix first 3 ingredients. Spoon onto crepes, top with grated cheese and fold in half. Place 2 or 3 on each plate and spoon gravy or sauce over.

MUSHROOM SPINACH CREPES

Jack cheese
Cashew Gravy or White Sauce
Basic Crepes
Topping:
1 lb. mushrooms, 1 large, chopped onion, 1 large, or 2 small bunches of cleaned, dried and torn spinach, and 3 T. SunButterBlend

Roll pre-made crepes around fingers of Jack cheese. Lay side by side in oiled oblong pan. Prepare one recipe Cashew Gravy or Basic White Sauce; pour over crepes and heat in 325° oven for 15 minutes while you prepare topping. Topping: Saute mushrooms, onion and spinach in SunButterBlend. Spoon over crepes and serve when cheese is soft.

Variation: Substitute asparagus or broccoli for spinach.

DESSERT CREPES: Fill crepes with applesauce, fresh mashed berries or other fruit, chopped nuts, dates, melted butter and cinnamon and honey. Fold in half or roll and dollop with yogurt or whipped cream. Or stack in layers, pile whipped cream around top and garnish with whole fresh fruit and mint leaves.

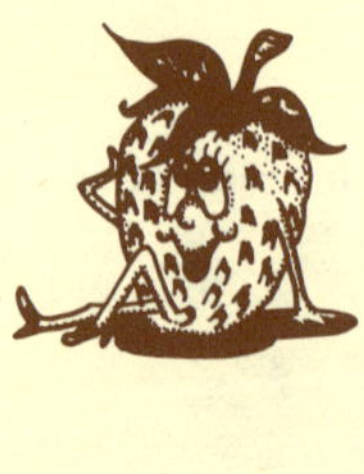

ORIENTAL OFFERINGS

FOR SUCCESSFUL STIR-FRYS OR WOKS

1. Quickly stir-fry sliced onions, mashed garlic cloves, and herbs.
2. Add hard vegetables; after a few minutes add medium veggies; then in the last few minutes of cooking, add soft veggies.
3. Stir in the sauce until thickened: Sauce is 1 c. cold water or broth mixed with 1-2 T. arrowroot, dash powdered ginger, 2-4 T. tamari-soy sauce and a little honey.
4. Add mung bean sprouts and mixed sprouts the last few minutes of cooking and cover and steam for a few minutes.
5. Serve over hot brown rice.

HARD VEGGIES: (12-15 minutes cooking time) green beans, celery, carrots, broccoli, cabbage, cauliflower, kale, bok choy, green tomatoes, potatoes.

MEDIUM VEGGIES: (8-10 minutes cooking time) asparagus, mushrooms, snow peas, green peas, zucchini, yellow summer squash, eggplant, radishes, corn, red tomatoes.

SOFT VEGGIES: (3-4 minutes cooking time) spinach, chinese cabbage, beet greens, Swiss chard, scallions, sprouts, green peppers, onions, water chestnuts, edible-pod peas.

NUTSY ORANGE AND GREEN RICE

½ cube butter
2 stalks chopped celery
6-8 sliced green onions
3 large, finely chopped mushrooms
1 t. vegetable salt
dash garlic powder
1 grated carrot
4-6 sprigs fresh, chopped parsley
1 handful chopped walnuts
1 handful cashews
2 T. each oil and tamari-soy sauce
2-3 cups cooked brown rice

In a skillet, melt butter and saute celery, onions and mushrooms. Add seasonings when mushrooms are tender; then add carrot and parsley. Stir in nuts and saute in a little more butter in 1 section of skillet while other veggies are pushed to one side. Remove everything from skillet and spoon into a large bowl. Now add oil and tamari sauce to skillet and stir-fry rice until it browns. After 5 minutes, add the veggie-nut mixture; stir together and serve. Makes a chewy, colorful main dish.

Variation: Substitute millet for rice.

AWARENESS WOK

1 sliced onion
2 minced garlic cloves
¼″ piece fresh ginger
½ sliced green pepper
½ to 1 cup chopped broccoli (flowers and stalks)
½ cup chopped Jerusalem artichoke
1-2 stalks chopped celery
1 diagonally sliced carrot
1 small cubed yam
1 cubed potato
½ cup cauliflowerets
3-4 sliced green onions
Sauce:
1 cup stock, ¼ cup tamari-soy sauce, ⅛ cup honey, 2-3 T. arrowroot, ⅛ t. dry mustard
sesame seeds
bean sprouts

Peel the root vegetables. Cut all veggies on the diagonal. Slice the *hard* veggies thinner than the *soft* veggies so that cooking time will be equal. Peel the ginger, then slice and mince. Saute ginger, garlic and onion in skillet or large wok in hot oil. Add other veggies. Stir and flip veggies, adding enough water to steam. Cover and steam, stirring occasionally, until barely tender. Add sauce to wok: Mix sauce ingredients and stir with veggies until thickened. Top with sesame seeds and serve with bean sprouts over rice.

Variation: Add bean sprouts to vegetables during steaming.

H2O-CRESS AND H2O-CHESTNUT SALAD: If you have access to fresh water or overland cress, you will delight in this zesty accompaniment to any Oriental main dish. Prepare ½ cup *each:* sliced clelery, diagonally cut tender green beans, edible-pod peas, sliced fresh mushrooms, chopped water chestnuts, chopped watercress, shredded jicama and mung bean sprouts. Toss with a tamari-oil mixture or dollop with seed yogurt. Sprinkle lavishly with toasted sesame seeds.

LANI'S EGGPLANT EGG ROLLS

1 bunch grated celery (2½ cups)
4-6 sliced mushrooms
2 sliced green onions
½ diced green pepper
½ can sliced and chopped water chestnuts
¾ to 1 cup adzuki-mung-lentil sprouts (2 day old)
1 handful 5 day old mung bean sprouts
oil
2 cups cubed eggplant (about half eggplant)
3 T. tamari-soy sauce
1/3 cup celery water
½ t. ginger
2-3 t. arrowroot
2/3 cup water
dashes garlic powder, kelp, cayenne
Egg Roll Skins:
2 cups sifted whole wheat pastry flour, 2 beaten eggs, 2 cups water plus 2 T.

In a food processor or grater grate one bunch of celery. Place celery mixture in boiling water (½-¾ cup) and cover for 5 minutes. Drain through strainer, pressing out liquids. *Reserve* liquid. Saute next 6 ingredients in oil in large skillet or wok, adding celery when veggies begin to soften. Add eggplant, tamari, ginger, spices and arrowroot that has been mixed with water. After mixture is tender-crisp, remove from heat and cool slightly. (Be sure there is very little liquid left in wok.)

In a blender prepare Egg Roll Skins by blending eggs, water and flour until smooth. Heat a 7" or 8" cast iron skillet and with a spatula, spread about ¼ t. butter around a pan. Turn burner to medium. When butter is melted, pour in about ¼ cup batter or just enough to spread to the sides when pan is tilted. Batter and egg roll is thicker than a crepe. When sides look dry, turn egg roll over and cook other side. Do not brown or they will become too stiff. Every few egg rolls, butter skillet.

To assemble: Lay an egg roll skin on a plate. Using slotted spoon place about 2 T. of veggie mixture in center of roll and spread slightly. Begin to roll up, tucking ends inside roll as you roll. Place seam side down on well-oiled shallow pan. Bake at 350° for 30 minutes. If desired, brush tops with oil or butter before baking and bake until hot and browned.

Variation: Quickly fry in small amount of hot oil until golden. Drain and serve. Egg Roll recipe makes about 1½ dozen 7" rolls. Make a double batch for more rolls, ahead of time, cover well, and refrigerate until time to assemble.

FOR ITALIAN "ROME-ANTICS"

GRILLED EGGPLANT STEAKS

1 eggplant
½ cup olive oil
½ cup sunflower oil
3-4 crushed, minced garlic cloves

Slice unpeeled eggplant into ¾" slices. Brush both sides of each slice with a mixture of the oils and garlic. Place slices on grill and grill each side about 5-8 minutes, or until browned.

BAKED STUFFED EGGPLANT

2 medium eggplants
butter or olive oil
2 crushed garlic cloves
1 medium, chopped onion
½ cup chopped mushrooms
1 cup cooked brown rice
1 cup cottage cheese
1 cup grated Jack cheese
¼ cup ground nuts
¼ cup toasted sun seeds
sea salt/kelp to taste
½ t. crushed basil
paprika
Crumbly Topping

Slice eggplants in half lengthwise and bake them face-down on an oiled cookie sheet at 350° for 20 minutes. Scoop out the insides, leaving ¼" around edges and mash or mince the insides in a large bowl. In a skillet, saute garlic, onion and mushrooms in oil or butter. Then add the eggplant pulp and saute a little longer. Add rice, cheeses, nuts, seeds and seasonings. Stuff eggplant shells with mixture; dust with paprika, and sprinkle with Crumbly Topping. Bake at 350° for 35-40 minutes. Serves 4 hearty appetites or scooped out as a side dish will serve 6.

Variation: Substitute Cheddar for Jack cheese, and ricotta for cottage cheese.

IT'S-A BEST-A LASAGNA

1 recipe Hearty Spaghetti Sauce
2 T. *each* flour and water, mixed
2 cups diced eggplant OR
sliced baby zucchini (opt.)
8 oz. whole wheat or spinach lasagna noodles
1 cup grated Parmesan or Romano cheese
1 lb. ricotta or cottage cheese
¼ cup chopped parsley
2 eggs, beaten
½ lb. Mozarella cheese, sliced

Prepare Hearty Spaghetti Sauce and thicken with flour/water mixture, stirring constantly. Add eggplant or zucchini, if you choose; cover and keep warm. Cook noodles in boiling, salted water until tender; drain. Mix eggs and parsley with ricotta cheese. Spread a thin layer of sauce on a 9″x13″ baking dish. Using ¼ of each, build up lasagna in layers: noodles, sauce, ricotta mixture, Mozarella slices, grated Parmesan. Repeat, ending with Parmesan. Bake at 350° for 40 minutes and allow to cool for 10 minutes for easier cutting. Cut in squares to expose layers and serve with a tossed green salad and thick slices of garlic-buttered toast.

Variation: Substitute steamed spinach for veggies and mix with cheeses. Spread on noodles and roll up like a pin wheel; stand on edge in pan and pour sauce over all.

DIANE'S NOODLES ROMA

¼ cup SunButterBlend
½ cup finely chopped parsley
8 oz. cream cheese
¼ cup vegetable stock (onion is best)
1 t. basil, rubbed between fingers
2 dashes *each* vegetable salt and fresh grated pepper
8 oz. thin wh/wheat or spinach noodles
3 minced garlic cloves
1/3 cup SunButterBlend
1 cup grated Romano or Parmesan cheese

Combine first six ingredients in top of double boiler and mix with a whip until well blended; keep warm. Cook noodles in boiling, salted water until tender; drain. Saute garlic in SunButterBlend and pour over noodles, tossing lightly to coat well. Sprinkle with ½ of Romano cheese and toss again. Pile noodles on hot serving platter; spoon parsley sauce over the top and sprinkle with remaining Romano. Serve with Unforgettable Fresh Spinach Salad.

SATURDAY NIGHT MUNG SPROUT SPAGHETTI (NO PASTA!)

2 sliced green onions
4 chopped mushrooms
1 chopped stalk celery
1 T. tamari-soy sauce
butter
¼ to ½ cup water
½ to 1 cup Mixed Sprouts
4 loose cups fresh mung bean sprouts
Hearty Spaghetti Sauce
2 t. chili powder

In a large skillet, saute onions, mushrooms, celery in butter and tamari sauce. When tender, add water and Mixed Sprouts. Cover skillet and steam for 8-12 minutes or until tender with a slight crunch. Prepare Spaghetti Sauce, adding chili powder for added spiciness. To serve, place a handful of mung bean sprouts in each bowl. Using a slotted spoon dish out the sprout-veggie mixture into each bowl. Spoon some sauce over all and eat with chopstix. Optional: If you wish the sprouts to have a spaghetti-like texture, steam them with the mixed sprouts, but they are more nutritious uncooked.

Variation: Add diced eggplant or cooked garbanzo beans for "meaty" texture.

MUNG SPROUTS FOR SATURDAY NITE MUNG SPROUT SPAGHETTI

For salads, mung beans can be sprouted in 2 to 3 days to a sweet, tender crunchiness. But for this recipe and many Chinese dishes, you may want them nice and fat. If you just let them grow longer, the roots would get long and spindley instead of plump. Follow these directions for growing plump and crisp bean sprouts:

1. Soak 1/3 cup mung beans in a large 1½ quart jar (a 46 oz. peanut butter jar works fine) overnight. In the morning rinse, drain and keep the jar inverted all day, with a piece of nylon attached to the opening by a rubber band or canning jar ring. Rinse 3 times this first day.
2. On the second day, rinse, drain, and place a tall, thin jar filled with water inside the jar of sprouts (serves as a weight). Rinse only mornings and evenings now, and keep sprouts in a dark cupboard (making sure to drain well after each rinse).
3. By the fifth or sixth day, they will be long, thick, white, crispy and delicious.

MIXED SPROUTS

1. Soak ¼ cup of a mixture of adzuki, lentil and soy beans overnight.
2. In morning, drain, rinse, drain and invert. Rinse twice daily. By the second or third day, when the sprouts are as long as the beans, rinse, drain, and refrigerate.

ALMOST AS QUICK AS A PIZZA PARLOR PIZZA

1 recipe Super Duper Refrigerator Biscuit dough (See *Labor of Love Lunches*) OR
2 cups Snappy-Quick Mix mixed with 3 T. oil, ½ cup milk, up to 2 T. water
Easy Pizza Sauce (See this Chapter) but add 1 small can tomato paste and 1 extra t. Italian Herb Mix to Sauce
Mozzerella or Jack cheese
Parmesan cheese
Toppings: chopped black olives and green onions, mushroom slices and green pepper strips, circles of thinly sliced zucchini and tomato, sun sprouts and mixed sprouts (opt.)

Prepare Super Duper Biscuit dough OR Snappy-Quick Mix as stated above. After adding oil, milk and water to Snappy-Quick, the dough should be consistency of pie crust dough and not too sticky. Oil a round pizza pan or cookie sheet *and* your hands. Roll or press dough to make a thin crust. Spread Pizza Sauce evenly over crust. Add your choice of toppings (see above) and lay thin slices of Mozzerella or Jack cheese on top. Sprinkle with Parmesan cheese. Bake in a preheated 425° oven for 15 minutes or until bubbly. Garnish with sun sprouts and mixed sprouts if desired. Serves 6 average appetites or 4 super-hungry persons.

OTHER FANTASTIC TOPPINGS: Thinly sliced eggplant OR grated eggplant, grated carrot, grated zucchini, red onion slices, sliced tomatoes, broccoli, tofu.

MEXICAN PIZZA: Use Enchilada Sauce (See this Chapter) and top with refried beans, diced green chiles, chopped onions and grated Cheddar cheese. After baking, garnish with chopped tomatoes, shredded lettuce and alfalfa sprouts and dollop with sour cream.

Variations: For individual pizzas, prepare Super Duper Refrigerator Biscuit dough. Roll into a long roll, about 2″-2½″ in diameter. Slice into ¾″-1″ rounds and place up to 6 rounds of dough on a *large* oiled cookie sheet. Using an oiled glass, roll out each round to a 4″-6″ flat circle. Spoon Pizza Sauce onto each pizza. Top with favorite toppings, sprinkle with grated cheese and bake at 400° for 8-10 minutes. Makes 10-12.

SOUTH OF THE BORDER FIESTA

FRIJOLES REFRITOS

2 T. oil
1 chopped onion
4 minced garlic cloves
5-8 cups of cooked pinto beans
1 small can chopped green chiles
1 6 oz. can tomato paste
1-2 T. chili powder
1 T. sea salt
¼ to ½ t. cayenne
2 T. butter
1½ t. cumin

Saute onion and garlic in oil in a large skillet. Add beans and mash with a potato masher, adding a little bean broth so mixture doesn't get too dry and burn. Add chiles, tomato paste, seasonings and butter. Stir well and heat until hot, adding additional bean broth if necessary. Serve as a side dish, stuffed in pocket bread with grated Jack cheese, or on whole wheat chapatis or corn tortillas for burritos and tacos. Freeze leftovers in small containers.

QUESADILLAS: Melt slices of Jack cheese between chapatis. Cut in wedges to serve as an accompaniment to dinner or as a light lunch.

NACHOS: Place crisp tortilla chips on a large platter close together. Sprinkle with shredded Cheddar cheese. Place under broiler about 2 minutes or until cheese melts. Remove from oven and serve immediately with guacamole, hot sauce or sour cream.

MEXICAN BEANS AND RICE

2¼ cups cooked brown rice
2¼ cups cooked beans
3 minced garlic cloves
1 large chopped onion
1 small can chopped green chiles
1½ cups cottage cheese
milk
1 t. sea salt and/or
1 T. tamari-soy sauce
½ to 1 cup grated Cheddar cheese

Mix beans, rice, garlic, onions and chiles in a large bowl. In a blender, blend cottage cheese with just enough milk to make creamy, sea salt and/or tamari sauce. Stir into rice-beans mixture. Bake in a buttered casserole dish at 350° for 30 minutes. Sprinkle grated cheese over casserole and return to oven for 5-10 minutes more. Garnish with black olives, chopped green onions, parsley. This makes a great buffet or pot luck dish.

COMPLEMENTARY CORNBREAD

3 cups corn meal
1 t. Vegesal
1½ t. baking powder
½ t. baking soda
2 t. herbs of your choice
2 cups buttermilk
2 eggs
2 T. oil
2 T. honey

Sift dry ingredients into large bowl and make a well in center. Beat wet ingredients together well and pour into dry mixture, stirring only until blended. Preheat oven to 400°. Bake in oiled 8″x8″ baking dish for 25 to 30 minutes or individual muffins for 20 to 25 minutes. Double recipe and freeze half. Makes excellent protein complement to Mexican Beans and Rice.

Variation: Add chopped onions, grated cheese or diced chiles to batter. OR place cheese cube in center of muffins.

GAZPACHO

2 minced garlic cloves
1 T. fresh, chopped parsley
3 T. olive oil
3 T. cider vinegar
OR 2 T. lemon juice
¼ t. cumin
¼ t. basil
½ t. sea salt/kelp
cayenne to taste
4 finely chopped tomatoes
1 chopped green pepper
1 chopped Spanish onion
OR 2-3 thinly sliced green onions
1 chopped, peeled cucumber
4 cups tomato or V-8 juice
optional herbs: thyme, tarragon, chervil
black olive slices
herb-buttered croutons

In blender, blend garlic, parsley, oil, vinegar or lemon juice and seasonings. In a large bowl, mix tomatoes, green pepper, onions, cucumbers and juice. Blend half of the vegetable mixture with the herb and oil mixture until smooth. Refrigerate in a jar. Cover and refrigerate remaining veggies. To serve: ladle liquid into bowls and float chopped veggie mixture on top. Garnish with olives and croutons.

CHILES RELLENOS

2 4 oz. cans whole green chiles
6 eggs, separated
½ t. sea salt/kelp
dash cayenne
½ t. cumin
2 T. butter
thin slices of Jack cheese

Split chiles and remove seeds. Butter a 9″x13″ pan and place chiles side by side in pan. Cover with thin slices of cheese. Beat egg whites until stiff. Beat yolks with seasonings; fold gently into whites. Spoon mixture over cheese and chiles. Bake uncovered at 350° for 20-30 minutes or until set. Serve immediately.

CASA FELIZ TOSTADAS: Start with your choice of a soft or crisp corn tortilla. Spread with Frijoles Refritos and heap (really *heap*) with shredded lettuce, diced tomatoes, alfalfa sprouts and shredded Jack cheese. Top with a dollop each of sour cream and guacamole.

FESTIVAL RICE: Using a pressure cooker, bring 3 cups vegetable stock to boiling. Add 8 oz. tomato sauce, 1 medium chopped onion, 1 t. *each* Vegesal and cumin, and ½ t. chili powder. In a cast iron skillet, dry-toast 1¼ cups *long grain* brown rice until it dances and pops. Add hot rice to boiling liquid and continue cooking 3 minutes. Turn burner OFF, place lid and regulator on pressure cooker and leave alone for twenty minutes while you prepare the rest of the meal. Remove lid from pan and allow any excess moisture to evaporate. Rice will be light and fluffy. Serve immediately.

ACAPULCO MELT

2 T. SunButterBlend
1 large chopped onion
1 recipe Enchilada Sauce
1 4 oz. can diced green chiles
2½ to 3 cups cooked, drained pinto beans
grated Cheddar and/or Jack cheese
Garnishes: guacamole, sour cream, chopped olives, diced tomatoes
tortilla chips

Saute onion in SunButterBlend until transparent. Stir in Enchilada Sauce, chiles and beans, mashing beans with spoon and stirring until hot and thick. On heat-proof platter spread bean mixture. Top with a thick layer of grated cheese and place in hot oven about 4 minutes until cheese melts. Garnish with your choice of above garnishes. Use tortilla chips to dip into bean-cheese mixture.

ZESTY ZUCCHINI BURRITOS

1 large, thinly sliced onion
2 minced garlic cloves
2 T. oil
½ lb. sliced mushrooms
1 large chopped green pepper
2 medium, thinly sliced carrots
4 medium, cubed zucchinis
2 large, peeled and cubed tomatoes
1 small can diced, drained green chiles
1 small can sliced, drained black olives
1 t. chili powder
½ t. cumin
½ t. sea salt
½ t. oregano
¾ cup grated Jack cheese
¾ cup grated Cheddar cheese
Chapatis (whole grain tortillas)

Saute onion and garlic in oil in a large skillet. Add next 5 ingredients and mix well. Stir in chiles, olives and seasonings. Bring to a boil and simmer, covered, until veggies are barely tender, about 10 minutes. Uncover and gently simmer, stirring often, until liquid has evaporated and the veggies are tender. Stir in the cheeses and mix well. To assemble: Spoon veggie-cheese mixture at one end of a chapati. Top with your choice of garnishes listed below and roll up like a burrito. Repeat with others.

Variation: Leave chapati flat like a tostada, spread with filling and top with garnishes.

Garnishes: taco sauce, guacamole, sour cream or yogurt, sliced green onions, chopped tomatoes, sun seed sprouts, alfalfa sprouts.

TAMALE PIE

½ cup chopped onion
1 minced garlic clove
½ chopped green pepper
½ cup chopped celery
2 T. oil
2 cups cooked, mashed beans
1 t. chili powder
1 t. tamari-soy sauce
3 T. tomato paste
½ cup water
¼ cup sliced olives
½ cup corn
Cornmeal Batter:
2½ cups cold water, 1½ cups cornmeal, 1 t. salt, ½ t. chili powder
¼ cup grated Cheddar cheese

Saute veggies in oil. Add beans, seasonings, tomato paste, water, olives and corn, mix well and cook over medium heat about 5 minutes, stirring often. In a saucepan, combine water, cornmeal, salt and chili powder. Cook mixture over medium heat, stirring constantly until thickened. Oil an 8″x8″ pan and spread 2/3's of the cornmeal mixture over bottom and sides. Pour bean mixture into crust and spread the remaining cornmeal on top. Sprinkle with cheese and bake at 350° for 30 minutes.

AVOCADO BUTTER: Place 2 large avocados, peeled and seeded, in blender with 1 cup butter and juice of 1 lemon. Add a dash of cayenne and herbs of your choice. Blend until creamy, then smooth on warm chapatis.

EGGPLANT ENCHILADAS

1 small-medium eggplant
2 minced garlic cloves
1 medium, coarsely chopped onion
1 large, coarsely chopped green pepper
2 T. sunflower seeds
¼ cup butter
1 small can diced green chiles
salt and cayenne to taste
1½ cups grated Cheddar cheese
1 recipe Enchilada Sauce
Corn tortillas
1 cup Cheddar cheese (topping)
sliced black olives
sour cream or yogurt

Peel eggplant and cut into ½" cubes. In a large skillet, saute first 5 ingredients. When eggplant is tender (10-15 minutes) add drained green chiles, salt and cayenne and 1½ cups cheese. Mix well. Heat Enchilada Sauce in a saucepan large enough to accommodate tortillas. To assemble: Dip each corn tortilla in sauce until slightly softened. (Tortillas may be oven-crisped at 350° for 10 minutes or fried quickly in a little oil, and drained, before dipping, so they won't break apart when dipped in sauce.) Spoon about 1/12 of the vegetable mixture at one end of tortilla. Roll to enclose filling; arrange filled tortillas, seam side down, in an oiled 9"x13" pan. Cover evenly with remaining sauce and top with 1 cup Cheddar cheese. Bake uncovered in a 350° oven for 20 minutes or until hot. Garnish with black olives and sour cream or yogurt.

CHILE CON QUESO

1 large chopped onion
1 minced garlic clove
2 T. SunButterBlend
1 T. Bakon yeast
1 T. whole wheat pastry flour
1 8 oz. can tomato sauce
2 cups Frijoles Refritos
1 4 oz. can diced green chile-salsa
1 lb. cubed Cheddar cheese
¼ t. each chili powder and cumin
dash cayenne
1 large diced tomato
tortilla chips

Saute onion and garlic in SunButterBlend. Stir in yeast and flour until paste forms. Add tomato sauce, chiles, beans and cook 5 minutes, stirring constantly. Reduce heat to low and add cubed cheese, spices and tomatoes. To serve: For a "fondue" dip, serve hot with tortilla chips.

Variation: For a cold dip, add 1 cup mashed pinto beans and refrigerate. Serve with cold Gaspacho.

AVOCADO ENSALADA: Tear enough of three kinds of greens to almost fill a large salad bowl. Peel 3 avocados and slice into ¼" rings, working carefully around seed. Slice 4 hard-cooked eggs and ¼ lb. fresh mushrooms into ¼" slices. Wash and remove stems from 1 pint cherry tomatoes. Arrange veggies atop greens and sprinkle with toasted sunseeds or chopped nuts and thin-sliced green onions or a few thin-sliced rings of sweet purple onion. Spike some mayonnaise with lemon juice, chili powder and cumin or garlic powder and drizzle over all.

HALF-SHELL ENSALADA: Dice 2 medium tomatoes, 2 hard-cooked eggs and 1 cucumber. Mince 2 stalks celery and slice 2 green onions or 1 heaping T. chives. Drain any excess juice from tomatoes and toss all veggies lightly with 1 qt. cottage cheese and 1 T. mayonnaise. Place peeled avocado halves on individual, lettuce-leaf lined salad plates. Heap centers with cottage cheese mixture and sprinkle with pepitas or toasted seeds of your choice.

AVOCADO CREAM PIE: Blend 2 large avocados, peeled and seeded, in blender with 1 cup honey, 3 T. lemon or lime juice, 8 oz. cream cheese and 2 t. vanilla. Whip 2 cups heavy cream until very stiff and carefully fold avocado mixture into whipped cream. Place in prepared pie crust and refrigerate OR freeze OR spoon into parfait glasses, alternating with crumbled cookies or cake crumbs and top with coconut and a mint leaf.

Variation: Replace vanilla with ¼ cup rum or 2 t. rum flavoring.

AVOCADO VELVET: Blend 2 large avocados, peeled and seeded, with 3 cups pineapple-coconut or peach-coconut juice (from health store). Add 2 T. *each* lemon and honey and 6 or 7 1-inch chunks of frozen banana. Blend until smooth as velvet and serve in chilled stemware with a mint leaf for garnish.

Variations: Add 1 pint homemade vanilla ice cream OR ¼ cup rum OR for texture, ¼ cup *each* ground walnuts and grated coconut.

RAMONA'S PINATA PIE

1 cup whole wheat flour
½ cup corn meal
1 t. baking powder
½ t. Vegesal
¼ cup butter
½ cup milk

2 cups Festival Rice
2 cups shredded Cheddar cheese
2 tomatoes, sliced thin
4 green pepper rings
chopped ripe olives
sour cream

Mix first 4 ingredients and cut in butter until crumbly. Add milk and form dough into ball. Oil a pizza pan or a cookie sheet and spread dough evenly over pan forming a slight ridge. Bake for 15-18 minutes in center of a 350° oven. Spread with *hot* Festival Rice and top with cheese. Return to oven to melt cheese then garnish with tomato slices, green pepper rings, olives and sour cream. Serve with Avocado Ensalada.

HEALTHSAVING HINTS

1. Nutritional yeast provides the B vitamin complex, 16 amino acids and 18 important minerals. Purchase in small quantities until you find one that appeals to your tastebuds, then keep plenty on hand for frequent use in juices, drinks, cookies, patties and loaves, breads and in fudges.
2. Use parsley often as it is high in vitamin C. It keeps well in a jar in the refrigerator or can be dried. Tie a bunch and hang upside down or place sprigs on cookie sheet and leave in a warm place until dry.
3. If you use the expression "vegetate" to scold children who sit around and do nothing, they may develop a misconception of the life of vegetables and a nagging psychological aversion to them. Help kids grow their own gardens so they will see that veggies really twist and wind and dart and grow and change constantly before their very eyes. In this positive light, the word "vegetate" is more closely related to "motivate."

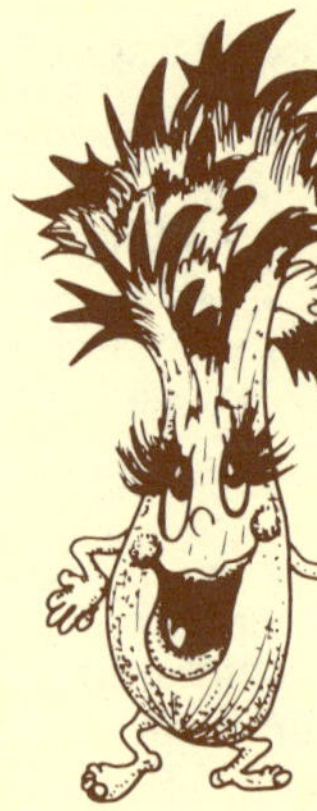

4. Do you know an elderly person or invalid who lives alone and finds it a hardship to cook his/her meals? Food from a can may be all s/he can handle. When you make a soup, loaf or casserole for your family, place a good-sized helping in a freezer container or zip-lock bag and freeze immediately. Deliver to your friend. S/he will be most grateful for the variety, flavor and nutrition contained in the packets. These frozen meals have more quality than the commercial frozen or canned foods and no preservatives or chemical additives. To prepare: partially thaw, heat quickly and serve.
5. Spread a little liquid lecithin on warmed cooking utensils with a paper towel and there will be less sticking of foods, less cooking fat calories added to the food, less greasy taste and less clean-up. Enjoy only the natural flavor of the food dish. Use lecithin on cookie sheets, for frying eggs or potatoes, in casseroles or souffles.
6. In a glass of water place a paper-thin, round slice of lemon. It looks elegant and makes the water taste sweet and delicious.
7. To add protein and eye appeal to a casserole, make some depressions in the top. About 15 minutes before casserole is done, break an egg into each. Continue baking until eggs are set to your liking and sprinkle with fresh parsley just before serving.
8. Perform the art of food preparation and serving the way you would expect an artist to paint — with enthusiasm and love for the person/s who will enjoy the finished product. If you are harried and frantic, those who partake of your meal will pick up nervous vibrations. Be calm, gentle and loving and you will transfer your attitude to those who will share your food and friendship in peace and harmony.
9. Yams are delicious grated into burger mixture. Or mash leftovers and add to beans and grains; saute onions and green pepper and shape into patties. Use yams whenever plentiful for they are high in vitamin A.

10. Eat veggie dishes in a bowl and use chopstix instead of a fork. You will surely slow your eating, chew thoroughly and enjoy a relaxed dinner.
11. If you would like to wean your family away from meat or at least from having the meat as the main portion of the meal, try adding a little cooked fish or chicken to some of our vegetable dishes. Your family will still have some meat (albeit in a smaller portion) while the vegetable dish becomes the main attraction on the plate.
12. When making any nut-seed-grain-bean patties, shape the mixture into hot dogs and bake or saute and place in whole wheat hot dog buns. Use condiments of pickle relish, mustard, mayonnaise and catsup.
13. Use vegetable stock whenever water is called for in casseroles, loaves, patties or other supper dishes.

TIMESAVING HINTS

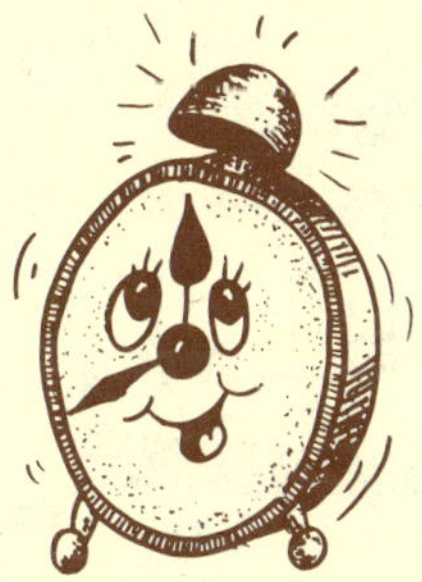

1. Protect pages of cookbook with a rack to support your open book while you stir and splash OR use a layer of clear plastic.
2. If a recipe calls for only 2 or 3 T. minced onion, go ahead and mince an entire onion. Keep the remainder refrigerated in a small glass jar to be used within the week or added to veggie stock for soup.
3. When possible, prepare recipes in quantity and freeze the unused amounts — especially loaves, soups, tomato or other sauces, pancakes, waffles, muffins, etc.
4. Fresh frozen mint and parsley, right from freezer are colorful and tasty additions to garnish or place in vegetable dishes.
5. When making a loaf or a casserole, make two and freeze one for those busy days when there's no time to prepare a meal. Defrost, heat and eat.
6. If your souffle falls, just use it as a cheese sauce for a grain or bean dish or fill center with sauteed veggies and pretend that was how it was supposed to be. No one will know the difference and you will receive lavish compliments for your "original creation!"
7. When you have an abundance of ripe produce (fresh or leftover), puree and freeze in ice cube trays. Veggies add zest to winter soup broth while fruits flavor and thicken smoothies and desserts.
8. Use a "lazy Susan" for garnishes. Place small containers that have lids on a revolving tray, so that at clean-up, the lids can be replaced and leftovers refrigerated. Use for dried fruit, seeds and nuts for a yogurt dessert, or chopped onions, hard-cooked eggs, tomatoes, coconut, toasted sun seeds and cashews for a curry.
9. Pizzas freeze well. Cook about 5 minutes less than recommended time. Cool quickly; wrap in clear plastic and freeze. Make and freeze individual-sized pizzas. They'll be ready for a hungry kid who needs a "quick" dinner. Place on cookie sheet and bake in preheated oven until bubbly.
10. Whack garlic cloves with bottom of heavy skillet; skin comes off and is easily removed. Then mash or chop with knife.
11. To make flour tortillas more pliable, wrap in foil and place in 350° oven for 15 minutes.
12. To use just a squirt of lemon juice, prick a hole in lemon with end of a large needle or tine of fork. Squeeze desired amount.
13. Ripen avocados in brown paper bag on top of refrigerator or other warm place in your kitchen. Check daily for ripeness. They should be slightly soft under mild pressure of thumb, near stem.
14. To make your own specialty cheeses, follow these instructions. For onion cheese, thinly slice Jack cheese and whole onions. Alternate layers of cheese and onion, wrap tightly and refrigerate for two days. Remove onions and enjoy the aroma and flavor of your specialty cheese. For dilly-onion, sandwich a few slightly crushed dill seeds between cheese and onion layers. For garlic cheese, slightly mash fresh garlic cloves and place between Jack or Cheddar cheese, wrap and refrigerate. Another time try caraway seeds.
15. Take the time to make your own Resourceful Recipe File and try the Rotating Menu Plan for a month, using your family's favorite converted recipes or the recipes in this book. You'll be amazed at how much time you'll save by being so organized.

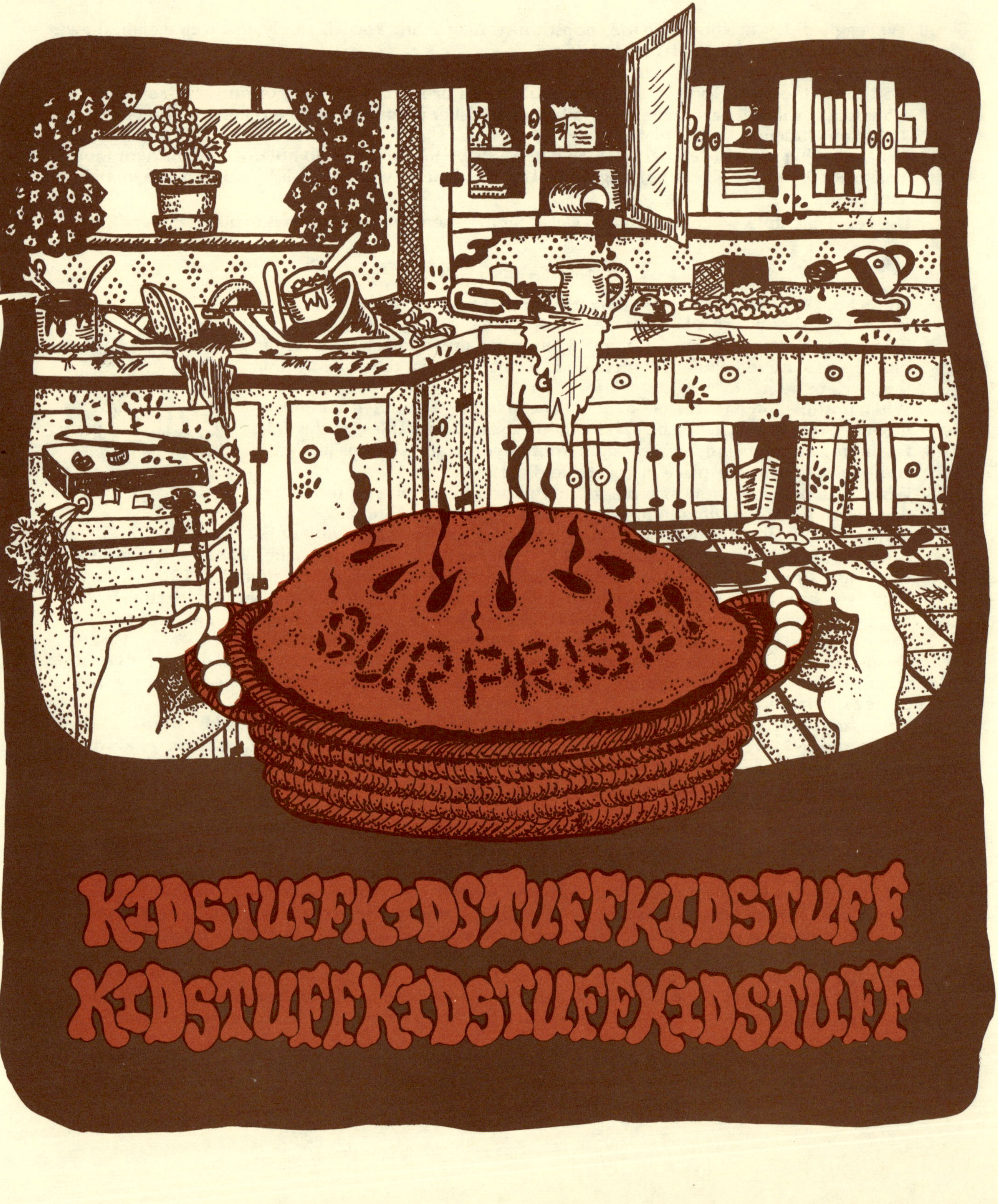
SURPRISE!
KIDSTUFFKIDSTUFFKIDSTUFF
KIDSTUFFKIDSTUFFKIDSTUFF

Kid Stuff

SEVEN SUPER-DUPER KIDS, no different than yourself
Took their mothers' recipes down from off the shelf.
Out they got the measuring cups; out they got the spoons;
Proceeded then to have themselves the WILDEST afternoon.

Some began to grate and grind, others mash and chop
(Their mothers, incidentally, had gone to town to shop!)
"I'll begin to wash and rinse, and you may peel and core.
Don't forget to measure well — better let me pour.

Sprinkle, garnish, sift and crush; read directions, do not rush.
Mash the 'tatoes, roll the crust; glaze the top with pastry brush."
Some were beating whites of eggs and some were whipping cream.
One was cooking vegetables, nutritionally, by steam.

"Chop the nuts, two teaspoonsful; flour, one-half cup.
Knead it well, punch it down and later roll it up."
They looked around the kitchen then and said, "We must confess,
That we have made an unbelievable, terrible, sloppy mess."

But, being Super-Duper Kids, they knew 'twas time to stop
To clean the table, wash the pans, and sweep and wipe and mop.
When the Moms returned from town, they couldn't believe their eyes!
Those Super Kids had prepared the most "fantastical" surprise!

"The table's set, the candles are lit, and let us say a prayer.
Please be seated, dearest Moms, for now it's time to share!"
And that's when they discovered that the kids who like to eat
Can make the KidStuffKidStuff foods for truly tasty treats.

The first course was concocted by the little boy named Chris
Whose Big Bionic Breakfast food was served with hug and kiss.
Mona made Fruit Pizza with samples as hors d'oeuvres —
A colorful creation — and the secret was all hers.

The main entree was Heidi's Mashed Po-Lentil Pie.
She made it perfectly the first time that she tried.
The Incredibly Edible Play Dough shaped by little Randy
Looked very much like animals, but tasted more like candy.

On top of yogurt-cottage cheese, Matt sprinkled dried fruit and seeds
While Wendy's Five-Layer Bars satisfied their sweet-tooth needs.
And then, at last, dessert was Dan's — called Dan's Delicious Fudge.
By now the Moms were delightfully full — so full they couldn't budge.

Now all you kids who like to eat can easily learn to cook.
Just follow the recipes in the KidStuffKidStuff Chapter of this book.

SillyStuffSillyStuffSillyStuffSillyStuffSillyStuffSillyStuffSillyStuff

FUNNY-LOOKING SNACKS YOU CAN MAKE

CELERY CARTS

Use carrot circles on toothpick axles for wheels and lay a piece of celery across toothpicks for cart bed. Spread cream cheese or peanut butter in the cart and fill with nuts or seeds.

SALAD-ON-A-STICK

Veggie: Thread zucchini slices, cherry tomatoes, avocado cubes, cheese cubes, mushrooms, cucumber slices, black olives, rutabaga slices, Jerusalem artichoke slices, green olives, etc., onto skewer sticks.
Fruit: Thread orange wedges, banana chunks, apple wedges, apricot halves, pears, pineapple chunks, grapes, cantaloupe or watermelon balls, nectarine slices and so on, onto skewer sticks.
For a special treat, dip fruit skewers in pineapple juice, roll in shredded coconut and/or ground nuts and freeze until solid. Then eat like a popsicle.

JAWBREAKERS

For individual jawbreakers, freeze green grapes, red or purple sweet cherries (not dyed marachino cherries), and watermelon and cantaloupe balls. To eat, chew or suck balls very carefully. They are delicious! Store a large container of them in your freezer.

MAKE THE MOST OUT OF TOAST

1. Sprinkle buttered toast with Parmesan cheese, kelp and onion powder. Cut into long fingers.
2. Spread toast with a honey-butter-cinnamon mixture and cut into long fingers.
3. Spread toast with soft cream cheese and sprinkle with ground walnuts, raisins and cinnamon and cut into fingers.

FUNNY FACES

On a slice of bread, spread peanut butter, Tahini, cottage cheese OR cream cheese. Now *you* are the artist! Design a funny face. Use sprouts or carrot curls for hair; radish sliver or apple slice for mouth; cherry tomato, strawberry or raisins for nose; almonds for eyes; olive slivers for eyebrows.

YAPPOLA

Yam + Apple + Granola = Yappola. Mash some leftover yam and add a sprinkle of cinnamon. Then scrub an apple really clean. Cut it in half through the equator and scoop out the seeds. Stuff the hollow with mashed yam stuff and spread it over the top surface. Dip in a bowl of granola so the top looks frosted.
Variation: If you are losing some teeth and the granola gets caught in your empty spaces, then dip your Yapple in shredded Jack cheese and make up your own name for it!

(Be sure to check *Holiday Harmony* for additional snack recipes.)

GO BANANAS WITHOUT SUGAR

1. Peel and cut bananas in half. Dip in pineapple juice and roll in your choice of coconut, ground sunflower seeds, Almond-Cinnamon Mixture, dried, grated orange peel with cinnamon, OR toasted wheat germ.
2. Peel bananas and cut in 1″-2″ chunks. Heat peanut butter just enough to soften and dip or spread chunks with peanut butter. Roll in granola. Use a toothpick to pick up and eat!
3. Halve 5-6 ripe bananas lengthwise. Lay in a single layer in a shallow pan. Warm 2 T. SunButterBlend and mix with ½ t. cinnamon and a small can crushed pineapple in its own unsweetened juice. Pour mixture over bananas and sprinkle with coarsely chopped walnuts or filberts. Heat through, but do not cook, for 5-8 minutes at 275°.

SILLY STUFFINGS FOR DATES, PRUNES, CELERY, HOLLOWED-OUT APPLE HALVES OR ?

1. A whole almond or walnut.
2. A mixture of: 2 T. orange juice, 4 oz. softened cream cheese, ¼ cup chopped, sun seed sprouts.
3. Cream cheese, mixed with nuts and raisins OR crushed pineapple OR toasted sesame seeds.
4. Cottage cheese, mixed with grated carrots and raisins OR chopped cucumber OR finely chopped, mixed raw veggies.
5. Peanut butter, mixed with wheat germ and sun seeds (sprouted or half toasted and half raw).

ChipStuffDipStuffChipStuffDipStuffChipStuffDipStuffChipStuff

DO NOT DISTURB HERB DIP

½ cup mayonnaise
2 T. snipped chives
2 T. fresh, chopped parsley
¼ t. dried basil leaves
¼ t. dried tarragon leaves
¼ t. dried thyme leaves
½ t. sea salt/kelp
a dash of cayenne
a dash of Tabasco
1½ cups plain yogurt

In a blender, blend mayonnaise and seasonings. Remove from blender and place in a bowl with the plain yogurt. Stir gently but thoroughly, then chill.

KIDS SUPER DIPPER

2 cups cottage cheese
¼ cup grated carrot
2 T. sliced green onions
2 T. chopped green pepper
2 sliced and diced radishes
¼ t. dried dillweed
1 scant t. sea salt/kelp
a dash cayenne

In a blender, blend 2 cups cottage cheese. Remove from blender and place in a bowl. Stir in the veggies and seasonings. Cover bowl and chill. Serve with your favorite veggies or crackers.

WHAT TO USE FOR CHIPS FOR DIPS

Whole grain crackers, Green Crackers (See *Labor of Love Lunches*), stone-ground corn tortilla chips.
Make your own tortilla chips by crisping corn tortillas in a moderate oven (350°) and breaking up into chips when cool.
Slice zucchini very thin and sun-dry or warm oven-dry the chips. Season with sea salt/kelp and use as chips for dipping. Also try:

apple wedges, carrot sticks, celery sticks
sliced jicima, cherry tomatoes, celery cut in diagonal wedges
thin slices of turnips, beets and rutabagas
raw yams, sliced in long sticks or in thin circles
cauliflowerets, broccoli flowers and thinly sliced broccoli stalk
Jerusalem artichoke slices, cucumber sticks and carrot circles
zucchini slices or sticks and whole or sliced mushrooms
green onions, carrot circles and green pepper strips

OUTER SPACE SENSATIONS

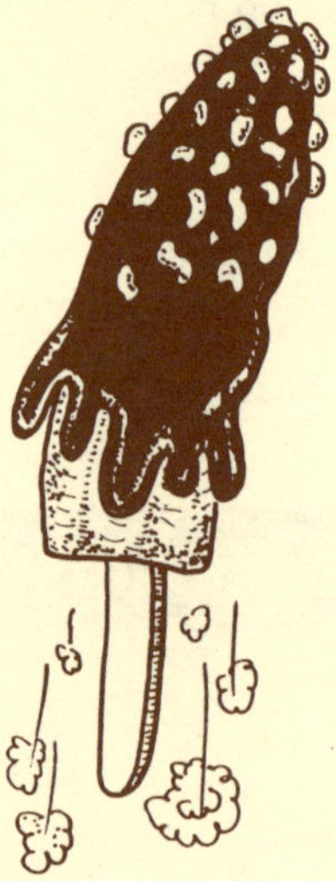

LASER BEAMS: Peel bananas and cut in half. Insert a popsicle stick in cut end of each half. Lay on cookie sheets and freeze until firm. Then dip bananas in Carob Sauce until coated, letting excess sauce drip off. Roll immediately in one of the following: ground walnuts, ground sesame seeds, ground sunflower seeds, granola, Almond-Cinnamon Mixture. Wrap in sandwich bags and freeze until firm or eat and enjoy!

CAROB SAUCE

1 cup carob powder
½ cup water
½ cup honey
½-1 cup instant powdered milk
½ t. vanilla

In a pan, heat carob, water and honey, stirring constantly. Add powdered milk, a little at a time, stirring until blended smooth. Cool, then stir in vanilla. Sauce should be thick.

ALMOND-CINNAMON MIXTURE: To 1 cup of finely ground, shelled almonds, stir in 1 T. cinnamon. Store in covered glass jar in refrigerator.

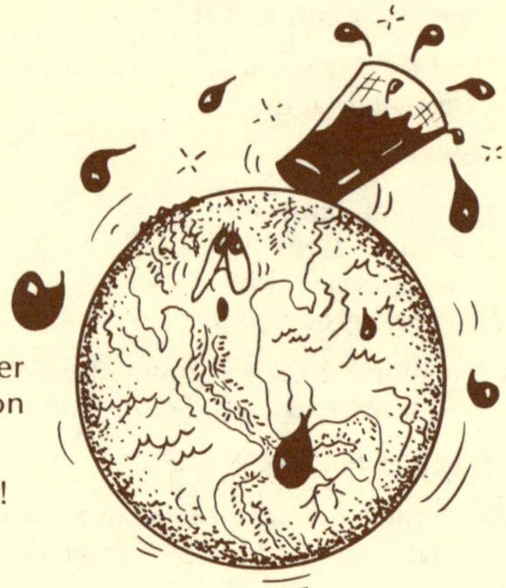

EARTH SHAKING SHAKE

1. Fill your glass with frozen banana chunks.
2. Pour milk in around the bananas.
3. Pour milk and bananas from glass into blender and add 1 to 2 teaspoons of Almond-Cinnamon Mixture.
4. Blend until thick and smooth. You'll love it!

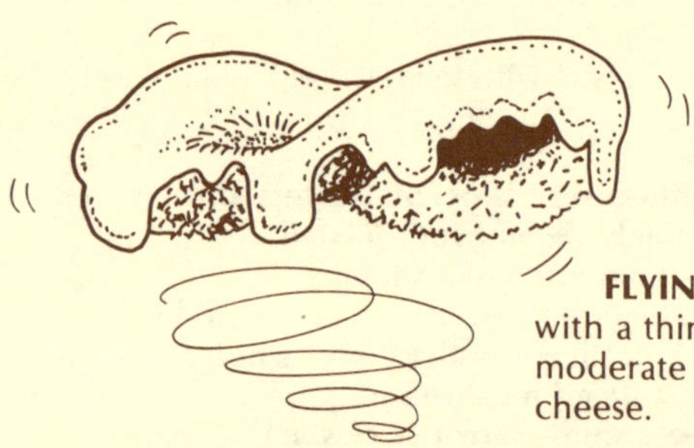

FLYING SAUCER: Top a whole wheat pretzel with a thin slice of Jack cheese. If desired, place in a moderate oven (350°) for just a few minutes to melt cheese.

JUPITER BALLS: Select a red apple and an orange. Wash well. Stick toothpicks with the following tidbits all around the apple: cheese cubes, grapes, melon balls. Stick the orange with pineapple chunks, dates stuffed with peanut butter or cream cheese, small slices of stuffed celery, or banana chunks that have been dipped in orange juice and rolled in coconut, granola or wheat germ.

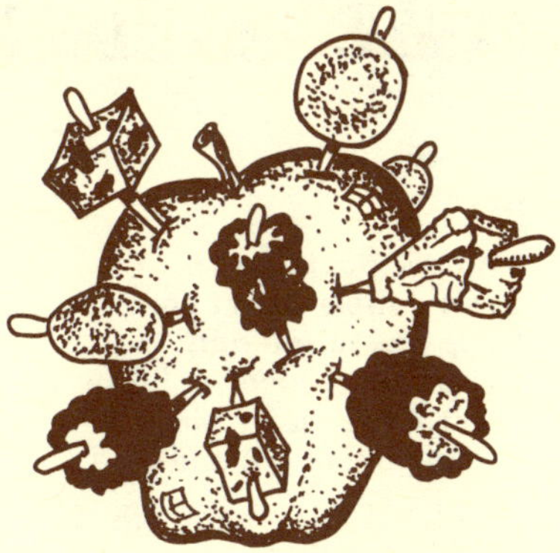

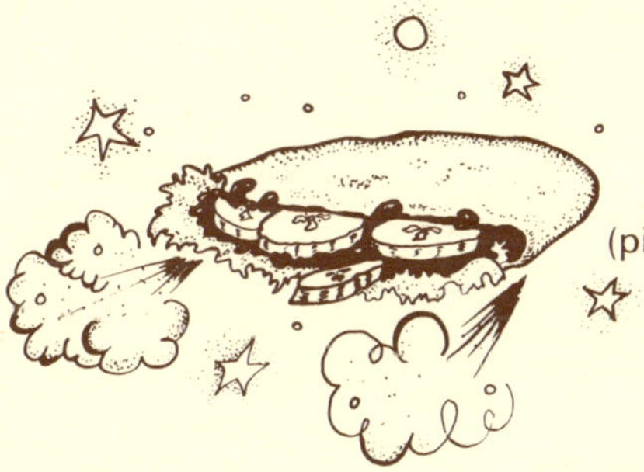

SATELLITE SANDWICH: Spread pocket bread (pita) with peanut butter. Fill with banana slices.

U.F.O.'s

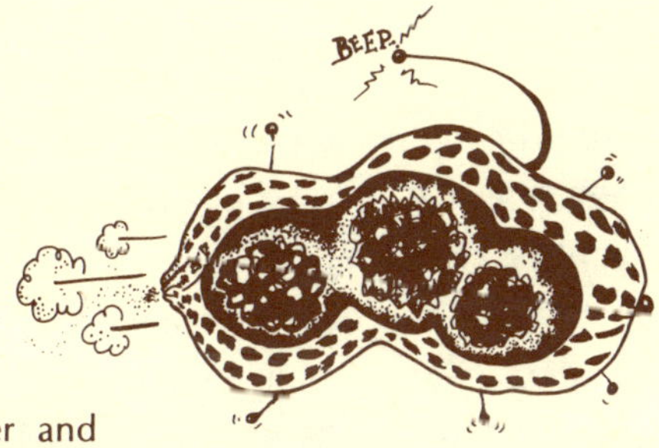

4 cups instant powdered milk
3 cups peanut butter
1½ cups honey
1 cup granola

Mix powdered milk with peanut butter and honey. Knead well. Then add granola and mix again. Form into walnut-sized balls and place in a pan. Keep refrigerated or frozen.

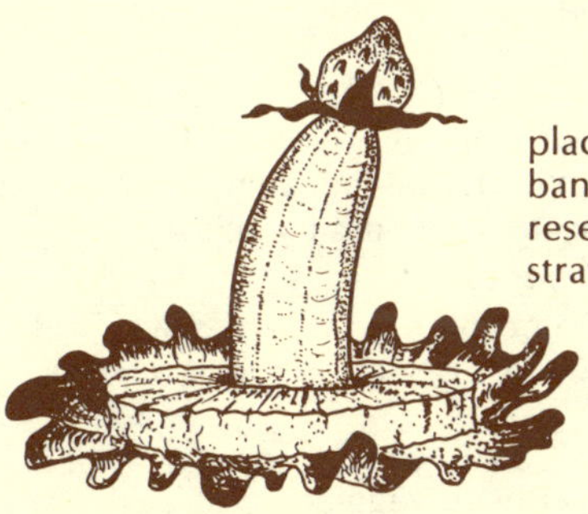

SPACESHIP SALAD: On a red-green lettuce leaf, place one slice of pineapple. Set one-half of a peeled banana, upright in the center of the pineapple — to resemble a rocket. Top with a cherry or an inverted strawberry.

FOR ALL YOU NUTS OUT THERE

ZIPPITY-DO-DAS

4 quarts, popped popcorn
2 cups whole wheat pretzel sticks
1 cup raw mixed nuts
1 cup raw, shelled sunflower seeds
(opt.) 1 cup puffed rice
½ cup SunButterBlend
1 t. tamari-soy sauce
1 minced garlic clove
1 heaping T. very finely chopped onion OR 1 t. onion powder
1 t. vegetable salt OR lemon pepper OR Gomazio

In a large bowl, mix together the first 5 ingredients. In a saucepan, mix the SunButterBlend and seasonings until melted and blended. Pour this mixture over the mixed nuts and popcorn and toss together. Spread mixture in 2 large cake pans or cookie sheets and toast in the oven at 275° for 30 minutes, stirring at 10 minute intervals. Eat right away or cool and store in covered containers.

JACK-IN-THE-BAGS*

1½ cups peanuts
4 quarts popped popcorn
½ cup SunButterBlend
2/3 cup honey
dash sea salt

Toss peanuts with popcorn in a large bowl. In a saucepan, mix SunButterBlend, honey and salt until well blended. Drizzle honey-butter over popcorn and nuts and toss to coat well. Allow to cool, then fill individual lunch sacks 2/3's full and tuck in your own special surprise. Marbles, barrettes, funny erasers, key chains, squeeze-type coin holders, pencils, pens, toothbrush, combs, rubber bugs, etc., can be wrapped in foil to add an element of excitement to opening the surprise. *Moms — if children are used to watching the ball game while munching on caramel corn that has a surprise in the bottom, keep them happy with these!

ENCORE POPCORN: Toss 4 quarts buttered popcorn with any vegetable seasoning or Gomazio.

EASY CHEESEY: Toss buttered popcorn with ¼ c. Parmesan cheese.

LEMON TANG: Toss buttered popcorn with 1 t. lemon pepper.

YEAST FEAST: Sprinkle buttered popcorn with good-tasting nutritional or brewer's yeast.

OTHER POPCORN TOPPINGS: Toss buttered popcorn with honey OR taco seasoning mix.

CUP O' CRUNCH: Mix raw almonds, cashews, walnuts, sun seeds, roasted peanuts, pumpkin seeds, and/or any other nuts. Roast and season half the mixture with sea salt/kelp; then toss together with the raw mixture.

SWEET TOASTED TREAT: Drizzle a mixture of melted butter, date sugar or honey and a dash of cinnamon over almonds, cashews, peanuts and walnuts. Roast at 300° on a cookie sheet until browned.

SAVORY TOASTED TREAT: Drizzle a mixture of melted butter, sea salt/kelp and tamari-soy sauce over almonds, cashews, peanuts and walnuts. Roast at 300° on a cookie sheet until browned.

TAHINI STUFF

Tahini is sesame seeds ground in a nut grinder or blender to a fine powder with a few drops of oil added to hold it together. Sesame butter is Tahini with more oil. It can take the place of peanut butter in sandwiches or be used in salad dressings, dips or treats. Tahini is a rich source of calcium, protein and unsaturated fatty acids.

TAHINI DIP: For Humus, place 2 cups cooked garbanzo beans with some bean liquid in a blender. Add 3 T. lemon juice, ¼ cup Tahini, ¼ t. cumin, and 1 garlic clove. Blend. Refrigerate. Use as a raw vegetable-crisp cracker dip.

TAHINI DRESSING: In a blender, blend 1/3 cup Tahini, 2 T. lemon juice, 2/3 cup yogurt, and a dash of garlic powder. Store covered, in refrigerator. Spoon over salads, cottage cheese or cooked veggies.

TAHINI SAUCE: Blend 1 ripe banana, ¼ cup Tahini and a little fruit juice to make a thick sauce. (Apple juice is great!) Pour sauce over a bowl of sliced bananas. Garnish with soaked raisins or apples and a dash of cinnamon.

TAHINI SPREAD: Mix together ¼ cup Tahini and 2 T. peanut butter. Add ¼ cup finely chopped nuts (any kind). Store in refrigerator. Use on crackers, in lettuce leaf Roll-Arounds or in sandwiches with sprouts.

TAHINI TOPPING: Mix 1/3 cup Tahini, 2 T. honey, ½ t. cinnamon, 2 T. apple juice. Chill in covered container. Use as a topping or dip for fruit, or spread on bread and top with sliced apples.

TAHINI BALLS

#1.

½ cup Tahini
1-2 T. honey
1 heaping T. peanut butter

#2.

¼ cup Tahini
¼ cup honey
¼ cup rolled oats (blender-ground)
⅛ t. pumpkin pie spice

#3.

2 T. Tahini
½ cup sun sprouts
½ cup peanut butter
¼ cup carob powder
¼-½ cup honey

Mix well and knead. Form into balls. Roll balls into the following: #1 — granola, #2 — Almond-Cinnamon Mixture, #3 — sesame seeds. Chill.

LunchStuffLunchStuffLunchStuffLunchStuffLunchStuff

PACKING COLD LUNCHES

Packing lunches for children may take a little imagination and pre-planning, but should be kept simple yet varied from day to day. Most elementary school children eat in an atmosphere not conducive to good digestion. They're usually more interested in the activities on the playground than the food in front of them. Sandwiches may be gulped down with liquid, rather than carefully chewed and swallowed. Often part of the lunch is left uneaten so that as much of their short lunch period as possible can be spent in the gym or playground.

As long as your child begins the day with a good breakfast and enjoys a nutritious, relaxing dinner at home, you need not be over-concerned about lunch. A half sandwich, a piece of fruit with some cheese or raw vegetables with a dip, plus milk or juice will be sufficient to keep the child's energy level high and will be easily digested. An older child might enjoy a thermos of hot, homemade soup with crackers or a salad with a sandwich. On a day when sports events follow school and extra energy will be required, tuck in an extra fresh fruit.

Pretzels, whole grain crackers, puffed rice cakes, fruit n' nut breads, chapatis, and pita bread, can replace bread in a sandwich for lunch. Choose snacks and healthy lunch ingredients from recipes in this chapter; check *Labor of Love Lunches* for recipes for sandwich fillings and spreads.

HELPFUL TIPS FOR KIDS WHO HELP PACK THEIR LUNCHES

1. If packing a fruit or vegetable salad, yogurt, dip or sandwich made with mayonnaise that must be kept cold, make an insulated container: The night before, wrap a damp wash cloth around the empty container, then freeze. In the morning, fill container with food and slip frozen cloth back in place. Food should remain cool until noon. This works for lunch buckets only; will not work in paper sacks.
2. Bananchaladas, Roll-Arounds and pocket-bread sandwiches pack well and provide a change from the traditional sandwich while piquing the curiosity of classmates, who might convince their moms to make one for them.

3. Raw carrot, celery and yam can be cut like chips for dipping, placed in a glass jar filled with lemon-water, and refrigerated overnight, then drained and wrapped in paper towels and aluminum foil to keep crisp until noon.
4. Cheese cubes, olives and hard-cooked eggs are easy to pack and will be safe to eat without refrigeration for a few hours.
5. If you're packing a sweet dessert, nuts, raisins, or other dried fruit, it's a good idea to pack a toothbrush too!
6. Prepare a batch of "trick" cookies especially for school lunches. For example, you could prepare Easy Half Cup Cookies, but use less honey, more nuts and add 1 or 2 T. nutritional yeast to batter before baking. Extra nuts and seeds add extra protein. The kids at school will think you're eating "junk food," but you will know that your power-packed cookies are good for ya!
7. When you get the urge to doodle, display your talents on lunch sacks, then bring them home to be recycled or saved for the memory box. How many people do you know who have a collection of art-deco lunch sacks?
8. Suggest to your principal that lunch be served AFTER play time. This gives you an opportunity to work up an appetite and prevents you from inhaling your food just to get out onto the playground.
9. Nut and seed burgers or patties taste great cold with mayonnaise and sprouts. For hot lunches at home on holidays or week-ends, see *Labor of Love Lunches* and *Serendipity Suppers* for soups and loaves and patties.
10. Plan your menus for lunches around fruits and vegetables that are in season.

TIPS TO MOMS AND DADS OR WHOEVER PREPARES THE LUNCHES

1. Tuck little "love" messages into your child's lunches, like, "Good luck at your game today. I know you'll do just great!", or "You're a terrific kid! I love you!" It is guaranteed to cheer them up if they've had a bad morning. Be creative! If you're packing a mock tuna sandwich, tuck in a stick fishing pole with the line attached to a note, "Nice catch! Somewhere there's a tuna who loves you."
2. Let your children select and prepare their favorite cold lunch ingredients. They choose things they like so you can be reasonably certain they eat what they take.
3. Although we have seen improvement in some school lunch programs (sandwiches with one slice whole wheat and one slice white bread plus the addition of a few fresh fruits and vegetables), we still feel that cafeteria lunches provide too much refined carbohydrate. Just because a lunch is HOT does not automatically mean that it is nutritious. Take the time to observe your school's cafeteria. Eat there, then compare the quality with what you can send from home. Do not compare price, however, for schools get many foods free from the government. Just because something is *free* doesn't mean it is healthy!

On the following pages are helpful menu suggestions and inexpensive, easy-to-prepare nutritious snacks and lunches. Many of the recipes are in this Chapter, but be sure to check *Labor of Love Lunches* for sandwich fillings, salads, soups and whole grain breads and crackers. Also see *Serendipity Suppers* for burger and loaf recipes — the leftovers make super sandwiches and/or dips for veggies.

Fear less, hope more; eat less, chew more;
whine less, breathe more; talk less, say more;
hate less, love more; and all good things are yours. *Swedish Proverb*

DAY	SNACK	LUNCH	SNACK
Monday	UFO's	Funny Face Salad	Hot Carob Cocoa Cinnamon Breadstix
Tuesday	Mixed Fruit Juice	Earth Shaking Shake poured over a bowl of granola	Pear Halves Peanuts in Shell
Wednesday	Chris's Bionic Breakfast Salad	Tooty McFruity Roll-Around	Zippity-Do-Das
Thursday	Hi Protein Seed Bars Milk	Mona's Fruit Pizza	Apple Banana Smoothie
Friday	Celery Carts	Super Sprout Salad	Fantastic French Fries
Monday	Tray of raw veggies: slices of carrot, celery, turnip, cherry tomato, jicima	Guacamole spread on bread or crackers and heaped with sprouts	Honey Lemonade Appley Muffin
Tuesday	Orange juice (squeeze it fresh and let kids eat pulp out of orange skins	Satellite Sandwich Milk	Let children pop corn. Toss with melted butter and Parmesan cheese.
Wednesday	Yappola	Tofu sandwiches cut in diagonals twice and shaped in flower or pinwheel or butterfly, with carrot stick stem or body	Randy's Incredibly Edible Play Dough. Let kids make and shape. Milk
Thursday	Frozen Yogurt-Sicle	Salad-on-a-Stick, with cottage cheese. Let kids make own skewers Example: cube of cheese, avocado slice, cherry tomato, black olive.	Watermelon slices OR fresh fruit in season
Friday	Cup O' Crunch	Heidi's Mashed Po-Lentil Pie Wedges	Jawbreakers — frozen green grapes or cherries
Monday	Cheese cubes on skewers with apple slices	Hard-cooked egg on bed of alfalfa sprouts and grated carrots V-8 juice	Orange wedges and chunks of whole fresh coconut. Demonstrate how to cut and drain milk from coconut
Tuesday	Bread Fingers	Fruit Skewers — orange wedges, banana chunks, cherries, apricots, grapes. Serve with cottage cheese	Peanut butter and wheat germ and sun sprouts on celery sticks
Wednesday	Fruit Yogurt: mix plain yogurt with mashed fruit. (Use honey only if needed)	Flying Saucers Fresh pear	Carrots and celery sliced diagonally in chip size to dip in favorite dip
Thursday	Mixed nuts in shell. Use hammer and block of wood. Each child gets to crack and learn names of a variety of nuts.	BanappleBerry Shake Cinnamon toast	Steamed caulifloweret sprinkled with grated cheese and ground walnuts. Serve hot.
Friday	Fresh pineapple slices. Demonstrate how to cut and slice the fruit, then share the results.	Bananchalada Milk	Yogurt-Cooler

BROWN BAGGERS

avocado-tomato-cottage cheese-mixed sprout salad
carrot stix
V-8 juice

cheese and sprouts on pocket bread
easy half cup cookie
milk

yogurt w/fruit
mixed raw nuts
grape juice

any bean spread sandwich
waldorf salad
milk

appley muffin
peanuts
fresh pear
apple juice

hard-cooked egg
alfalfa sprouts on whole grain crackers w/cheese
tomato juice

whole wheat pretzel
vegetable soup
cole slaw
milk

tofu sandwich w/sun sprouts
stuffed celery
V-8 juice

herb-yogurt dip
raw veggies
mock crab sand.
honey lemonade

Bananchalada
carob milk
raw almonds

egg salad sandwich
carrot and celery sticks
milk

mock tuna sand.
stone-ground corn chips
pineapple-carrot juice

MORE BROWN BAGGERS

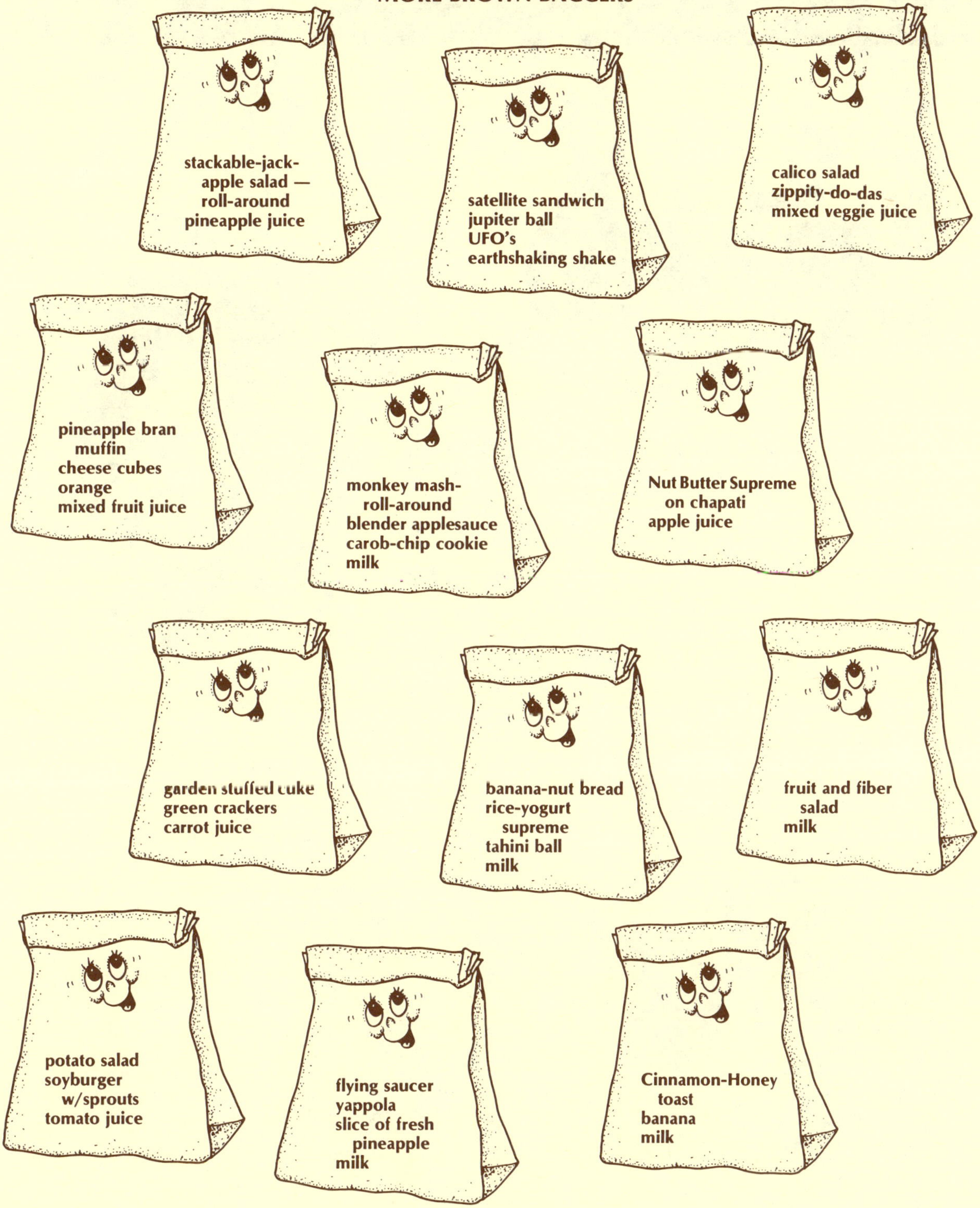
stackable-jack-apple salad — roll-around pineapple juice
satellite sandwich
jupiter ball
UFO's
earthshaking shake
calico salad
zippity-do-das
mixed veggie juice
pineapple bran muffin
cheese cubes
orange
mixed fruit juice
monkey mash-roll-around
blender applesauce
carob-chip cookie
milk
Nut Butter Supreme on chapati
apple juice
garden stuffed cuke
green crackers
carrot juice
banana-nut bread
rice-yogurt supreme
tahini ball
milk
fruit and fiber salad
milk
potato salad
soyburger w/sprouts
tomato juice
flying saucer
yappola
slice of fresh pineapple
milk
Cinnamon-Honey toast
banana
milk

Sprouts

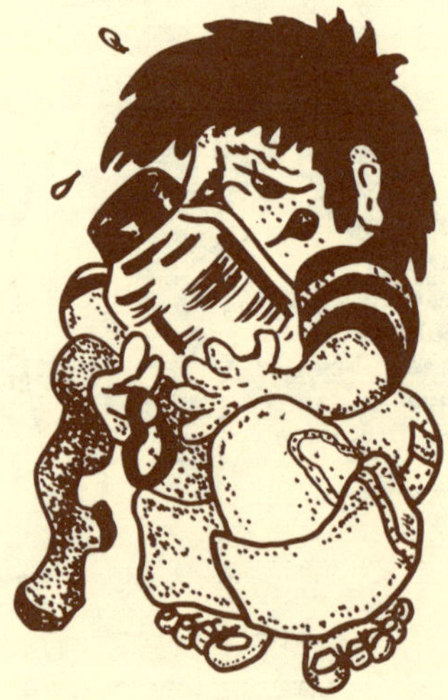

GROW YOUR OWN LIL' SPROUTS! You will need a quart jar, a piece of nylon (from panty hose) and a rubber band or canning jar ring.

1. PLACE 2 Tablespoons of alfalfa seeds in your jar. OR 4 T. of shelled sunflower seeds OR 4 T. of wheat berries, OR 4 T. of mixed beans (lentil-mung-adzuki).

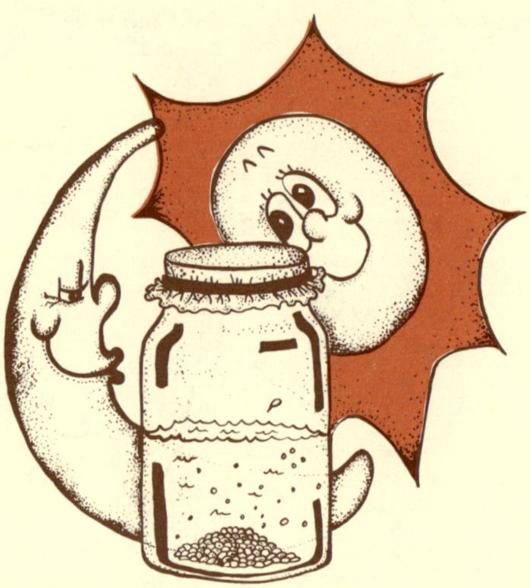

2. FILL the jar half full of water and attach the nylon with the rubber band or jar ring.

3. SOAK the seeds overnight.

4. DRAIN water in the morning. Rinse seeds in cool water and drain again.

5. INVERT jar and place in a bowl; cover with a towel or keep in a dark place.

6. RINSE the sprouts two or three times a day, draining well each time. The sun sprouts, wheat sprouts and mixed sprouts will be ready to refrigerate the second or third day when the sprout is the same length as the bean or seed.

7. SET the jar in front of a window or under a light when alfalfa sprouts have two little leaves on them. They will develop chlorophyll within a few hours and turn a lovely green!

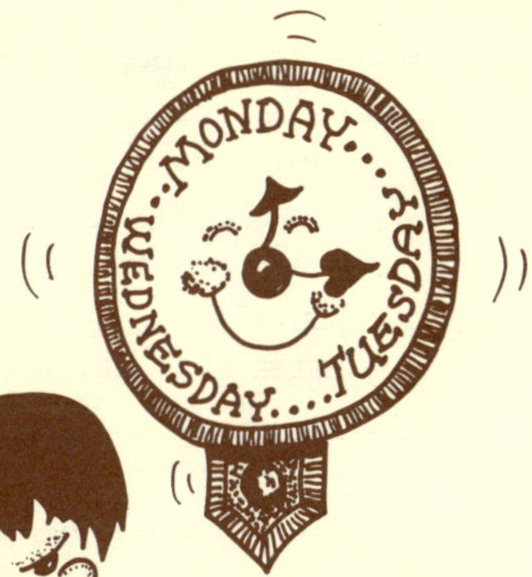

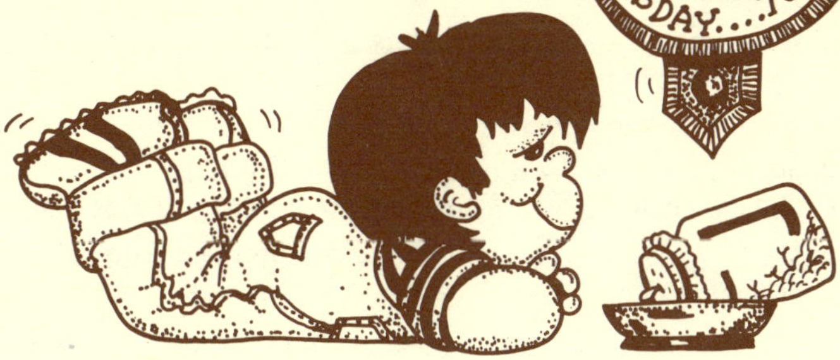

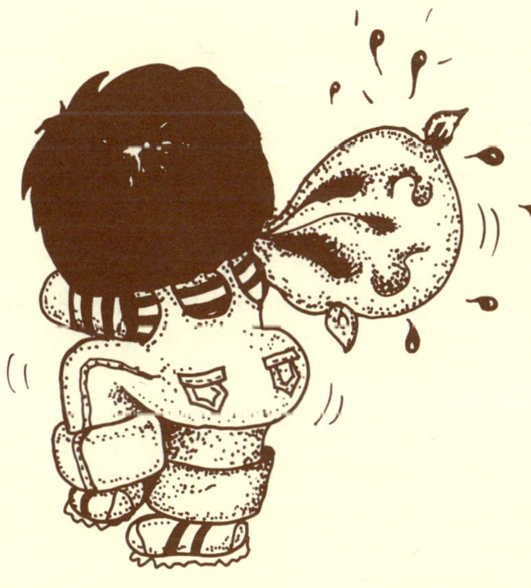

8. PLACE sprouts in a bowl of cold water; skim hulls off the top and drain.

9. FLUFF dry in a clean pillowcase: holding the top of the pillowcase tightly, wind arm around as if winding up for a pitch. Keep spinning until all the water is out. Store covered in refrigerator.

10. When ready to use, SPRINKLE sprouts on top of a salad or sandwich; eat and enjoy!

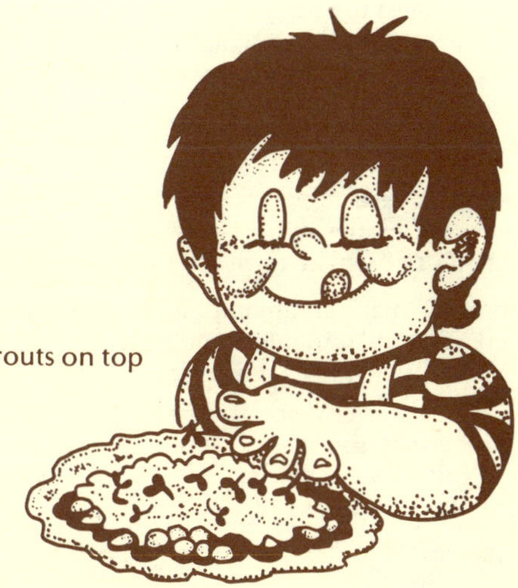

A ZILLION (WELL, ALMOST) USES FOR SPROUTS!

DRIED: Powdered in drinks, soups, patties, pancakes, they add nutrition and flavor.

DRINKS: Sun seed sprouts, wheat sprouts, mixed sprouts or alfalfa can be juiced or blended into fruit or vegetable juices, smoothies or shakes.

EGG ROLLS: Egg rolls and stir-fry wok dishes are delicious with mung bean sprouts or mixed sprouts steamed into the dish at the very last moment, or sauteed with other veggies before adding.

MARINATED: Marinate garbanzo bean sprouts or soy sprouts in vinegar, oil, honey and your choice of herbs and serve on a fresh green salad or add steamed green beans and onion slices for a piquant bean salad.

OMELETS: For souffles, scrambled eggs or omelets, use mung bean sprouts or mixed sprouts. Add at last minute or saute first with onion and green pepper.

PANCAKES: Any sprouts can go in batter or be toasted on one side of pancake or waffle.

SALADS: Add alfalfa, sun or mixed sprouts to tossed, three-bean, waldorf or fruit salads. Wheat sprouts taste great in fruit salads; cabbage-alfalfa-radish sprouts are great in tossed green salads.

SANDWICHES: Try sun seed sprouts with peanut butter, mung sprouts with egg, and heap alfalfa sprouts over any loaf, veggie, egg or cheese filling.

SNACKS: Rye, wheat and sun seed sprouts mixed with raisins and/or dates are delicious. Or top whole grain crackers with Jack cheese and alfalfa sprouts.

SOUPS: Add fresh sprouts just before serving. Rye sprouts taste like wild rice.

STEAMED: Serve as a vegetable dish — steamed with other veggies and a little tamari-soy sauce. (Use green pepper, mushrooms, onions, celery.)

SWEETS: Wheat or sun seed sprouts are great in nut butter-honey balls. Chop or run them through a food grinder before mixing in.

SPROUT SNACKS

NUT AND SEED: Mix 1 8 oz. package of cream cheese with 1 cup ground walnuts, 3 T. honey and ½ cup sun seed sprouts. Form into balls and chill.

AFTER SCHOOL: Soak 1 cup raisins in 1 cup very hot water and let sit until cool. Pour the raisin juice into a cup of herb tea or mix with any fruit juice. Toss the raisins with 1 cup sun seed sprouts (2-day old). Add a dash of cinnamon and enjoy!

SPICY SPROUTS: Toss together ½ cup wheat sprouts, ½ cup raisins, 1 t. date sugar and ½ t. cinnamon. Store in covered jar in refrigerator and toss again before eating.

HAIRY CREAM CHEESE BALLS

8 oz. cream cheese
2 T. honey OR maple syrup
½ cup alfalfa OR wheat sprouts
1/3 cup raisins OR chopped dates
1/3 cup chopped nuts
¼ t. nutmeg

In a medium bowl, mash cream cheese and honey together with a fork. Add sprouts, raisins or dates, nuts and nutmeg and blend well. Roll into bite-sized balls and coat with coconut, sesame seeds OR poppy seeds. Chill and eat!

SPROUT SURPRISE

1 cup wheat sprouts
2 cups pitted dates or raisins
1 cup chopped nuts
¼ cup sesame or sun seeds
¼ cup honey
¼ cup coconut or wheat germ

Grind sprouts and dates in a meat grinder. Add nuts, seeds and honey, and mix well. Form into balls and roll in shredded coconut. Chill.

Variation: Add ¼ cup peanut butter.

TRIPLE SPROUT SALAD

alfalfa sprouts
radish sprouts
sun seed sprouts
grated carrot
grated beet
fresh lemon juice
kelp
Pineapple-Cream Dressing
Cheddar cheese and avocado

Get your own wooden salad bowl and place a small handful of alfalfa sprouts in bowl (more if you want). Place 1 t. radish sprouts around alfalfa sprouts. On top of the sprouts, place about 1 T. sun seed sprouts (more if you like). With a hand grater, grate desired amount of carrot and beet (peel the beet) onto your salad. Cut a lemon in half and squeeze a small amount of juice over salad. Sprinkle with kelp and drizzle with Pineapple-Cream Dressing. Garnish with grated Cheddar cheese and chopped avocado.

Pineapple-Cream Dressing: Blend 1 small can crushed pineapple and 3 T. plain yogurt in blender until blended.

PHONY PHOOD

The world is phull of phony phood,
It's up to you to phigure it out.
Don't let phlashy labels inphluence you,
Discover what whole phood is all about.

Real phood grows on a plant or a tree,
Phull of nutrients to help you grow strong.
With phirm and steadphast energy,
To phorge you through when the day is long.

Play the phollowing game and see if you can phind,
The best natural alternative phor your phamily and yourselph.
Select the real phood that you know is the best kind,
And leave the phony phood on the grocery store shelph!

PHONY PHOODS		REAL FOODS
Chocolate Phudge	example	Lentil "Sausage" Links
Greasy Phrench Phries		Fresh Fruit Juice
Phroot Loops		Mashed Whole Potatoes
Phrankphurters		Nut and Seed Fudge
Phluffy Phrosting		Fresh or Frozen Fruit
Phizzle Pop		Garden Fresh Produce
Phrozen Popsicles		Cream Cheese 'N' Honey Icing
Phruit-Phlavored Punches		Baked Potato
Phortified Phlour		Apple Thirsty
Phritos		Granola
Phake Ice Cream		Tofu Patties
Phogna Bologna		Whole Grain Flour
Phluffo Instant Potatoes		Home-baked Corn Crackers
Phactory Phood		Homemade Banana Ice Cream

Draw a line from the phony foods in the first list, to the healthy alternatives in the second list. There are 41 misspelled words; see if you can find them.

SUPER SIMPLE SANDWICHES

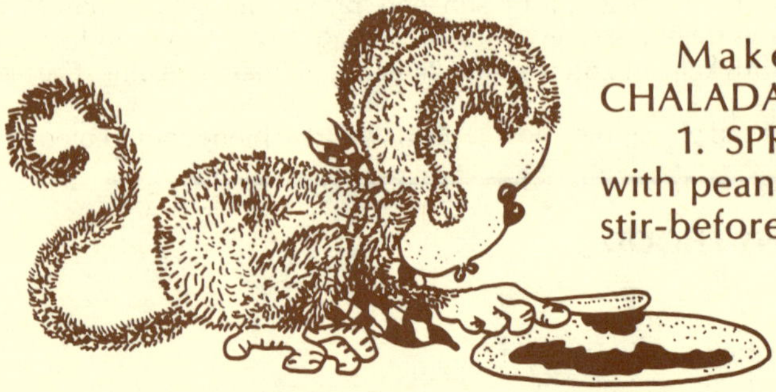

Make yourself a BANANCHALADA!

1. SPREAD a whole grain chapati with peanut butter (The old-fashioned stir-before-using kind.)

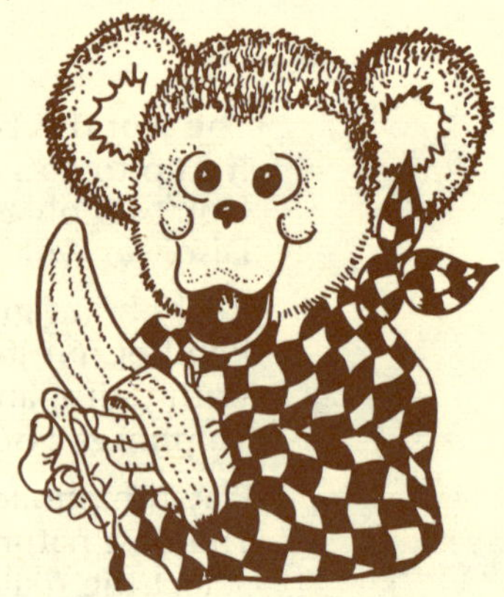

2. PEEL a banana and lay it at one edge of the tortilla.

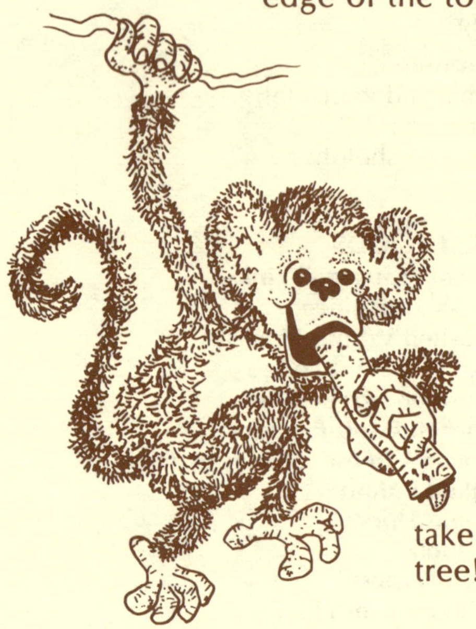

3. ROLL up the banana just like a burrito.

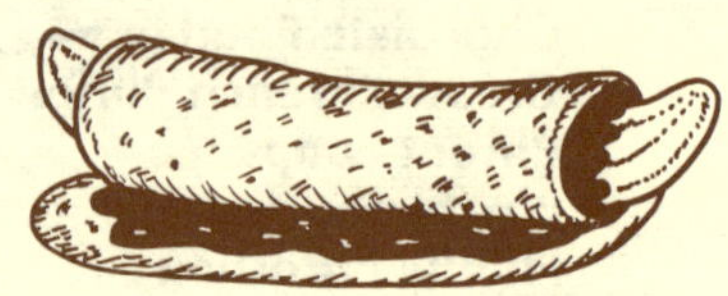

4. EAT it now, or wrap in foil and take with you as you swing from tree to tree!

OVEN-BAKED BANANCHALADA: Spread peanut butter onto a chapati. Lay a peeled banana across center. Drizzle with honey and sprinkle with cinnamon. Roll up and place seam side down on a cookie sheet. Cover with foil and bake at 350° until thoroughly heated.

PASADENA QUESADILLA: Using 6 chapatis, alternate chapatis with grated Cheddar cheese, beginning and ending with a chapati. Wrap in foil and place in oven at 375° for about 15 minutes or until cheese is thoroughly melted. Cut into wedges like a pie and serve with a salad or as a snack.

OVEN CRISPIES: Moms: Crisp a dozen corn tortillas, 6 at a time, by laying them directly on the middle rack, in a 300-350° oven. Turn once with tongs, tucking any curled edges under grating. Takes about 5-10 minutes. Check often so they won't burn — you just want them crisp, not browned. (Use room temperature tortillas; frozen ones curl.) When cool, store at room temperature in tightly covered containers. They'll keep for weeks — are ready for any filling at anytime.

Kids: Spread an oven-crispie (crisp tortilla) with mayonnaise and any leftover bean-nut-loaf spread, or egg salad mixture. Sprinkle grated cheese over filling. Place for 3-5 minutes in a preheated 400° oven. Then garnish with sprouts, tomatoes, lettuce, green onions, cucumbers, or olives. (See *Labor of Love Lunches* for spreads.)

CHEESE-APPLE APPLE-CHEESE: Sandwich 1 thin slice of Jack cheese between 2 round, thin slices of apple OR Sandwich 1 round, thin slice of apple between 2 thin slices of Jack cheese!

ROLL-AROUNDS

REGGIE McVEGGIE ROLL-AROUND: Spread a chapati with mayonnaise or Do Not Disturb Herb Dip. Spoon on your favorite bean, egg, tofu, or vegetable filling and top with grated carrots and sprouts. Roll up chapati around filling and eat out of the hand.

TOOTY McFRUITY ROLL-AROUND: Spread a chapati with cream cheese or honey-sweetened yogurt. Spoon on your favorite mashed fruit (bananas, strawberries, applesauce, peaches); sprinkle with nutmeg, anise, cinnamon, and sun seed sprouts OR chopped nuts. Roll chapati around filling and eat out of the hand.

KIDS: Be creative! Roll-Arounds can be different every time you make them. They are so easy to wrap and take with you to sports events, hikes or school activities. Leftover bean and loaf spreads keep well as do fruit Roll-Arounds.

FRUIT WALK-AWAYS: For delicious fruit pies or turn-overs that you can eat from your hand, follow this simple recipe: Slice 1" slices from Super Duper Refrigerator Biscuit Dough. (See *Labor of Love Lunches).* Use an oiled glass to roll out rounds to 6" circles on oiled cookie sheets. Spoon 2 T. fruit mixture in center of each circle. Fold circles in half and pinch sides together — like a turn-over. Make 2 slits in top for air to escape. Bake at 400° for 12-15 minutes or until bubbly and golden brown. Eat warm or cold.

Filling ideas: Diced bananas and crushed pineapple sprinkled with cinnamon. (Heat 1 cup pineapple juice with 1 T. arrowroot until thickened; then stir into fruit). Applesauce with cinnamon and honey added, homemade fruit jam, chopped apples, walnuts, raisins and cinnamon. (Make a thick sauce out of some apple juice and arrowroot flour. 1 T. arrowroot to 1 cup juice). Peaches or cherries. (Make a thick sauce from juice and mix into peaches or cherries).

SUPER SIMPLE SALADS

QUCK AND EASY CALICO SALAD (Main Dish Salad)

2 cups cooked small red beans OR pinto beans
1 grated carrot
5-6 sliced green onions
1 cup cubed cheese (your choice)
1 large chopped apple
3 finely chopped celery stalks
¼ cup chopped green pepper
¼ cup sun seed sprouts OR mixed sprouts
sea salt/kelp to taste
1 T. health catsup to 3-4 T. mayonnaise
Romaine lettuce or iceberg lettuce cups

Place beans in a large bowl. (Remember those freezer baggies of cooked beans in some liquid?) Add remaining ingredients except catsup, mayonnaise and lettuce. Mix well. Mix mayonnaise and catsup together and stir into salad. Use enough to hold it together — like any macaroni or potato salad. Cover bowl and chill several hours. To serve, spoon desired amount into lettuce cups or Romaine leaf; top with a sprinkling of alfalfa sprouts. Serves 8-12 as a salad or could be a main dish with crackers, raw vegetables and a dip.

Variation: Spoon salad into a Romaine lettuce leaf for a Roll-Around. Add sprouts and roll up.

STACKABLE-JACK-APPLE SALAD

5 apples
½ cup raisins
½ cup slivered almonds
OR ½ cup sun seed sprouts
1 cup cubed Jack cheese
plain yogurt

Wash, core and slice the apples. In parfait glasses, layer a spoonful of yogurt, a spoonful of apple slices, a spoonful of almonds or sun sprouts and a few cheese cubes. Continue to layer, ending with yogurt on top and garnish with a couple of nut slivers. Looks lovely for a beautiful dessert or salad.

Variation: To take to school, combine all ingredients in a large bowl and stir in enough plain yogurt to make a dressing for fruit, cheese and nuts. Cover bowl and refrigerate overnight. Spoon into individual containers for sack lunches.

YOU CAN TAKE IT WITH YOU FRUIT SALAD: Cut the top off an apple. Carefully scoop out center and save whatever apple shavings you can. Toss apple shavings with We Love Your Body Trail Mix and stuff apple. Take with you on a walk, hike or bike ride for quick, chewy nourishment. (See *Travel Stuff* this Chapter.)

HONEY-CINNAMON YOGURT: To 1 cup plain yogurt add 1 T. honey and cinnamon to taste.

(See *Better Beginnings: Breakfasts* and *Labor of Love Lunches* for additional salad recipes.)

MONA'S FANTASTIC FRUIT PIZZA

1. MEASURE 2¼ cups Snappy-Quick Mix into a large bowl. (See *Labor of Love Lunches.)* Add 1 cup water. (If you need to, add a little more water.)
2. MIX with a fork until dough is stiff and pulls away from sides of bowl.
3. SPREAD a generous layer of oil on a pizza pan. Push and press dough from center to outsides of pan and form a ridge around outside.
4. BAKE in a 400° oven or a pizza maker for 10-13 minutes. Check for doneness, and when done, allow to cool to room temperature.
5. MASH 1. T. pineapple juice into 1 8 oz. package of cream cheese. Spread this mixture onto cooled pizza crust just as you would spread tomato sauce.
6. SPOON drained, crushed pineapple in a 6″ circle in center of the pizza and make rings around the pineapple circle using any 3 of the following fruits, selecting them for their color contrast: strawberries, raspberries, blueberries, blackberries, boysenberries, cherries (pitted and sliced), seedless grapes, sliced apricots, peaches, red apples, mandarin orange segments, avocado slices, banana slices.
7. SPRINKLE a mixture of 2 T. coconut and 2 T. chopped nuts over fruit. Cut pizza in wedges with a *clean* pair of scissors.

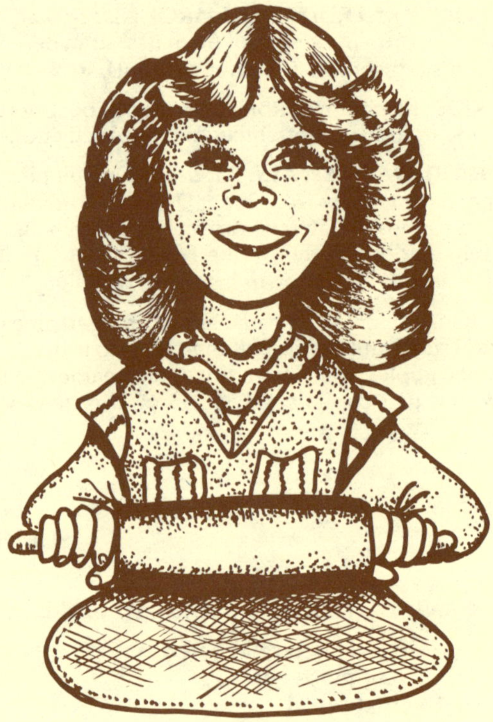

Variation: Slice 1″ slices of Super-Duper Refrigerator Biscuit Dough (make sure Mom keeps some wrapped in the refrigerator at all times for pizzas and Walk-Aways). Roll with an oiled glass into 6″ circles on an oiled cookie sheet. Make individual fruit pizzas as directed above.

CHRIS' BIONIC BREAKFAST SALAD

1. SLICE and mix the following ingredients in a large bowl:
   a. 2-3 bananas, peeled
   b. 2 apples, unpeeled
   c. 1-2 oranges, peeled
2. SPOON mixture into individual bowls.
3. Blend the following in a blender:
   a. 1½ cups chunk pineapple
   b. ½ cup orange juice
4. POUR sauce over salads.
5. GARNISH with your choice of the following:
   a. finely chopped almonds
   b. sunflower seed sprouts (2-day)
   c. chopped dates
   d. a few dashes of cinnamon or nutmeg

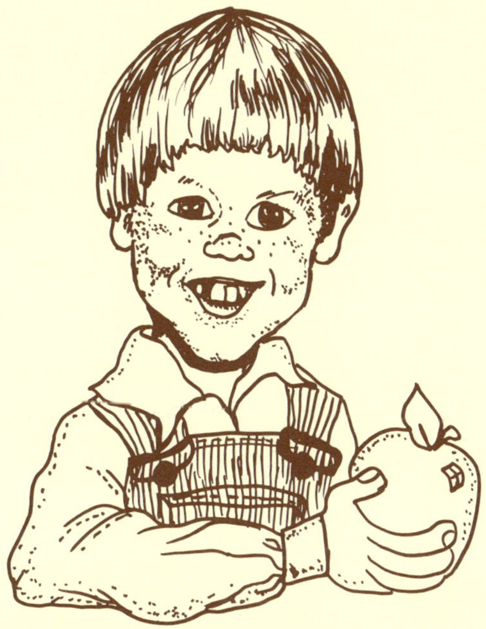

HotStuffHotStuffHotStuffHotStuffHotStuffHotStuffHotStuff

FANTASTIC FRENCH FRIES

1. Scrub potatoes. (Do not peel.) Cut in half lengthwise and slice into ⅜" slices. Immerse in ice cold water to which a few t. of lemon juice have been added. (Place ice cubes in a bowl of water for ice cold water.) Leave for 5 minutes. Then drain and pat dry.
2. Toss potato strips with about 2 T. oil per 6 potatoes and place on oiled cookie sheet in preheated 450° oven for 8 minutes or until golden-brown; then lower oven temperature to 400° and bake until tender.
3. Sprinkle with sea salt/kelp, an herb seasoning or paprika.

EGG IN A BASKET

1. Oil heat-proof bowls or ramekins and fill 2/3's the way full with hot mashed potatoes. Make a well in the center of each.
2. Break an egg into each well. Using the tongs of a fork, scratch the nest of the potatoes to look like a nest or a basket.
3. Bake at 300° for 15 minutes or until done. Sprinkle paprika and grated cheese over egg and potatoes and serve on plate with a green salad.

YANKEE DOODLE MACARONI

3 cups boiling water
2 cups vegetable macaroni
1½ cups tomato sauce
¼ cup finely chopped celery
1 cup shredded Cheddar cheese
¼ cup finely chopped mushrooms
½ t. sea salt/kelp
dash of cayenne

Bring water to boiling, add vegetable macaroni and stir constantly for 3 minutes on medium-high heat. Turn burner off, cover and let sit while you prepare the sauce. When pasta has absorbed all the water (15-25 minutes), drain any remaining liquid and return to burner. Stir in tomato sauce, veggies, cheese and seasonings. Heat until cheese is melted and sauce is blended. Serve.

Variation: Just before serving, add 1 cup chopped, steamed broccoli.

A DROP IN THE BUCKET: Allow 1 slice of whole grain bread and 1 egg for each serving. Using a doughnut cutter or the rim of a glass, cut a circle out of the center of the slice of bread. Butter both sides of bread and hole. Place in a medium-hot, buttered skillet. Break an egg into hole and toast on one side. With spatula, flip egg-toast and round hole and brown other side. When egg is done to your liking, transfer carefully to plate.

Who wants the last drop out of the can gets the lid on his nose.

HEIDI'S MASHED PO-LENTIL PIE

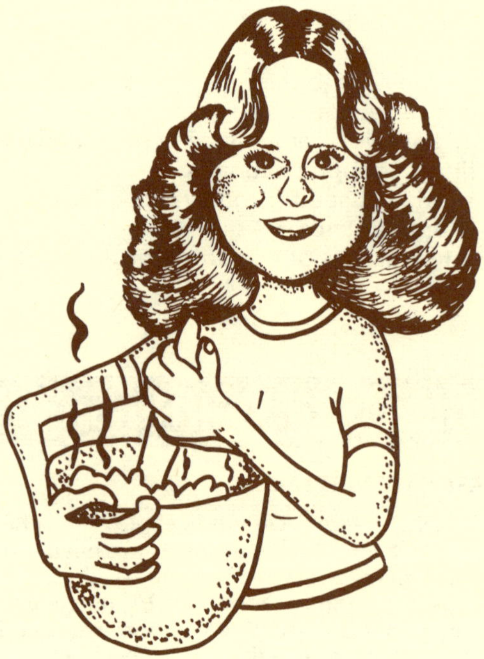

1. MASH 3 cups cooked lentils in a large bowl.
2. ADD the following:
   a. 1 chopped onion
   b. 1 t. sage
   c. 1 scant t. sea salt/kelp
   d. a dash of cayenne
   e. ¼-½ t. oregano
3. MIX onions, seasonings and lentils. Place in an oiled 10″ pie plate.
4. SPOON 1 layer of a steamed vegetable onto the lentil mixture. (Corn, carrots, broccoli, zucchini, peas, green beans.)
5. MASH about 6 cooked potatoes with some milk and butter. Spread on top of lentil-vegetable mixture.
6. DOT potatoes with SunButterBlend and sprinkle paprika over all.
7. BAKE at 350° for about 20 minutes or until hot and browned.

SLOPPY JOSES

1 medium, chopped onion
2 minced garlic cloves
1 cup chopped celery
½ cup chopped green pepper
1 cup ½″ cubed eggplant
3 cups tomato juice
2 t. sea salt/kelp
2½ t. chili powder
1 t. cumin
1 T. butter
2 T. honey
2 T. vinegar
2 cups cooked lentils
4 cups slightly mashed, cooked pinto beans

In a large cast iron skillet saute first 5 ingredients until barely tender. Use oil or butter. Add tomato juice and seasonings. Bring to a boil and simmer, uncovered, for about 20 minutes. Add lentils and beans and continue to simmer until beans absorb flavorings and juices cook down to desired consistency. To serve, spoon mixture onto buttered whole grain buns. This is a great patio dinner dish for a teen crowd or any group of hungry kids! Serve with a tossed green salad and stone-ground tortilla chips. Serves about 12-14 people. If you don't have so many hungry mouths to feed, prepare the entire recipe anyway and freeze what you don't use for another dinner.

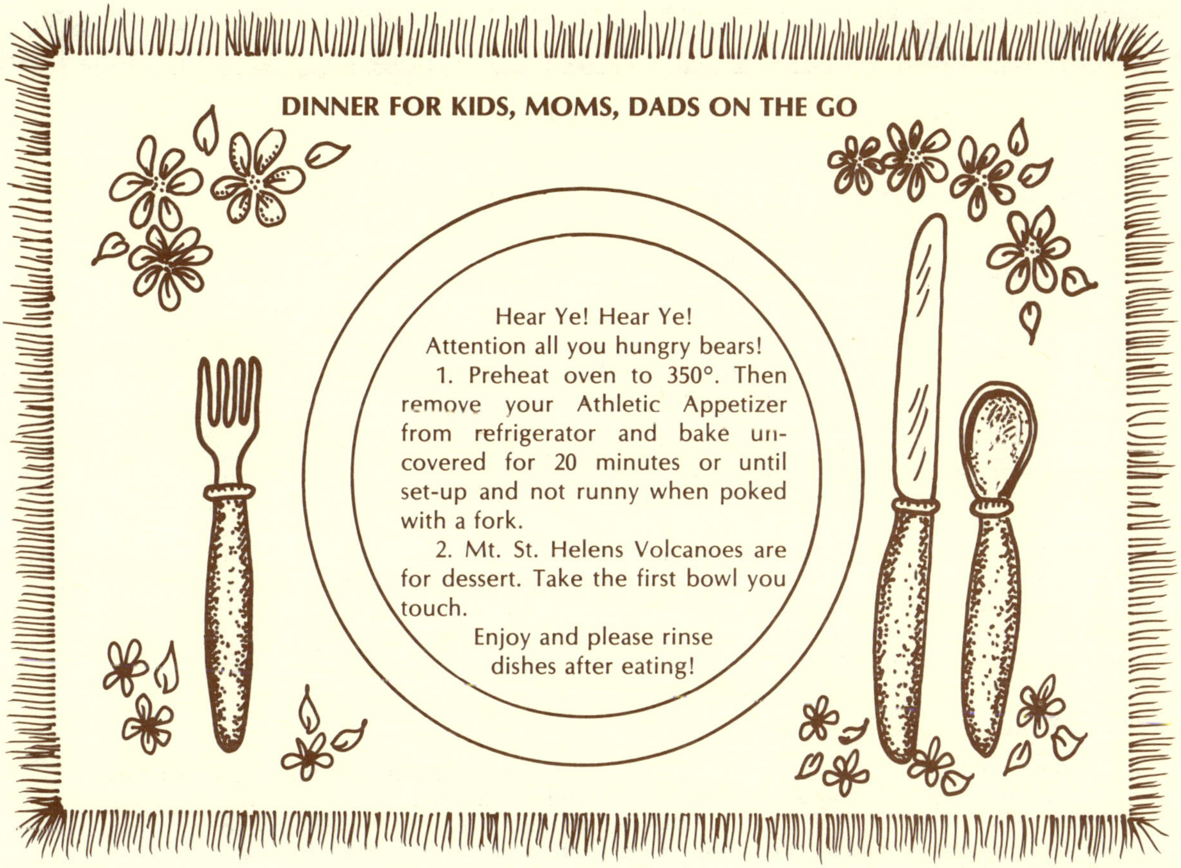
DINNER FOR KIDS, MOMS, DADS ON THE GO
Hear Ye! Hear Ye!
Attention all you hungry bears!
1. Preheat oven to 350°. Then remove your Athletic Appetizer from refrigerator and bake uncovered for 20 minutes or until set-up and not runny when poked with a fork.
2. Mt. St. Helens Volcanoes are for dessert. Take the first bowl you touch.
Enjoy and please rinse dishes after eating!

When your children are on the go and must eat at different times and/or you won't be home for dinner, prepare the following recipes and place in individual containers in the refrigerator. Then, using the back of a paper placemat or an 8½"x11" piece of paper, draw the above picture, writing your own set of instructions for dinner. Using magnets, place picture on refrigerator door for all to see, so that each child can prepare his/her dinner when needed. Keep salad and vegetable in refrigerator.

ATHLETIC APPETIZER

10 oz. tofu
1 cup milk
½ cup cottage cheese
4 eggs
¼ t. garlic powder
1 t. dry mustard
1 t. sea salt/kelp
dash cayenne
1 T. tamari-soy sauce
1 T. Parmesan cheese
½ chopped onion
5-6 chopped mushrooms
½ t. crushed basil
2-3 T. butter
3 slices whole grain bread
1-1½ cups grated Jack cheese

In a blender, place the first 10 ingredients. Blend until smooth. In a small skillet, saute the onion, mushrooms and basil in the butter until clear. To prepare, butter 6 large stoneware soup mugs. Using ½ slice of bread per mug, break into small pieces and place in bottom of mug. Divide saute mixture into 6 portions and place a spoonful of the mixture in each mug. Then pour the blender mixture evenly into the mugs. Top with grated cheese; cover with foil and place in refrigerator. When ready to eat, place in preheated 350° oven and bake 20 minutes or until set.

Variation: Place a spoonful of steamed spinach, broccoli or asparagus in bottom of mug before adding blender mixture and omit bread.

MT. ST. HELENS VOLCANOES

1 6 oz. can frozen apple juice concentrate
½ cup water
1 cup strawberries
3-4 T. arrowroot
3 cups sliced strawberries
3 bananas, sliced
3 T. honey
1 pint whipping cream
1 recipe graham cracker crust
(See Labor of Love Lunches)

In a blender, blend the apple juice concentrate, water, strawberries and arrowroot until smooth. Place in a saucepan and stir constantly over medium-high heat until clear and thickened. Cool. In a separate bowl, place sliced strawberries and bananas. Pour cooked mixture over strawberries-bananas and stir.

Prepare a graham cracker pie crust, following recipe in *Labor of Love Lunches,* making these substitutions: increase honey to ½ cup; omit nutmeg and Almond-Cinnamon Mixture, adding ¼ cup each of blender-ground sunflower seeds and almonds. Press crust mixture firmly into bottom of 6 or 7 large custard cups. Bake at 375° for 5-10 minutes or until browned. Cool. Prepare whipped cream, by whipping the cream and drizzling in the honey, until desired consistency.

To assemble volcanoes, divide whipped cream into cups, then with a spoon, make a crater in center of each volcano, almost down to the crust, with only ½-¾" whipped cream along sides of cup. Spoon the cooled strawberry-banana mixture into crater. Refrigerate. For the final touch, a flambeau, place a lemon extract-soaked sugar cube (recycle your old ones) on top of each volcano. Light and enjoy the eruption!

Variation: Use Baby Birds' Nests in place of graham cracker crust.

EASY BREEZY FRUIT SHERBETS

1. Choose from a variety of fresh fruits (bananas, strawberries, peaches, nectarines, cherries, etc.)
2. Freeze the fruit — either whole, chopped, or pureed and poured into ice cube trays.
3. When solid, put a little fruit juice into the blender (apple, orange, lemon, pineapple, grape, etc.). Add frozen fruit cubes or chunks and blend on high until mixture is of sherbet consistency.
   EASY BREEZY SHERBETS are really very thick Fruit Smoothies.

EASY BREEZY ICE CREAM

1. Freeze banana chunks.
2. In a blender, pour about 1 cup very cold milk, cream or half and half. Add flavoring (almond, vanilla, peppermint or maple extract) OR add carob powder, ground nuts, high protein powder.
3. Add frozen banana chunks and blend everything until of ice cream consistency. Add more banana chunks if necessary. Eat immediately.
   Variation: Add frozen peaches, orange juice cubes, strawberries or cherries for a fruit-flavored ice cream.
   EASY BREEZY ICE CREAMS are really very thick Shakes.

FOR HOME ICE CREAM MAKERS

In a blender, blend ½ cup orange juice, ½ cup lemon juice, frozen banana chunks equivalent to 2 bananas. Blend until smooth and thick. Mix this mixture in a large bowl with 4-5 cups half and half. Freeze as directed on ice cream freezer.

TAKE-A-LOOK: NO-COOK STRAWBERRY ICE CREAM

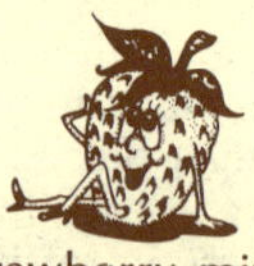

1. Separate 3 eggs. Whip the whites until stiff and mix yolks into 1 cup warm honey.
2. Mash 1 quart strawberries and partially strain before mixing in honey-egg mixture.
3. Whip 1 pint whipping cream and fold in egg whites. Then fold this mixture into strawberry mixture. Freeze 1 hour. Eat and enjoy!

FRESH FLASH-FROZEN YOGURT-SICLES

1. Mix any amount of plain yogurt (amount depends on how many popsicles you want to make) with any amount of frozen fruit juice concentrate (amount depends on how fruity and sweet you want it to taste).
2. Add 1 cup mashed bananas, ½ cup applesauce, OR 1 small can crushed pineapple. Whiz everything in the blender until smooth.
3. Spoon mixture into paper drinking cups or muffin cups and freeze until thick and slushy; then insert a stick in center. Freeze until hard.
4. Peel off cup or run under hot water for a few seconds and it will come right off. Eat outside!

Variations:

a. **Strawberry-Banana Popsicles:** Blend 1 pint fresh strawberries, 2 bananas and 1½ to 2 cups orange juice in a blender until smooth. Stir in 1-2 cups plain yogurt. Pour into cups and freeze.

b. **Apple Pops:** Blend ½ cup frozen apple juice concentrate, ½ cup water and 2 bananas in a blender until smooth. Stir in 1-2 cups plain yogurt. Pour into cups and freeze.

c. For a surprise for any flavored popsicle, place a fresh strawberry, grape or cherry in the bottom of each cup.

SELECT 'EM YOURSELF SUNDAES AND SPLITS

BASE: homemade ice cream, frozen yogurt, plain yogurt, cottage cheese
FRESH FRUIT: berries, peaches, bananas, pineapple, cherries, melon balls
SAUCE: carob, homemade preserves, maple syrup, honey, molasses

Toppings

DRIED FRUIT: raisins, dates, apricots, prunes, apples.
NUTS: peanuts, walnuts, almonds, pecans, cashews (chopped or ground).
OTHERS: sun seeds (sprouted or toasted), peanut butter, carob chips, granola, shredded coconut, toasted wheat germ, cinnamon, whipped cream.

TO MAKE A SUNDAE

1. PLACE 1 scoop of a BASE in a bowl.
2. SPREAD some FRESH FRUIT around the BASE.
3. POUR your favorite SAUCE over all.
4. TOP with any of the TOPPING suggestions.

TO MAKE A SPLIT

1. PLACE 3 scoops of any BASE in a long dish.
2. PLACE a split banana along each side.
3. SPREAD 3 different fruits around the 3 BASES.
4. TOP each BASE with your choice of SAUCES.
5. ADD your favorite TOPPINGS.

SATURDAY NIGHT SUNDAE

This is a great after-the-ballgame-treat! Mom can prepare the topping while the kids get the yogurt and applesauce ready.

1. Stir 3-4 T. maple syrup into 1 quart yogurt; divide into bowls for your family.
2. Stir 1 t. cinnamon into 2 cups applesauce; spoon over yogurt.
3. Sprinkle with Crunchy Butterscotch Topping.

Crunchy Butterscotch Topping: Dry-toast ½ cup ground nuts in a large cast-iron skillet at medium-high heat (Filberts are outstanding!) for 3-5 minutes, stirring constantly. Add 1 cup wheat germ and continue stirring another 2 minutes. Add ½ cup shredded coconut and toast 3 minutes more, being certain to stir constantly. Remove to a bowl and keep handy. Melt 2 T. butter in the hot skillet and add 2 T. honey. When bubbly, turn heat off and stir in toasted mixture.

This is a sticky one; serve it with a spoon and follow with a toothbrush!

BABY BIRDS' NESTS

1. Crumble 6 large, shredded wheat biscuits into a large bowl with 1 cup shredded coconut, ½ cup ground almonds and ¼ cup wheat germ.
2. Melt ¼ cup honey with ½ cup SunButterBlend and drizzle over dry mixture. Stir well and divide into 12 equal portions.
3. Press into buttered muffin cups and toast in 275° oven for about 10 minutes or until golden brown. Cool and remove carefully, then fill with fresh fruit and/or homemade ice cream or yogurt.

EAGLES' NESTS

Crumble 6 large, shredded wheat biscuits into a large bowl with 1 cup shredded coconut, ½ cup sunflower seeds and ¼ cup finely chopped walnuts. In a saucepan, heat ½ cup honey with ¼ cup butter until it begins to bubble. Continue to bubble and stir for 1 minute, then remove from heat. Stir in ¼ cup crunchy peanut butter and 1 t. vanilla. Mix well with the dry ingredients and then press into 6 large custard cups or ramekins which have been buttered well. Form a hollow as for a nest and bake in a 275° oven for 10-12 minutes or until browned. Serve stuffed with a fruit salad with yogurt dressing or with banana ice cream.

JIFFY JAM TOPPING AND FILLING: Heat 1 cup mashed berries with 1 6 oz. can frozen apple juice concentrate, ½ cup water and 4 T. arrowroot. When thickened, add 3-4 cups fresh sliced and slightly mashed fruit, such as strawberries, blackberries, boysenberries or peaches. Continue to heat until desired consistency. Store in covered, sterile jars in refrigerator and use within a few weeks OR freeze in covered containers.

MATT'S BLUE RIBBON FORMULA FOR TURNING A PLAIN BOWL OF YOGURT INTO AN UNFORGETTABLE-EDIBLE-AFTER-SCHOOL-SNACK

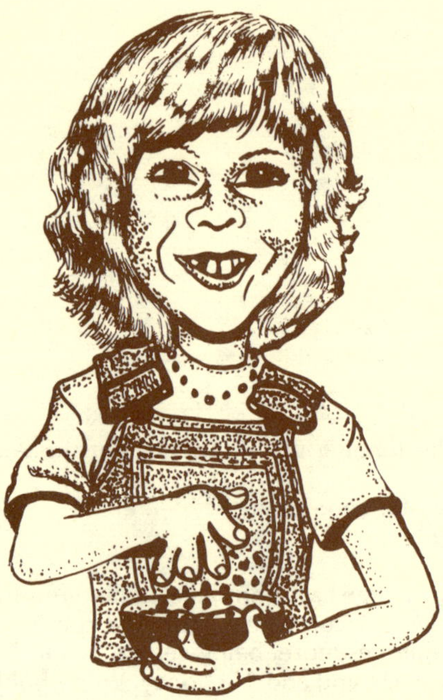

1. SPOON ½ cup plain yogurt into a soup bowl. Yogurt is from the DAIRY group.

2. SELECT one from each of the following food groups and SPRINKLE 1 t. each on top of your yogurt:

PROTEIN GROUP
cashews
filberts
almonds
peanuts
sun seeds
sesame seeds
chia seeds
other nuts or seeds

CEREAL GROUP
granola
grape nuts
wheat germ
shredded wheat
bran flakes
puffed millet
puffed rice

FRUIT GROUP
raisins
chopped apricots
chopped dates
chopped apples
chopped peaches
chopped pears
chopped pineapple
dried or fresh berries

EXTRAS
shredded coconut
carob chips
date sugar & cinnamon
honey
maple syrup
homemade jam or jelly
peanut butter 'n' honey mix

RANDY'S INCREDIBLY EDIBLE PLAY DOUGH

This recipe is so fun and easy that a toddler can do it with just a little help.

MEASURE AND MIX in a large bowl:
1. 1 cup peanut butter
2. ½ cup honey

MEASURE AND MIX in a medium bowl:
1. 1 cup instant powdered milk OR 2/3 cup non-instant
2. ½ cup wheat germ
3. 1 t. vanilla protein powder (opt.)

Spoon dry mixture into peanut butter-honey mixture and stir until almost blended. With VERY CLEAN HANDS, mix dough well and divide play-dough in half. MIX 1 heaping T. carob powder into ½ the dough. You now have 2 colors of play dough.

You can roll some out flat and cut with cookie cutters and add eyes, noses, buttons, or other trim with the contrasting color. You can form shapes: circles, squares, triangles, rectangles, spheres, cubes, cylinders and stars. Make 1 shape of each color of dough, then play a matching game. Form snakes, turtles, snails, lady bugs, mice with long tails and whatever your imagination wants to form.

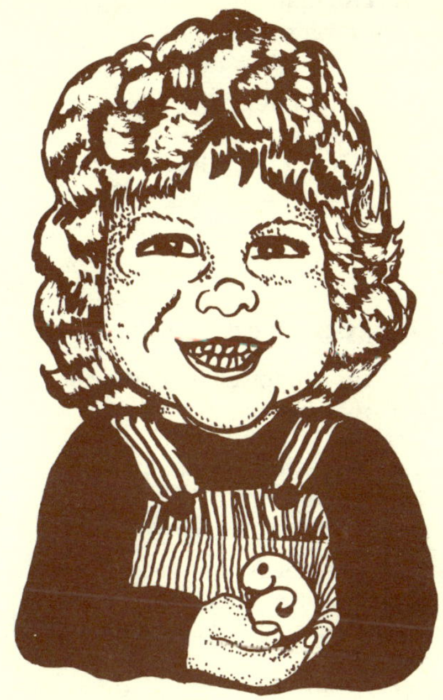

Add chopped nuts, raisins and shredded coconut to your creations before you put them on a wax-paper-lined cookie sheet to refrigerate until after dinner. Won't your family be pleased when you share with them? And you did it all by yourself!

ANY FRUITS AND ANY NUTS DELIGHT

1 cup cooked brown rice (leftover rice is great!)
1 cup nut milk (whiz ¼ cup favorite nuts in blender with ¾ cup water)
2 beaten eggs
2 T. honey, as desired
1 cup fresh, frozen or dried-reconstituted fruit
Honey-Cinnamon Yogurt

In a saucepan, mix together the rice, nut milk, eggs and honey. Cook over low heat until thick, stirring constantly. Spoon into dishes and top with fruit. Drizzle Honey-Cinnamon Yogurt over pudding. (See this Chapter.)

Variation: Substitute honey-vanilla whipped cream for Honey-Cinnamon Yogurt.

BOX-LESS VANILLA OR CAROB PUDDING

¼ cup honey
3 T. arrowroot flour
¼ t. salt
2½ cups milk
1 beaten egg
1½ t. vanilla

In top of a double-boiler, mix together honey and arrowroot and salt. When smooth, gradually add milk. Stir in egg and cook until pudding is thickened, then cook 2-3 minutes more. Remove from heat and add vanilla.

Variation: Divide pudding in half and add 1-2 T. carob powder to 1 half. Serves 4.

CHUNKY 'N' CHEWY COLD PUDDING

1½ cups leftover whole grain (brown rice, millet, wheat berries)
1 diced apple
1 cup raisins soaked in ½ cup hot water
¼ t. salt
½ t. cinnamon
¼ cup honey
½ cup chopped walnuts
½ cup plain yogurt

In a large bowl, mix grains, apple, drained raisins, salt and cinnamon. Stir in honey and yogurt until well-mixed. Mix in walnuts. Serve in bowls and dollop with additional yogurt if desired. (Drink raisin juice.)

Variation: (For hot pudding breakfast) Steam raw rice or millet for 25 minutes. Then add apple, raisins and spices and simmer 10-15 minutes longer. Cool; remove from heat and add honey and yogurt. Top with whipped cream or yogurt.

NUTRITIOUS COOKIES

RICE-ALMOND SPICE COOKIES

2/3 cup sunflower or safflower oil
½ cup honey
2 eggs
1 t. orange juice concentrate
1 t. vanilla
3 cups brown rice flour
½ cup blender-ground sunflower seeds
2 T. rice polish
1 T. arrowroot flour
1½ cups blender-ground almonds
½ t. cinnamon
½ t. nutmeg

Mix oil, honey, eggs, orange juice and vanilla in an electric mixer. In a large bowl, sift together brown rice flour, sun seeds, rice polish, arrowroot flour, ground almonds, cinnamon and nutmeg. Add liquid ingredients to dry ingredients and stir or mix well. Shape into 2 long rolls 1½" in diameter. Refrigerate overnight or freeze for a couple of hours.

Slice very thin. Place on oiled baking sheet and bake at 350° for 5-6 minutes. Makes 6-7 dozen cookies. *Important:* After baking 3 minutes, flip each cookie with a spatula so they will brown on both sides.

Variation: Bake like a pancake on a lightly oiled griddle or cast iron skillet on top of stove and flip so both sides can brown.

HI-PROTEIN SEED BARS

1½ cups whole wheat flour
2 t. baking powder
1 T. cinnamon
3¼ cups blender-ground oats
2 cups sesame seeds
2 cups sunflower seeds
1 cup blender-ground walnuts
3 eggs
½ cup oil
1 cup honey
2 t. vanilla

In a large bowl, sift together flour, baking powder and cinnamon. Add and stir blender-ground oats, sesame seeds, sun seeds and walnuts. In a blender, blend eggs, oil, honey and vanilla. Pour over dry ingredients and stir well. Dough should be stiff. Oil 2 cookie sheets, divide mixture in half and roll each half on a separate cookie sheet to ¼" thickness with a floured rolling pin. Bake at 350° for 12-15 minutes or until golden brown. Cut into bars and keep refrigerated.

40-CARAT COOKIES

½ cup boiling water
½ cup raisins
½ cup honey
½ cup oil
1 egg
1 t. lemon juice
½ cup finely shredded carrots
1 2/3 cup whole wheat flour
2 t. baking powder
½ t. sea salt

Pour boiling water over raisins. Soak for 5 minutes, then drain. (Reserve juice for drinking.) Beat together honey, oil, egg and lemon juice. Stir in carrots and drained raisins. In a separate bowl, sift together the flour, baking powder and salt. Add to the first mixture and blend well. Drop by teaspoonfuls onto oiled cookie sheet. Bake at 350° for 8-12 minutes. Makes 40 cookies.

TUTTI-FRUTTI BARS

- ½ cup SunButterBlend
- ½ cup honey
- 1 egg
- 1½ cups mashed bananas
- ½ t. salt
- 1 t. cinnamon
- 4 cups rolled oats OR barley flakes OR half oats and half barley
- ½ cup chopped dates OR raisins (soaked in hot water until plump and drained)
- ½ cup chopped walnuts
- ½ cup sprouted or plain sun seeds

Mix SunButterBlend, honey, egg, bananas, salt and cinnamon with an electric mixer. In a separate bowl, mix oats or barley, dates or raisins, walnuts and sun seeds. Combine liquid and dry mixtures and spread in an oiled 9"x13" baking pan. Bake at 325° for 45-50 minutes or until toothpick inserted in center comes out clean. Cut in bars.

Variation: Try mashed ripe peaches or mashed berries, reducing amount to 1 cup for very wet fruit. Use in place of bananas.

DANDY BARS

- 1 cup shredded coconut
- 2 cups rolled oats
- 2 cups barley flakes
- 1 cup rye flakes
- 1 cup wheat germ OR ½ cup wheat germ and ½ cup whole wheat flour
- ½ cup sesame seeds
- ½ cup raw sunflower seeds
- ½ cup whole, raw almonds (shelled)
- ¾-1 cup raw cashews (washed and drained)
- ½ cup flaked bran
- 1 cup chopped dates
- 1½ cups raisins (opt.)
- ¼ cup non-instant or ½ cup instant powdered milk
- 1½ cups honey or part honey/molasses
- 2/3 cup oil

In a very large bowl, mix together all the dry ingredients. Use your hands or a wooden spoon. Heat the honey and oil in a saucepan. Pour over the dry ingredients and stir until well-coated — like a granola. Spread and pack into large cake pans or large cookie sheets if they have a rim. You want to have granola bars that are at least ½" high. Be sure to oil the pans first. Bake at 275° for 45 minutes to 1 hour, depending on thickness. Bars will be soft. Cut into squares while still fairly warm. Store in plastic bags or covered container. This is a great energy bar — take along for breakfast, snack, lunch, or dessert.

GADZOOKS! SUGARLESS-FLOURLESS-EGGLESS GEMS

- 3 mashed bananas
- 1 cup chopped dates
- 1/3 cup oil
- 1 t. vanilla
- ¼ t. kelp
- 2 cups rolled oats
- ½ cup chopped nuts OR Almond-Cinnamon Mixture plus chopped nuts to make ½ cup

Mash bananas with a fork. Add dates, oil, vanilla and kelp and mix well. Stir in oats and let sit for a few minutes. Add nuts and drop by spoonfuls onto ungreased cookie sheet. Bake at 350°-375° for 10-15 minutes or until golden.

HOMEMADE CAROB CHIPS (CIRCLES OR SQUARES)

- ½ cup coconut oil
- 1 cup honey
- 1 T. liquid lecithin
- 2 t. vanilla
- ¾-1 cup carob powder
- ½ cup soy milk powder
- 2/3 cup non-instant or 1 cup instant powdered milk
- ¼ t. sea salt
- 1 T. vanilla hi-protein powder (opt.)

Melt first 4 ingredients in top of a double boiler, just until blended together. In a large bowl, sift together dry ingredients twice for thorough mixing. Pour liquid mixture into dry mixture and mix and stir until all lumps are out. The thick mixture should pull away from the sides of the bowl. Roll "dough" into ¼" diameter "snakes" OR spread ¼" thin on an oiled cookie sheet. Refrigerate and when hard, cut snakes into tiny discs or the cookie sheet spread, into tiny squares. Must be refrigerated. Use as you would carob chips.

*Note: Coconut oil is highly saturated fat and we do not recommend its frequent use, but it works well in the carob chips which we hope you will be using sparingly. Commercial carob chips contain brown sugar, so we feel these are preferable to the commercial chips. They taste good too!

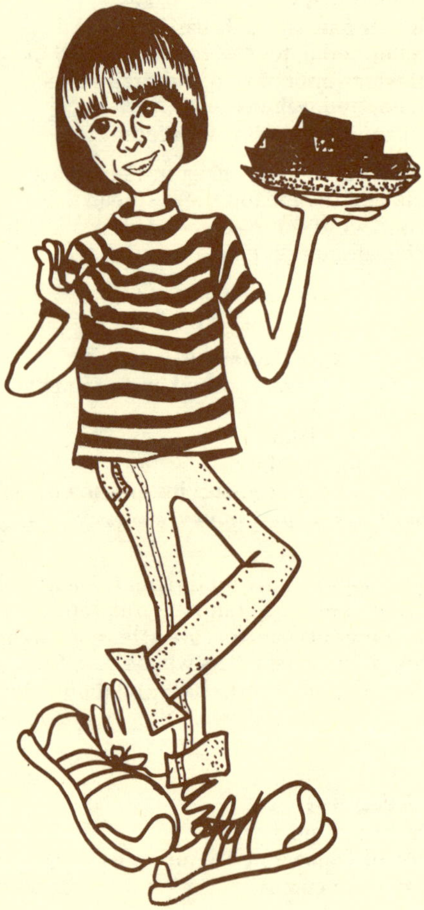

DAN'S DECIDEDLY DELICIOUS FUDGE

1. HEAT 1 cup honey and 1 cup peanut butter in a saucepan until well-blended.

2. MIX in ¼-½ cup carob powder. (Amount depends on your taste.)

3. REMOVE from heat and stir in the following:
   a. 1 cup blender-ground sesame seeds
   b. 1 cup blender-chopped sunflower seeds
   c. ½ cup or more of shredded, unsweetened coconut
   d. ½ cup dates or dried apples all diced up (opt.)
   e. ½ cup chopped walnuts (opt.)

4. SPREAD into an oiled 8″x8″ pan or spread thinly in a 9″x13″ pan. Refrigerate.

5. CUT into squares. Makes from 25-40, depending on thickness of fudge. Keep refrigerated. Wrap individually for school lunches or back packs.

EASY HALF CUP COOKIES

½ cup peanut butter
½ cup honey
½ cup blender-ground sesame seeds
½ cup blender-ground sunflower seeds
½ cup blender-ground rolled oats
½ cup whole wheat pastry flour
½ cup blender-chopped walnuts
½ t. baking powder
½ t.-1 t. vanilla
1 egg

In a large bowl, measure all ingredients except baking powder, vanilla and egg. Using a wooden spoon, mix well. In a small bowl, beat an egg, vanilla and baking powder together; then add to large bowl and mix well. Drop by t. on an oiled cookie sheet. Flatten each cookie with an oiled fork. Bake for 10-12 minutes at 300°. (Just until very light brown) Do not over-bake.

BETTER PEANUT BUTTER SANDWICH COOKIES: Mix 4 parts peanut butter to 1 part honey. Spread mixture on Easy Half Cup Cookies, then sandwich them together.

BETTER PEANUT BUTTER-CAROB CREAM SANDWICH COOKIES: Make Easy Half Cup Cookies, adding 3-4 T. carob powder to dough. When cookies are cooled, spread with a mixture of cream cheese, honey and vanilla. (See Frosting recipes.) Sandwich them together by 2's for a delicious cream-filled cookie.

DELECTABLE DATE BARS ALIAS FABULOUS FIG NEWTONS

2 cups chopped fresh or dried dates	**3 T. honey**
1½ cups water	**1 t. vanilla**
½ cup orange juice	**¼ t. allspice**
½ cup oil	**½ t. nutmeg**
½ cup whole wheat flour	**½ t. cinnamon**
½ cup wheat germ	**dash salt**
2 cups oats	**½ t. baking powder**
1 egg	

Date Filling: In a blender, blend dates with water and orange juice, a little at a time.

Date Bar Mixture: Mix together the oil, flour, wheat germ, oats, egg, honey, vanilla, spices and baking powder. Add 1/3 of the Date Filling to this mixture.

To assemble: Spread half of the Date Bar Mixture (with 1/3 Filling added to it already) in the bottom of an oiled 9"x9" pan. Spread the remaining Date Filling as the second layer, and top with the rest of the Date Bar Mixture. Bake at 350° for 30 minutes or until Bar Mixture is browned on top. Cool; then cut into squares.

Variation: Between the Date Filling and the top layer, sprinkle 1 cup chopped walnuts. To make FABULOUS FIG NEWTONS, substitute figs for the dates.

WENDY'S WONDERFUL FIVE-LAYER BARS

1. CRUMB 20 honey graham cracker squares in the blender, a few at a time OR roll them between 2 sheets of wax paper with a rolling pin.

2. MELT 1 cube butter in a small pan. (1 cube = ½ cup).

3. POUR butter into a 9"x13" pan and spread evenly.

4. SPRINKLE graham cracker crumbs over the butter evenly and press down, like for a pie crust.

5. CHOP 1¼ cups walnuts in a nut-chopper or blender. Arrange evenly over the crumbs.

6. SPRINKLE 1 to 1¼ cups Homemade Carob Chips over the nuts.

7. SPRINKLE 1½ cups shredded, unsweetened coconut evenly over the crust-nut-chips mixture.

8. POUR the following mixture evenly over everything: In a saucepan, heat 1½ cups milk, ¼ cup non-instant OR 1/3 cup instant powdered milk, and ¼ cup honey. Blend until smooth.

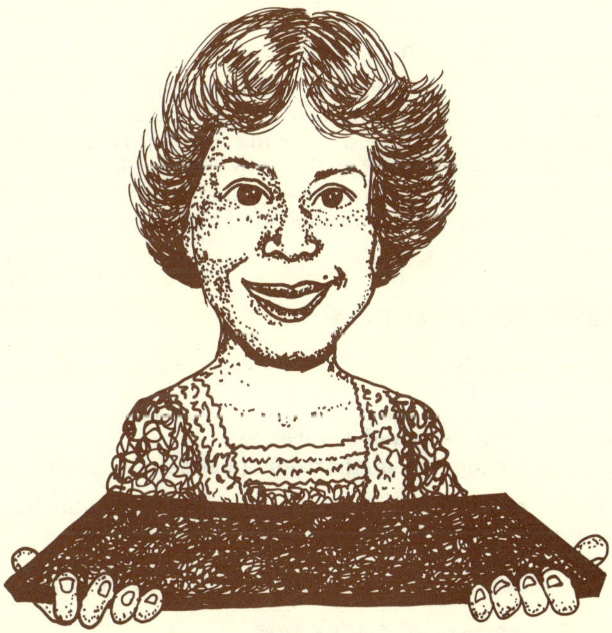

9. BAKE at 375° for 20-25 minutes or until browned and set.

10. CHILL and cut into squares. Wrap individually for school lunches or special occasions.

COCO-CABANA COOKIES

½ cup butter
½ cup peanut butter
1 cup honey
2 eggs
3 T. carob powder
1 t. vanilla
¼ t. sea salt
½ t. baking powder
½ t. baking soda
½ cup soy flour
3 cups whole wheat flour
1½ cups shredded coconut
1½ cups carob chips
1 cup toasted, unsalted sun seeds
¼ cup chopped, roasted peanuts

In an electric mixer, beat butter, peanut butter and honey. Cream in eggs, carob powder and vanilla and beat until all is creamy. In a separate bowl, sift together salt, baking powder, baking soda, flours and coconut. Add to creamed mixture and stir well. Add carob chips, sun seeds and peanuts and stir well. Chill batter; then roll into large marble-sized balls; place fairly close together on an unoiled cookie sheet. Bake at 325° for 10 minutes. Makes about 10 dozen cookies.

MARS BARS

1½ cups chopped dried dates
1¼ cups hot water or apple juice
1 cup SunButter blend OR butter
¾ cup honey
2 eggs
2 cups whole wheat flour
1½ t. baking soda
1 t. vanilla
¾ cup carob chips (or ¼ cup carob powder)
½ cup carob chips
¾ cup chopped walnuts, pecans OR almonds

Stir dates with hot water or juice. Allow to cool. Set aside. In an electric mixer, beat together the SunButterBlend, honey and eggs until creamy.Gradually add the flour which has been sifted with the soda. Beat well. Add the cooled date mixture, vanilla and ¾ cup of carob chips OR ¼ cup carob powder into the butter-flour mixture. Mix the batter well, then spread it across the bottom of an oiled 9"x13" pan. Top with ½ cup carob chips and ¾ cup chopped nuts. Bake at 350° for 25-30 minutes or until a toothpick comes out clean. Then cool and cut into squares.

Variation: Frost with a blended mixture of 8 oz. of cream cheese, 2-3 T. honey, 1 t. vanilla and ¼ t. cinnamon.

QUALITY CAKES

BETTER BIRTHDAY CAKE

1 cup honey
4 eggs
1½ cups oil
4 cups grated carrots
2 cups whole wheat flour (may be half pastry)
2 t. baking soda
1 t. salt
1 t. cinnamon
1 cup broken walnuts

In an electric mixer, beat honey, eggs and oil. Stir in carrots. In a separate bowl, sift together flour, soda, salt and cinnamon. Add dry mixture to liquid along with 1 cup broken walnuts. Pour into a 9"x13" oiled pan and bake at 325° for 30-35 minutes or until sides of cake come away from pan.

Variation: Substitute 1 cup crushed pineapple for half carrots and bake as cupcakes.

SUE'S APPLESAUCE DATE CAKE

2 cups whole wheat pastry flour
2 t. baking soda
¼ t. salt
1 t. cinnamon
½ t. allspice
½ t. nutmeg
¼ t. cloves
½ cup butter
½ cup honey
2 eggs
2 cups hot applesauce
1 cup chopped dates
1 cup chopped nuts

In a large bowl, mix flour, soda, salt and spices together. Then add eggs, honey, butter and 1 cup of the applesauce, beating well with an electric mixer until well-blended. Add remaining cup of applesauce, nuts and dates and stir well. Pour into a 9"x9"x2" pan and bake at 350° for about 50 minutes or until done. Frost with Ooey-Gooey Honey-Butter Frosting.

HEAVENLY CHEESE CAKE

16 graham crackers (blender-ground)
1 cup finely ground walnuts
1 t. cinnamon
½ cup melted butter
8 oz. cream cheese
2 cups cottage cheese OR half cheese and half tofu
2-3 T. honey
1 t. cinnamon
4-6 cups ripe banana slices

In a 9"x13" pan, press crust made of graham crackers, walnuts, cinnamon and melted butter. (Reserve some for topping.) Blend cream cheese, cottage cheese, honey, cinnamon in a blender or electric mixer. Fold in banana slices. Spread creamy-banana mixture over crust. Sprinkle with remaining crumb-topping. Refrigerate for at least 2 hours.

Variation: Add 1 T. carob powder to creamy mixture and top with shredded coconut.

BEST APPLE WALNUT CAKE EVER

3 large apples
2 t. cinnamon
2 cups whole wheat pastry flour
1 t. baking soda
½ cup butter
½ cup buttermilk or kefir
2 t. vanilla
¾ cup honey
walnut pieces
maple syrup

Slice apples and sprinkle them with cinnamon. Set bowl aside. Mix flour and soda. Using a pastry blender, cut in the butter until mixture is crumbly and in small pieces. Make a well in flour-butter mixture and pour in buttermilk or kefir, vanilla and honey. Stir all together just enough to combine. Butter a 9" cast iron skillet or pie pan. Spoon in enough batter to thinly cover pan and spread around. Add a layer of the apples, then a handful of walnut pieces. Drizzle a few T. of maple syrup over all. Then add more dabs of batter and spread as best you can. Continue layering apples and batter until everything is gone, ending with batter on top. Don't fill pan over 2/3 full. Bake at 350° for 35-40 minutes or until golden brown. Serve with Honey-Cinnamon Yogurt. Best warm.

ORANGE YOGURT SHORT CAKE (For fresh berries or other fruit)

1 cup butter
1 cup honey
1 t. vanilla
½ t. grated orange peel
3 eggs
2 cups unsifted whole wheat flour
¼ cup wheat germ
¼ t. baking soda
½ t. salt
1 cup plain yogurt
½ cup orange juice

In an electric mixer, cream butter and honey until fluffy. Add vanilla and orange peel. Beat in eggs, one at a time. Mix flour, wheat germ, soda and salt in a separate bowl. Add dry mixture to liquid mixture alternately with the yogurt-orange juice. Pour into a greased and flour-dusted small bundt pan. Top with Nutty Topping (see Frostings) and bake at 325° for 35-40 minutes or until toothpick inserted comes out clean. Cool on rack 20 minutes. Then remove from pan. Eat sliced with bowls of fresh, mashed fruit and whipped cream.

FROSTINGS AND TOPPINGS FOR QUALITY CAKES

TROPICANA FROSTING: Blend 1 8 oz. package softened cream cheese, ¼ cup honey, 1 T. lemon juice plus 1 t. grated lemon peel and ½ cup drained, crushed pineapple. Spread on a cooled cake or cupcakes. Mix ¼ cup shredded coconut and ¼ cup chopped filberts, pecans or macadamia nuts and sprinkle on top.

PEANUT BUTTER AND BANANA FROSTING: Cream together ½ cup crunchy peanut butter, ½ cup honey, 1 mashed banana, 1 T. oil or butter and 1 t. vanilla.

ZESTY ORANGE ICING: Cream together 1 8 oz. package softened cream cheese, ¼ cup honey and 1 T. frozen orange juice concentrate.

FRUIT FLUFF: Soak 1 cup chopped dates in hot apple or orange juice. (Just enough for dates to absorb.) Add 1 small can, drained, crushed pineapple. Fold in 1 cup of whipped cream very carefully. Spread.

ALMOND-CINNAMON: Mix 1 cup Almond-Cinnamon Mixture (see Space Stuff for recipe), 1 T. butter, 1/3 cup honey, 1 T. or so of milk and ½ t. vanilla. Stir until thick and smooth.

CAROB ICING: Mix 6 T. instant powdered milk, 1-2 T. carob powder, 1-2 T. honey, 1 t. vanilla and a small amount of cream. Blend until smooth.

CAROUSEL CABARET CARAMEL COATING: Blend ½ cup honey, ½ cup ground cashews, 1 T. Tahini, 1 t. Almond-Cinnamon Mixture (see Space Stuff for recipe), 1/3 cup shredded coconut, and a few drops of vanilla. Then spread on a baked cake and broil for a couple of minutes until browned and bubbly.

Variation: Try baking it with the cake batter for a crunchy bake-on-frosting.

CO-CO-NOATS: Mix together ¾ cup oats, ¾ cup shredded coconut, and ¼-½ cup chopped nuts. Sprinkle evenly on top of cake before it is baked.

Variation: Mix above ingredients with ¼ cup melted SunButterBlend, 1-2 T. honey and 1 t. vanilla. Spread on fruit cobbler before baking.

OOEY-GOOEY HONEY-BUTTER FROSTING: Blend ½ cup butter, 4 T. honey, 1 t. vanilla, 3 T. non-instant powdered milk, 1 8 oz. package cream cheese and ¼ t. cinnamon. When smooth and creamy, spread on slightly cooled cake. Keep refrigerated.

Variation: Omit cinnamon and add 1-2 T. carob powder for a carob-cream cheese frosting.

NUTTY TOPPING: Mix 1 cup oats, 1 cup shredded coconut, ¾ cup chopped nuts, ½ cup butter, 1 t. vanilla and ¼ cup honey. Spread on fruit cobbler or cake before baking.

Variation: Spread on baked cake and broil for a couple of minutes.

BIRTHDAY PARTY MENUS

For 2-5 year olds

1.
Randy's Incredibly Edible Play Dough
Earth Shaking Shake
Banana Bread

2.
Stackable-Jack-Apple Salad stuffed into whole wheat ice cream cones
Date-Cashew Shake

3.
Baby Birds' Nests with Homemade Ice Cream

For 6-8 year olds

1.
Better Birthday Cake
Homemade Ice Cream or Sherbet
Mixed Fruit Juice

2.
Jack-in-the-Bags
Hot Spiced Cider

For 9-12 year olds

1.
mixed raw nut cups
cupcakes
BanappleBerry Shake
Fresh Fruit Skewers

2.
Dandy Bars
Hot Carob Cocoa
Banana Splits

Teen-Age Mini Dinners

(Before the traditional cake and ice cream)

1.
raw veggie tray with dip
oven-crisped corn tortillas with melted cheese served with Guacamole and alfalfa sprouts
Zippity-Do-Das
carrot or V-8 juice

2.
Sloppy Joses with whole wheat buns
stone-ground corn chips
fruit salad bowl

3.
Whole Wheat Pizza
Honey Lemonade with Perrier water

1. Have a progressive dinner (contact parents for approval).

2. How about a potluck? (Kids can bring ethnic dishes). For a Mexican potluck, hang a pinata that you've filled with nuts and wrapped 'candies' from SWEET STUFF; use colorful paper flowers, place settings and recipes from South of the Border Fiesta Food — *Serendipity Suppers).* Serve fruit juice in punch bowl with fresh floating fruit — oranges, lemons, limes.

SUPER SIMPLE SMOOTHIES SUPER SIMPLE SHAKES

KIDS! Here's how to make a Super Simple Fruit Smoothie or a Super Simple Shake that will earn First Place in Thickness, Flavor and Nutrition.

ASK YOUR MOM TO HELP YOU MAKE IT THE FIRST FEW TIMES!

BASIC DIRECTIONS FOR SMOOTHIE OR SHAKE

FOR ONE TALL GLASS

1. FILL glass about 2/3's full with frozen banana chunks and/or other fruit (fresh or frozen).
2. POUR fruit juice OR milk around frozen fruit in glass until filled. Then pour all into blender.
3. ADD any of the flavorings or nutritious additions that follow.
4. BLEND on high until thick and smooth.

FOR SEVERAL GLASSES

1. POUR desired amount of fruit juice or milk (less 1 cup) in blender.
2. ADD frozen banana chunks and/or other fruit until they are 2/3's the level of the liquid.
3. ADD any other flavorings or nutritious additions.
4. BLEND on high until thick and smooth — adding more banana chunks if necessary.

NUTRITIOUS ADDITIONS

MILK BASES: milk, soy milk, buttermilk, kefir, homemade ice cream, powdered milk, yogurt, any nut milk.

FLAVORINGS: cinnamon, nutmeg, mint, vanilla, almond extract, mace, anise, etc.

SWEETENERS: frozen banana chunks, honey, real maple syrup, carob powder, peanut butter, Tahini, molasses.

HIGH ENERGY: dates, raisins, sun seed sprouts, raw egg, coconut, wheat germ, nutritional yeast, sesame seeds, ground nuts, flavored hi-protein powder, etc.

INVENT-A-DRINK: ADD WHAT YOU LIKE AND GIVE YOUR OWN SPECIAL NAMES TO YOUR OWN SPECIAL DRINKS.

HERE ARE JUST A FEW SAMPLES TO GET YOU STARTED

ORANGE PEACH SMOOTHIE: In blender, place 1 sliced peach, about 1 cup orange juice and some frozen banana chunks. Blend on high until smooth and thick.

APPLE PEACH SMOOTHIE: In a blender, place 6-7 frozen banana chunks, ½ cup apple juice, 1 chopped fresh or frozen peach, 5-6 T. plain yogurt and 1 small handful raisins. Blend on high until smooth and thick.

BANAPPLEBERRY SHAKE: Fill your glass half full of frozen bananas and half full of frozen strawberries. Pour pineapple juice to cover fruit. Place all in blender and blend until pink and smooth. For Quantity: In a blender, place 2 frozen bananas (cut in chunks), one half a package of frozen, unsweetened strawberries, and one half a large can of unsweetened pineapple juice. Blend until smooth.

STRAPPLE SMOOTHIE: In a blender, place 1 handful fresh or frozen strawberries, 1 handful frozen banana chunks, 3 heaping T. plain yogurt and 1 cup apple juice. Blend until smooth and thick.

APRICOT SMOOTHIE: Soak ½ cup dried apricots in 1½ cups water. Add 1 cup Mixed Fruit Juice and 1 cup frozen banana chunks. Blend until smooth and thick.

(See *Better Beginnings: Breakfasts* for many more Smoothies, Shakes and drink recipes.)

MAKE A DATE WITH A NUT SHAKE: In a blender, blend 3 T. cashews with ¼ cup water. Add 2-3 T. chopped dates, 1 cup milk and enough frozen banana chunks to blend into a thick milkshake.

Variation: Add ½ t. vanilla or a dash of cinnamon. For Quantity: Blend 1 cup cashews in 4 cups cold water. Add ¼ cup soaked, chopped, pitted dates and enough frozen banana chunks to make a thick shake. Blend until smooth.

OTHER DRINKS

MIXED FRUIT JUICE: Blend 3 parts fresh apple juice, 3 parts fresh orange juice, 1 part fresh or canned pineapple juice and a few squeezes of fresh lemon juice. Chill.

APPLE THIRSTY: To 1 quart of apple juice, stir in about 1 T. of liquid acidophilus. Cap loosely and let sit at room temperature overnight. Chill. It will be tangy and bubbly like a carbonated beverage, and a good source of friendly intestinal bacteria.

BUBBLY: Any fruit juice can be combined with a small amount of Perrier or sparkling mineral water for a bubbly.

HERB TEAS: Mix herb teas half and half with fresh fruit juices for refreshing drinks. Apple juice goes well with peppermint tea or lemon tea. Honey Lemonade goes well with mint or lemon tea.

HONEY LEMONADE: Stir the juice of 1 lemon, 3-4 cups of warm water and honey to taste. Chill.

CAROB MILK: Blend 1 cup milk, ¼ t. vanilla, 1 t. carob powder, 2 t. honey and a dash of cinnamon.

HOT CAROB COCOA: In a saucepan, heat and stir 1 quart of milk, 2-4 T. carob powder, 3 T. honey, 1 t. vanilla and a few dashes of cinnamon.

You must chew your drinks and drink your foods. — *Mahatma Gandhi*

BabyStuffBabyStuffBabyStuffBabyStuffBabyStuffBabyStuff

FIRST FOODS: Mother's milk is recommended for the first 4-6 months of baby's life. For foods, use a baby food grinder, or chop, mash, blend or puree, depending upon baby's age, readiness, and digestive system.

FRUITS: banana, papaya, avocado, apples, peaches, apricots, pears. All fruit must be very ripe to prevent gas. Banana skins should be speckled.

DRINKS: pure water, fresh fruit or vegetable juices, kefir, nut and seed milks, goat's milk.

VEGETABLES: squashes, beets, yams, carrots, peas, green beans.

DAIRY PRODUCTS: cottage cheese, yogurt.

CEREALS: Variety is important so allergies don't develop. Millet is excellent for a first cereal as are barley, oats, wheat, cornmeal, brown rice. Serve with milk or yogurt, soaked and mashed raisins or dates in small amounts, OR fresh, mashed fruits.

SOUPS: With whole grain or vegetable noodles, barley, cracked beans, lentils, split peas, steamed or simmered vegetables.

NUTS AND SEEDS: Whizzed with water to make milk, or blender-ground into peanut butter, cashew butter, almond butter or Tahini (sesame seed butter.) (See *Better Beginnings: Breakfasts* for recipes.)

OTHER PROTEIN: wheat germ, cooked, scraped egg yolk.

FINGER FOODS: dried whole grain toast, whole grain unsalted crackers or rice cakes, cheese cubes, sliced or cubed fresh fruit, carrot sticks.

*Avoid the addition of honey to any baby food. Besides the possibility of honey being harmful to babies under age 1, it is pointless to train baby to have a sweet tooth, only to have to break the habit later.

VITAMINS AND MINERALS: For extra nourishment try any of the following:

1. Sprouts: Alfalfa or sun sprouts (1 T.) blended into juices. Provides protein, vitamins and minerals.
2. Mineral Drink: A handful each of almonds, raisins and oat groats soaked for a couple of days in one quart of water in refrigerator. Strain and add 1 t. of unsulphured molasses if desired to the liquid. Use the nuts, raisins and oat groats for older child's cereal topping. Provides minerals.
3. Brewer's Yeast: Start with ½ t. and add to orange juice. Provides vitamin B complex, amino acids.
4. Cod Liver Oil: ¼ to ½ t. Provides vitamins A,D,E.
5. Rose Hips: Blended into fruit juices. Provides vitamin C complex.
6. Wheat germ and/or oil from pierced vitamin E capsule: Added to drinks. Provides vitamin E and unsaturated fats.
7. Bran Drink: Cover one cup of flaked bran with two cups boiling water. Allow to cool. Strain and mix liquid half and half with fruit or veggie juices. Provides minerals and vitamins.
8. Raw Blender Applesauce: In blender, blend 4-6 apples (cored and chopped), 1 orange (peeled and chopped), and 1/3 cup fresh apple or orange juice. Blend to desired consistency. Stir in 1-2 t. cinnamon and nutmeg to taste.

*Before you season your family's dinner, scoop some out, blend to a puree and freeze in ice cube trays. You can then take out as many as you need for single servings for baby. This gets baby used to the kind of meals your family eats instead of the commercial kind in the jars. As teeth come in and digestion improves, mash with a fork (rather than blend to a puree) to encourage chewing.

TravelStuffTravelStuffTravelStuffTravelStuffTravelStuff

BY AIRPLANE, TRAIN OR SHIP:

Bring along your choice of:
sun sprouts or sun seeds for garnish
home-bagged raisins, nuts, dates, sun seeds
homemade nut and seed fudges, fruit leathers
fresh fruit — banana, orange, apple, cookies
(most airlines will accommodate special diets if you call a day ahead of your flight.)

BY CAR:

Bring along any of above plus:
gallon jug of water — for rinsing sprouts, drinking
seeds, nylon, rubber band, jar, for sprouts

An ice chest for your choice of:
fresh fruit and vegetable juices
fresh vegetables — carrot and celery sticks
salad greens, onions, mushrooms, tomatoes
hard cheeses, yogurt
kefir, milk, butter, peanut butter, mayonnaise
lemon — for water or salad dressing
sandwiches from home

A basket for:
whole grain bread, crackers
homemade cookies
granola, other dry cereals
large thermos of homemade soup

IF STAYING IN A MOTEL:

Bring along any of above OR
Purchase groceries and make your own.

IF CAMPING BY TENT, VAN, CAMPER OR TRAILER:

Bring along any of above, plus your choice of:
campstove with pans and utensils
hot cereal, eggs, Snappy-Quick Mix
frozen patties for cooking at campsite
whole grain buns
oil, tamari-soy sauce, honey
a tub of yogurt to mix with fresh fruit
popcorn to pop over the campfire
homemade dried soup mix and seasonings
scrubbed vegetables for adding to soup pot
frozen beans/grains in packets for soup pot

IF BACKPACKING:

Bring along your choice of:
baggies of sprouts
seeds for more sprouting
some hard cheese
cracked grains and beans; pasta
herb-seasoning mix, dried veggies
ground/flaked grains for cereals
dried fruit; some fresh fruit, fruit leathers
homemade trail mix, popcorn
nut and seed fudges and cookies
water and purifier

SUN-BAKED BREAD AND GRAPE-NUTTY-CEREAL: Mix wheat sprouts with an equal amount of raisins and run them together through the meat grinder. Optional: add 1 t. malt. Form into flat patties and place on an oiled cookie sheet. Dry in the sun, turning several times. These can be eaten when still chewy or can be dried thoroughly and crumbled into grape nuts for your cereal. (Can also dry patties in a low oven.)

CAMP OUT SOUP

2 scrubbed, chopped carrots
4 sliced mushrooms
1-2 chopped onions
1 chopped green pepper
Seasoning Mix
4 small, scrubbed, cubed potatoes
1½ cups cooked lentils (brought frozen from home in plastic baggie)
1 can tomato paste
1 can tomato sauce
1-2 thinly sliced zucchinis
2-4 T. flour for thickening

Start with 2½ quarts of water. Bring to a boil and add carrots, mushrooms, onions and green pepper. Stir in Seasoning Mix. Cover and simmer 15 minutes. After 15 minutes, add potatoes. Then add lentils, tomato paste and sauce, and zucchini. Stir flour in some cold water and add. When veggies are tender, serve.

Variation: To use dried lentils, add along with first 4 veggies. For less tomato taste, omit the tomato sauce.

SEASONING MIX (FOR CAMP OUT SOUP): Mix all ingredients together and place in a covered container or plastic baggie until added to soup: ¼ cup pearl barley, 2 t. plus, chili powder, ¼ t. garlic powder, 1 t. plus, cumin, 1 t plus, crushed basil, 1 t. Italian Herb Mix, 1 t. dried parsley, 1 t. dried celery leaves, a dash of cayenne, and sea salt/kelp to taste. (See *Serendipity Suppers* for Italian Herb Mix.)

WE LOVE YOUR BODY TRAIL MIX: Raw mixed nuts tossed with 2-day sun seed sprouts, raisins and coconut.

POWDERED CAROB COCOA MIX: Mix together ¼ cup instant powdered milk, ⅛ t. barley malt sweetener, 1 T. carob powder and 1 T. vanilla hi-protein powder. Place in cup and add boiling water. For a large quantity: Mix 1 cup powdered milk, ½ t. barley malt, ¼ cup carob powder and ¼ cup vanilla hi-protein powder. Keep covered. Spoon about 6 T. mixture into cup before adding water.

(See recipes in *KIDSTUFF* and other chapters for recipe and menu ideas.)

DriedStuffDriedStuffDriedStuffDriedStuffDriedStuffDriedStuff

Dehydration is one of the oldest and safest methods of preserving foods. Dried food is delicious, easy to prepare, saves time and storage space and retains nearly all the nutritional value of the fresh food. Almost any food can be dehydrated, but two of our favorites are fruit slices and fruit leathers.

It certainly helps to have a food dryer, and once you discover the diversity of this kitchen addition, you may consider making, buying or trading your skills for a homemade dehydrator. We can't imagine being without this handy "appliance," that preserves not only fruit and vegetables, but herbs and spices, nuts and seeds (in shells), sprouts and sprout cakes, croutons and crackers, thick soups, and even cheese.

Until you have a dryer, you can make use of an oven, a wood stove, a drafty window or good old Brother Sun. Lay a thermometer next to your food to be sure the temperature does not go above 120° (you just want to dry it, not cook it). A shelf about two feet above a wood stove is ideal because of the rising warm, dry air. Whatever drying method you use, the preparation takes about one-half hour.

TO DRY FRUIT

Start with good quality, fresh, ripe fruit. Wash, peel, core, pit, or whatever is necessary to end up with nothing but edible fruit. Slice apples, pears, bananas, papayas, melons and pineapple in ¼" slices, either lengthwise or across the grain. Try some both ways to find out which you like best. Pit and quarter peaches and nectarines, halve plums, apricots and cherries, then lay on screen or tray, cut side up. Dry seedless grapes whole; most berries can be sliced once or left whole, depending on size. Dried berries are best reconstituted with a little hot fruit juice and used as a jam. All fruit can be dipped in either lemon, orange or pineapple juice to help retain color, but never use commercial sulphur preparations; they are unnecessary, and may be harmful to your health.

Lay fruit directly on clean screen of dehydrator or use a broiler tray with holes and ridges, which will shorten drying time. If any fruit overlaps another piece of fruit, neither will dry and both may mold or attract bugs. If flying friends are a problem (bugs know good stuff when they see it), simply make a frame or use an old picture frame a little larger than your cookie sheet or broiler pan and cover it tightly with nylon net or cheesecloth; then place on top of your tray of fruit or leather. It lets air in and keeps creatures out! Some fruits dry in one full day of sunshine, but some may require an overnight exposure to a drafty window. Store in clean glass jars with a cracker to keep dry.

FABULOUS FRUIT LEATHER

1. Prepare a cookie sheet as follows: Using plastic wrap 4" longer than your cookie sheet, lay over, smooth into corners, and fasten plastic wrap with masking tape. Tape will hold the plastic in place when you spread the puree.

2. Puree: Using fresh, ripe fruit, one kind or a combination, wash, cut, peel, core, or pit as with dried fruit. Place 1 T. lemon juice in blender and add 1 cup of cut-up fruit. Blend until pureed. Repeat until you have used all your fruit. Make as much as you wish, but use only 2 cups puree per large cookie sheet for best results. Add complementary spices or honey IF needed, remembering that the taste will be concentrated when it dries.

3. Spread pureed fruit on plastic covered cookie sheet a little less than ¼" thick and as even as possible. Begin drying your leather early in the day if you're using sunshine so you can take full advantage of the daylight hours. Bring it in at night and leave near a drafty window. Most leathers will take two days, with very juicy fruits possibly taking two and one-half days.

4. When dry, roll up like a Roman scroll. Or you may dollop puree onto tray and spread into individual 3" circles. When dry, roll up in cone-shapes and fill with cream cheese and nuts or spread with crunchy peanut butter and roll as for Roll-Arounds. You can even tear little pieces of leather and partially reconstitute (add moisture) with a little hot fruit juice to make delicious jam.

We have never made a fruit leather combination that we didn't like, so you really can't make a mistake. But here are some of the ones we liked the best, two of which were blue ribbon winners at the Oregon State Fair!

APPLE PIE LEATHER: 2 C. apple puree, 2 T. lemon juice, 1 t. cinnamon, dash nutmeg, dash cloves.

PLUM YUMMY LEATHER: 2 C. plum puree, 2 T. each lemon juice and honey.

STRAWBERRY CREAM LEATHER: 2 C. strawberry puree, 1 T. lemon juice, 1 T. honey, 1 t. vanilla protein powder.

CHEERY CHERRY LEATHER: 1 C. apple and 1 C. cherry puree, 2 T. lemon juice, ½ t. crushed anise.

JUST PEAR-FECT LEATHER: 2 C. pear puree, 1 T. lemon juice and ½ t. cinnamon.

NANABANANA LEATHER: 2 C. banana puree, 2 T. lemon juice.

PEACHES 'N' CREAM LEATHER: 2 C. peach puree, 1 T. lemon juice, 1 t. vanilla protein powder, honey to taste (some kinds of peaches need honey, some don't. Taste first.)

DRIED FRUIT COMPOTE: Pour 3 cups boiling water over 2 cups mixed dried fruits such as apples, pears, apricots, prunes, cherries, etc. Seal lid tightly and allow to reconstitute for two hours. Remove 1 cup liquid and mix with 1 T. honey, 2 t. arrowroot powder, 1 t. each, cinnamon and grated orange or lemon peel. Cook and stir just until thickened and bubbly. Add fruit and serve hot or cold in stemmed glassware with a dollop of orange-spice yogurt.

Common sense in an uncommon degree is what the world calls wisdom.
Samuel Taylor Coleridge

HEALTHSAVING HINTS

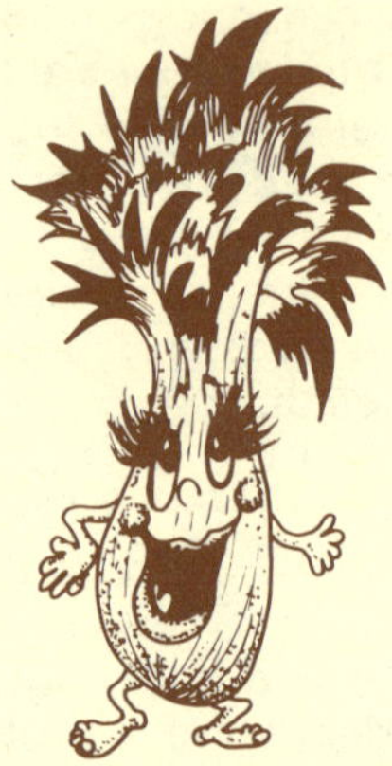

1. Always wash your hands before handling any food!
2. To avoid an electrical shock, always be sure your hands are dry before you plug in any small electric appliance.
3. Wash veggies like celery and carrot sticks and slices of Jerusalem artichoke and jicama, and place in a glass jar in the refrigerator. Place a dry paper towel in the bottom of the jar to absorb any excess moisture, so your veggies will be crisp whenever you want them.
4. Always wash all fruits and vegetables before eating them. Use a few drops of non-toxic vegetable cleaner in a bowl of water. Check with your mom for instructions.
5. Use a cutting board and a sharp knife to slice fresh, crisp, raw veggies. Be careful! Use a fork to hold vegetables when you get close to the end. Do not put sharp knives into a sink full of suds where the person washing dishes might have an accident.
6. For sprouts that aren't being used, spread on a cookie sheet in a single layer and dry overnight in a warm place, until dry. Blend to a powder in blender. Store in covered jar. This is a food concentrate of vitamins, minerals and protein that may be added to drinks, shakes, desserts, breads and casseroles. Will keep indefinitely.
7. When rinsing sprouts, save the soak or rinse water for your plants. The water is rich in vitamins and minerals.
8. You can refrigerate bananas. The skin will turn brown but the banana remains white.
9. Use color, shapes and your imagination to serve "new" foods. Utilize fancy dishes, candlelight or pretty placemats. A pleasant atmosphere can make different foods taste better.
10. To retain nutrients, always cook potatoes in their jackets before peeling for potato salad or mashed potatoes.
11. When a recipe calls for eggs, be sure to have an extra bowl handy. Break the eggs, one at a time, into a bowl. Check each egg for quality and bits of shells. Then slip carefully from bowl into ingredients.
12. Use pot holders whenever you use the oven, but be sure to keep pot holders away from the stove top when not in use. A hot burner with a pot holder lying too close could start a fire.
13. Don't let even a drop of water come in contact with your honey pot or it will sour.
14. Desserts don't always have to be super-colossal-all-day-in-the-kitchen baked goods. Simply combine two or three diced, fresh fruits in a pretty bowl. Sprinkle with coconut and garnish with a mint leaf.
15. Always turn the pan handle to the back of the stove so it won't be bumped by persons walking by. Use a spoon rest for spoons or spatulas so they won't get too hot to handle.
16. Remember to preheat oven, use potholders to remove hot pans and turn oven off when you are through baking.
17. Be sure to check *Holiday Harmony* for additional snack recipes.
18. Fresh vegetables and fruits are best for after-school snacks, but homemade, nutritious cookies are great for at the movies when everyone surrounding you is munching on a candy bar.
19. Dried fruit is highly concentrated. Always brush teeth after chewing dried fruit to remove sticky fructose from teeth. In fact, brush your teeth after eating *any* sweet food, including fresh fruit and juices.
20. Commercial citron contains sugar as well as synthetic dyes. Use unsulphured dried fruit for fruit-cake. Break walnuts in your hands, releasing essential oils and enhancing the flavor of the finished product.
21. Read the label on every food before you buy or use it. Avoid junk foods such as commercial candy, cakes and cookies, soda pop, dyed imitation fruit drinks, and anything that has white sugar or white flour in the ingredients. Instead, make your own from the tasty recipes in this Chapter.

22. If you think you don't like vegetables — it may just be the way they've been prepared. Try steaming any fresh vegetable until just tender but still crisp. Add a little butter and sprinkle with any of the following surprises: shredded cheese or coconut, ground seeds or nuts, a dollop of sour cream or yogurt, or a fine drizzle of honey.

TIMESAVING HINTS

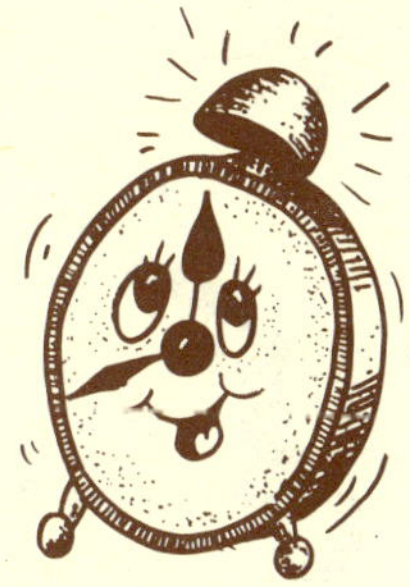

1. Assemble all utensils — bowls, measuring cups, spoons, etc. — and all ingredients before you begin. Before you put batter in to bake, double-check to make sure you have followed all instructions carefully and have added all ingredients.
2. The next time Mom prepares pizza crust for dinner, ask her to make extras for the freezer. Then, when you want to make Mona's Fantastic Fruit Pizza for breakfast or a special dessert, all you have to do is thaw the crust and add the toppings. It's fun and easy and looks like you spent all day making it!
3. Before measuring honey, measure the oil. Then place honey in same measuring spoon or cup; honey will slide right out of cup or spoon.
4. Whenever you bake cookies, stash a dozen or so in the freezer. Then when you make homemade ice cream, place a little of the cold, creamy mixture between two cookies; refreeze, and enjoy your own homemade ice cream sandwiches!
5. Most drop cookie dough can be shaped into a long roll, wrapped in wax paper and refrigerated or frozen. When ready to bake, slice dough thinly and bake, until browned, at designated time and temperature.
6. You will always be welcome in your family kitchen if you remember to clean up your mess! Soaking measuring cups, spoons, bowls and pans makes them easier to wash. Return ingredients to their cupboards, and wipe down all counters.
7. Keep plenty of Almond-Cinnamon Mixture on hand. To one cup of blender-ground almonds, add 1 T. cinnamon. Keep in a covered jar in the refrigerator.
8. Help your Mom find the ripe, spotted bananas whenever they've been reduced in price at the grocery store. Peel and slice into 1 inch slices on wax paper-lined pans. Freeze. When frozen, place in covered containers and keep frozen. Then they'll always be available when you want a shake or smoothie.
9. Wear an apron to keep drips from staining your clothes.
10. Do your best to be neat while preparing foods, but keep a wet dishcloth handy to wipe up those accidental spills that we all experience now and then.
11. Choose mixing bowls that are large enough to hold all your ingredients so you can mix without making a mess. Also select the right size saucepan to keep hot foods from dripping over edge onto a burner.
12. Use clean scissors to chop dried fruit, green onions, chives or parsley. Scissors also make quick work of cutting pizza.
13. If a recipe calls for melted butter, just place desired amount of butter in a heatproof pan and place in the oven while it preheats for the recipe.
14. Before you whip cream, place the whipping cream, bowl and beaters in the freezer for about ten minutes. Beat just until stiff peaks form. If you beat too long, don't worry; you can still use the butter and buttermilk!
15. Oven temperatures may vary — use an oven thermometer.

Good, Better, Best
Never let it rest,
Until your Good is Better
And your Better is Best!

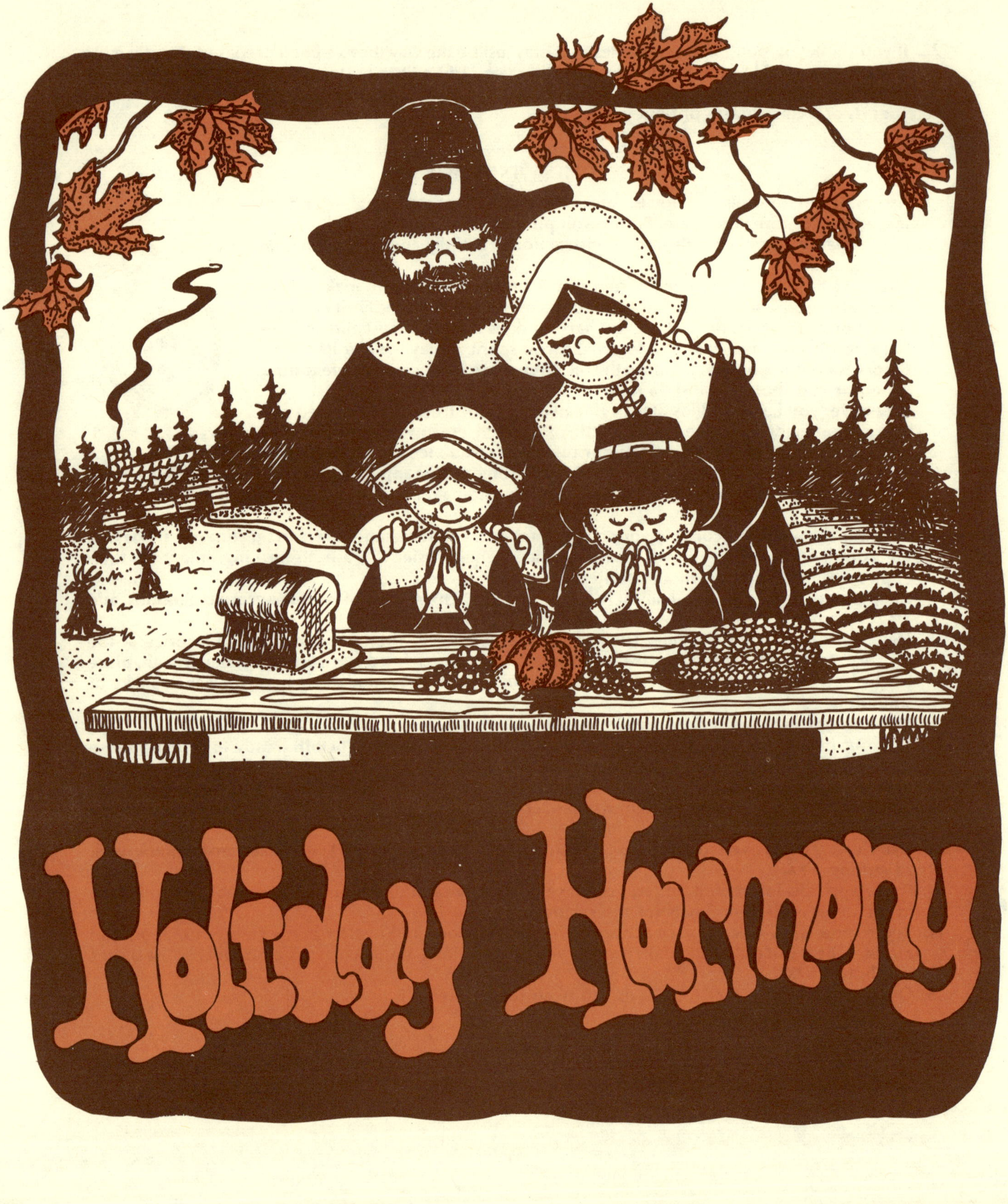
Holiday Harmony

Holiday Harmony

Especially during holidays children are exposed
To a variety of sweets put right under their nose.
Kids' clubs and school parties often serve snacks
Of food or drinks that "hype" — not relax.

This running stream of adult persistence
Only aids in "running" down the child's resistance.
After ingestion of candy, cookies or pops
Blood sugar rises, then abruptly drops.

The B and C vitamins stored inside them are used
To metabolize refined treats when sugar is over-used.
Consequently, a child is left with so few,
He becomes more susceptible to colds or the flu.

Some doctors state that after holidays their rooms are filled
With a greater number of children, "out of tune" and ill.
Many teachers dread classroom parties because they're aware
That hyperactivity increases with the festive food fare.

Peer pressure makes children want to affiliate;
If they say "no," someone might humiliate.
But there's no need for any activities to be missed.
We want you to remain on your kids' "favorite people" list.

There are several positive steps that you can take
So "Mikey" won't return with a stomach-ache.
The very next holiday is the time to start.
Your child CAN celebrate with a healthy-happy heart.

Donate home-baked natural goodies to the party of your choice.
You'll be surprised — other mothers might rejoice.
Suggest that prizes for games or races
Be non-food items like combs or shoelaces.

If the first two ideas can't be put to use,
Send your child to the party with a glass of fruit juice
And his own bag of peanuts or raisins to share.
S/he might really be pleased to see that you care.

If none of the above are possible for you;
Don't dispair — there's one more thing you can do.
The following food supplements will add extra protection.
When stirred into drinks, they might even escape detection.

Add brewer's yeast with its complex of vitamin B
And rose hip powder for vitamin C
Then if your child yields to temptations too great,
This army of nutrients will help assimilate.

Once you get into the daily habit
Of serving veggies to your little "Peter Rabbit"
And fruits, plain and simple for a terrific dessert
(They're the best foods to use when first trying to convert),

Then you're on your way to cavity and disease prevention,
And your kids will happily comply to junk food abstention.
Christmas, Easter, Halloween and Thanksgiving
Will become Holidays *in* Harmony *with your new natural way of living.*

A Celebration Of Life — Easter

You can enjoy the traditional Easter egg hunt and related activities without store-bought marshmallow eggs and chocolate rabbits. Following are some ideas a family can prepare together for the hunt.

WHAT YOU CAN DO

1. **Make UFO's (See *KIDSTUFF*); roll in coconut and freeze. Make Dan's Decidedly Delicious Fudge (*KIDSTUFF*) and refrigerate. Both these snacks can be placed in those plastic eggs that you may have saved from previous Easters. Make Silver Eggs (recipe follows); freeze.**
2. **Dye blown eggs or hand-cooked eggs in beet juice for red, red onion skins for purple (wrap skins around egg and secure with cheesecloth and rubber bands), a little saffron for yellow, and wheat grass juice for green; adding 1 t. vinegar to water or juice to set colors. Eggs can be decorated with glue and yarn scraps or recycle color crayons by melting down; either brush on or dip eggs into the melted colors.**
3. **Save the large eggs from panty hose and fill with special high-protein cookies or small gifts. Hide eggs outdoors if possible Saturday night. They'll be waiting for eager children to find at the crack of dawn.**
4. **A special use for those plastic eggs would be to include Bible verses and Celebration of Life messages (written by all members of the family), and hidden along with the others.**
5. **Take a basket of alfalfa sprouts to your favorite rabbit.**
6. **Select and/or make natural snacks, nuts, dried fruits or fresh fruits and little toys or finger puppets. Place on grass in hand-woven baskets, straw hats or a sand pail with shovel. For older kids, arrange combs, a pen, homemade cosmetics, jewelry, scarves, a belt, wild shoelaces, etc., in traditional Easter Baskets.**
7. **Check your local newspaper for the churches in your area that hold sunrise services. Some also show films depicting the Crucifixion and Resurrection.**
8. **Organize with others to bring spiritual films to your area. "The Cross and the Switchblade," "Brother Sun-Sister Moon" (the story of St. Francis of Assisi), and "The Hiding Place" are just a few possibilities.**

Easter Menu

Breakfast

Oregon Toast a la Cashew/SunButterBlend/Honey
Lentil "Sausage"*
Eggs Baked in Muffin Cups
Apricot Smoothie — Spearmint Tea

Lunch

Delicious Asparagus Protein Dish
Deviled Eggs* on Nest of Alfalfa Sprouts
Easter Bunny Salad
Lani's Mushroom Herb Health Bread*
Pineapple Plus Drink — Chamomile Tea

Dinner

Suzanne's San Francisco Quiche
Carrot-Cheddar Loaf*
Steamed Broccoli with Lemon Wedges
Scalloped Potatoes
Avocado-Orange Salad
Milk — Comfrey Tea

Late Dessert

Baby Birds' Nests* with
Strawberry Ice Cream and Fresh Fruit

*Can be prepared ahead of time.

EASTER BUNNY SALAD: On individual salad plates, place a nice crisp leaf of lettuce. Put a half of a home canned pear, hollow side down; place a scoop of cottage cheese for a bushy tail. Use almonds for ears, raisins or dates for nose and eyes. Shred cheese in long shreds for whiskers and lay a carrot slice along the side.

SILVER EGGS

1 pound carob chips
2 T. butter
½ to ¾ cup unsweetened, shredded coconut
½ to ¾ cup coarsely ground, raw almonds

Melt carob chips and butter in a double boiler. Add coconut and nuts. With hands, shape into small eggs. Freeze; wrap individually in foil.

DEVILED EGGS

6 hard-cooked eggs
chopped chives to taste
1 T. mayonnaise
1 T. yogurt
dash cayenne
1 t. lemon juice
1 T. crushed parsley
dash sea salt/kelp

Halve the eggs, scoop out yolks, and mash yolks with chives, mayonnaise, yogurt, cayenne, lemon juice, parsley and sea salt/kelp. Spoon filling back into egg-white halves and sprinkle with paprika. Arrange eggs on a nest of alfalfa sprouts.

VEGETABLE NUT LOAF

2 cups grated carrots
2 cups grated onions
2 cups sliced celery
2 cups walnut chunks
1 cup sunflower seeds
2 minced garlic cloves
¼ cup SunButterBlend
2 T. tamari-soy sauce
2 eggs
1½ cups bread crumbs

Saute first 6 ingredients in SunButterBlend and tamari-soy sauce. Place in a large bowl and add eggs and bread crumbs and mix all together. Put into oiled loaf pan and bake at 350° for 30-40 minutes.

DELICIOUS ASPARAGUS PROTEIN DISH

4-5 chopped mushrooms
1 medium, chopped onion
¼ t. garlic powder
1 T. tamari-soy sauce
dash cayenne
3 T. butter
¾ cup plain yogurt
¾-1 cup milk
5 oz. thin-sliced tofu
½ t. sea salt/kelp
25-30 stalks of young asparagus
1½ cups spoon-sized shredded wheat

Saute mushrooms, onions and seasonings in butter until just tender. In a bowl, mix yogurt, milk, tofu and sea salt/kelp. Stir in sauteed mixture and 1 cup of the shredded wheat and let sit while liquids partially absorb wheat biscuits. Steam asparagus; then cut in thirds. Mix with above mixture and spoon into an oiled, square pan. Bake at 350° for 15-20 minutes. Meanwhile, for topping, melt 2 T. butter with ½ t. tamari-soy sauce and a dash of garlic powder. Stir with remaining ½ cup shredded wheat. Sprinkle over casserole, then return to oven for 5 minutes or until sizzling hot.

Variation: Substitute fresh, steamed, green beans or butter-sauteed zucchini for asparagus.

CARROT CHEDDAR LOAF

¼ cup butter
2 cups chopped mushrooms
2 minced garlic cloves
1 chopped onion
4½ cups finely grated carrots
½ cup blender-ground sun seeds
1 cup coarsely ground walnuts
1 cup grated Cheddar cheese (total)
sea salt/kelp to taste
½ t. basil
½ t. thyme
4-5 eggs

Saute mushrooms, garlic and onion in butter. In a large bowl, add saute along with carrots, sun seeds, walnuts and seasonings, and ½ cup cheese. In a separate bowl, beat eggs. Then add to above mixture. Mix all well and pack into an 8"x8" oiled pan. Bake at 350° for 35 minutes covered, then at 375° for 15 minutes uncovered; then 10 minutes with remaining ½ cup cheese sprinkled on top.

Variation: Shape into 2 large ovals to resemble eggs; place on oiled cookie sheets and bake at 350° for about 45-55 minutes.

A Good Old-Fashioned Halloween

Here is a holiday that may be frustrating because it revolves around candy. School carnivals and trick-or-treating provide plenty of activity, but too many sweets. Children won't feel like they're missing out if you provide both the activities and the good treats.

WHAT YOU CAN DO

1. **Plan a scavenger hunt in costumes, and award non-food prizes.**
2. **Plan a treasure hunt. The first map clue leads to the next and so forth until the treasure is found. Fill treasure chest with goodies from** *KIDSTUFF.*
3. **Erect an obstacle course or "haunted walk" outside.**
4. **Older kids can have a pumpkin carving contest.**
5. **Many roller skating rinks have costume parties for the entire family.**
6. **Dress up in costumes and have a party — parents and kids with games geared to age levels.**
7. **For games, apples can be dunked or dangled from string on a clothesline strung at mouth's reach. Pin the tail on the cat can be played by young children. Run relay races such as carrying a peanut on a spoon.**
8. **If you are already involved with your local PTA, try to interest them in requesting cakes and cookies that are baked with wholewheat flour and honey for the cakewalk. Supply the recipes for them if you have willing volunteers to bake. Instead of candy prizes for the games, encourage a class to make UFO's, Jack-in-the-Bags or Zippity-Do-Da's. You may be surprised to discover many allies; mothers who have been wanting to remove the sugar but haven't had the courage to speak out. They just need motivation. You'll never know until you try.**
9. **If you stay home, give trick-or-treaters healthy foods from** *KIDSTUFF,* **individually wrapped and labeled with your name and phone number. Or use balloons or little toys.**

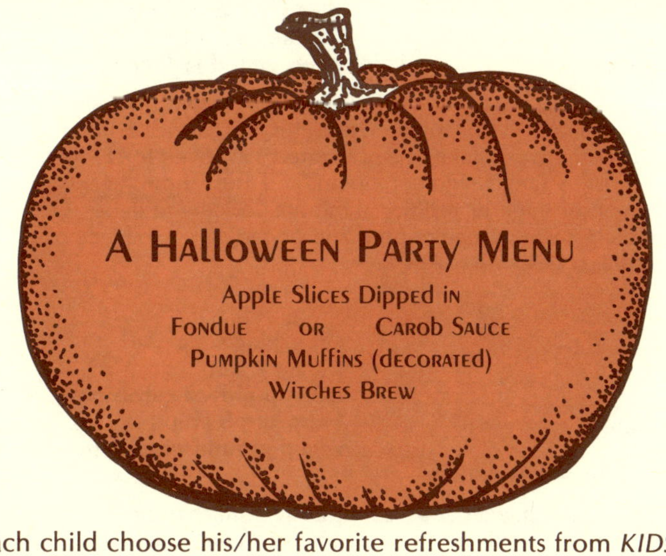
A Halloween Party Menu
Apple Slices Dipped in
Fondue or Carob Sauce
Pumpkin Muffins (decorated)
Witches Brew

Let each child choose his/her favorite refreshments from *KIDSTUFF.*

Follow suggestions in WHAT YOU CAN DO for games and party ideas. Decorations can include all the cats and goblins they've made at school and bring home daily. Spooky music or homemade rattles can provide the sound effects.

PUMPKIN MUFFINS

1 cup honey	**1½ t. baking powder**
½ cup safflower oil	**1 t. baking soda**
4 eggs	**½ t. salt**
1½ cups cooked pumpkin	**½ t. cloves**
3 cups sifted whole wheat flour	**½ t. nutmeg**
OR 2¾ cups dry Mama Bear's Porridge	**1 t. cinnamon**
(See *Better Beginnings*) plus	**1 cup raisins**
¼ cup soy flour	**1 cup chopped walnuts**

In a mixer, beat honey, oil and eggs. Add pumpkin. In a separate bowl, mix flour or Porridge flour and soy flour, and remaining dry ingredients. Add to pumpkin-honey mixture and mix well. Add raisins and nuts. Bake at 400° for 15 minutes in paper baking cups. Makes 2 dozen. Frost with any frosting. (See *KIDSTUFF*.) Kids can decorate with raisins, almonds, coconut, carob chips.

FONDUE FOR APPLE SLICES

1 cup peanut butter	**1 t. vanilla**
¾ cup honey	**1 T. oil**

Heat ingredients. When smooth and creamy, place in fondue dish over a candle to keep warm and creamy. Dip apple slices with fondue forks or skewers.

(For Carob Sauce Fondue, see *KIDSTUFF* for Laser Beam's Carob Sauce.)

ROASTED PUMPKIN SEEDS: Rinse and dry pumpkin seeds. Roast in a 300° oven until lightly browned.

WITCHES BREW

1 pint water	**1 quart apple juice**
1 cinnamon stick	**1 quart orange juice**
10 whole cloves	**1 quart cranberry juice**

In 1 pint water, boil cinnamon and cloves for 20 minutes. Remove spices and add juices. Heat, but do not boil.

GOBLIN-IT-UP RICE PIZZA

1 cup raw rice	**1 cup grated eggplant (peeled)**
2 cups water	**½ of a medium onion, chopped**
½ t. oil	**4-5 chopped mushrooms**
1/3 cup Parmesan cheese	**1 cup grated Jack cheese**
Easy Pizza Sauce (See *Serendipity Suppers*)	

Steam 1 cup rice in 2 cups water and ½ t. oil for 30-35 minutes. Stir Parmesan into rice. Spoon into an oiled 10" pie plate and press flat and up sides for a crust. Bake in a preheated 450° oven for 12 minutes. Remove from oven and spread Easy Pizza Sauce over crust. Arrange eggplant, onions and mushrooms evenly on crust; sprinkle with grated cheese and bake at same temperature for 10 additional minutes. Slice and eat.

Variation: Add chopped black olives, green pepper and grated carrot in place of above veggies. Add cubes of tofu and sprinkle with Mozarella cheese instead of Jack.

BLACK CAT COOKIES

1 cup butter	**1 t. baking soda**
¾ cup honey	**1 scant t. salt**
1 t. vanilla	**1/3 cup plus of carob powder**
2 eggs	**1 cup carob chips**
½ cup peanut butter	**½ cup ground or chopped nuts or seeds**
2 cups whole wheat flour or pastry flour	

Beat together butter, honey, vanilla, eggs and peanut butter. Sift together flour, soda, salt and carob powder. Add to butter-honey mixture and beat well. Stir in carob chips and nuts (opt.). Drop by teaspoonfuls onto slightly oiled cookie sheets. Bake at 350° for 8-10 minutes. Makes 100 2" cookies.

Variation: For crispier cookie, flatten with an oiled fork before baking.

A Time For Thanksgiving

Is Thanksgiving a conventional time of turkey, trimmings, and leftovers or can it mean something more than just food? Thanksgiving should be a "memory in the making." Build upon family traditions with new and different activities geared to enrich the spirit of Thanksgiving and prepare for the coming of Christmas. The following activities can become yearly events for your family that are eagerly anticipated by the children as the season approaches.

WHAT YOU CAN DO

1. **Take advantage of the holiday to take a family outing to the woods to gather wood for burning, or pine cones, nuts, and acorns to be made into a wreath for the door for the Christmas season.**
2. **Pack up those sleds, skis, inner-tubes, and Hot Carob Cocoa or Apple Cider and go to the nearest snow-covered hills or mountains for a "snow picnic."**
3. **Tree ornaments can be made at this time, so that new ones are added each year to the tree (even the youngest child can participate).**
4. **Thanksgiving is a time for thanks. Let people know how much you've appreciated their help, concern or time by personally thanking them, or as a family, putting together a fresh food basket for someone special.**
5. **For the months preceding November, family members can drop coins in a jar to be given to a world hunger program or a local food distributing organization for needy families. This can help children realize that not every family is fortunate to have a vast variety of food on their table.**
6. **Each member of the family can contribute to a special dinner by candlelight complete with festive table setting. Handmade place mats, napkins and napkin rings can brighten the plainest tablecloth. A centerpiece of dried seeds, flowers and pods, a fruit-filled cornucopia, or a funny-looking Jack-0-Lantern can be colorful and interesting.**
7. **Have children print a name card and menu card for each person, and fill individual nut cups with raw almonds, toasted pumpkin seeds (saved from Jack-o-Lanterns), cashews and peanuts.**
8. **Friends, family and relatives might discuss what they are especially thankful for or the special blessings that have been bestowed upon them throughout the year. For an unusual, but interesting way to liven up the dinner conversation, place notes under each plate with a humorous topic typed on each. Taking turns, each person gives a very short humorous speech on his/her topic.**
9. **For a vegetarian Thanksgiving, honor the turkey by having the children draw a large turkey on a poster. They can cut construction paper feathers and glue in place, and write underneath, "Turkeys Give Thanks to Vegetarians." Invite friends and relatives for a pot luck. "We Love Your Body" hostessed a Vegetarian Turkey Freedom Day attended by families, friends, couples, babies, teen-agers, and senior citizens. Everyone joined hands for a Thanksgiving prayer before dinner, which was a colorful and delicious variety of everyone's favorite vegetarian recipes. Then began an afternoon of conversation, music, volleyball, swimming and relaxation. The fellowship was wonderful and we knew that somewhere there was a turkey, alive and trotting, who appreciated the fact that he would not be served ten different ways for the next ten days. We discovered that it is really the colorful vegetable dishes, relishes, appetizers, salads, desserts, and pleasant company that everyone looks forward to at Thanksgiving rather than an over-stuffed bird. We would like to share some of the recipes that our guests contributed to that memorable day!**

If you feel that your minuses in life predominate, punctuate them with exclamation marks, transforming them into pluses. (+).

Lamder

Thanksgiving Day Menu

Breakfast

Diane's Versatile Harvest Waffles/Lemon Syrup
Sprouts and Cheese
Breakfast Salad
Cheese Wedges
Orange Juice — Orange Spice Tea

All Day Hors-d'oeuvres

Crunchy Toasty Spread* — Whole Grain Crackers
Raw Veggie Tray — Broccoli, Cauliflower, Carrots, Jerusalem Artichokes, Yams
Herb-Yogurt Dip* — Buffet Cheese Roll*
Fruit Tray — Apple Slices, Orange Wedges, Cheese Cubes
Bowl of Nuts in Shell with Nutcracker and Pick
Carrot Cocktails

Dinner

Fresh Fruit Skewers of Banana, Avocado, Papaya, Pineapple Chunks
Toasted Pumpkin Seeds and Almonds Nut Cup*
Thanksgiving Roast*
Stuffed Pumpkin
Mashed Potatoes — Mushroom Gravy
Whole Wheat Rolls — Cranberry-Orange Relish
Basil-Buttered Carrots in Parfait Glasses
Pumpkin Pie* — Whipped Cream
Float Frozen Lemon Slices in Stemmed Water Glasses — Milk

Evening Snack

Saturday Night Sundae

*Can be prepared ahead of time.

RECIPES FROM OUR FRIENDS AT TURKEY FREEDOM DAY, 1978

CURRY CREAM SAUCE

1 cup sour cream or yogurt
1/3 cup mayonnaise
8 oz. softened cream cheese
1 T. lemon juice or more to taste
sea salt/kelp and pepper to taste
1 T. curry powder
¼ t. ginger
1 minced garlic clove
2 t. minced onion

Mix all of the above ingredients; then chill. Serve with tray of raw vegetables.

NUTS AND CARROTS

5 cups of 3" carrot sticks
½ cup butter
2 t. honey
½ t. sea salt/kelp
¼ t. grated black pepper
2 T. lemon juice
½ cup coarsely broken walnuts

Steam carrot sticks just until tender. In a saucepan heat butter and remaining ingredients except walnuts. When melted and mixed, pour over the hot carrots. Toss with walnuts and serve hot.

CASHEW YAMS

yams or sweet potatoes
¾ cup broken cashews
¼ cup sunflower seeds
½ t. sea salt/kelp
½ t. ground ginger
2 T. butter
1½ cups home canned, sliced peaches

Cook desired amount of yams or sweet potatoes until just tender. Peel and slice. In a small bowl, mix cashews, seeds and spices and butter. In an oiled casserole dish, layer the yams, peaches and nut mixture. Bake, covered, at 350° for 30 minutes; then uncovered for 10 minutes.

SPINACH SOUFFLE

2 pounds fresh spinach
3 oz. softened cream cheese
¼ cup melted butter
1 small, chopped garlic clove
3 eggs (separated)
a dash or two of nutmeg
sea salt/kelp to taste

Steam spinach 6-8 minutes. Drain; then chop. Beat cream cheese with butter and garlic. Add egg yolks and beat well. Add spinach and seasonings. Whip egg whites until stiff and gently fold into spinach-egg yolk mixture. Pour into an oiled, 1 quart casserole. Bake, covered, at 350° for 20-25 minutes.

STUFFED PUMPKIN (You don't need a turkey to enjoy the dressing!)

1 medium-sized pumpkin
½ cup chopped onion
3 T. chopped green onions
½ chopped green pepper
½ cup plus, chopped celery
chopped parsley to taste
1 t. sea salt/kelp
1 t. sage
½ t. pepper
2 T. tamari-soy sauce
1/3 cup melted butter
½ cup water (more or less)
½ cup sunflower seeds
4 cups whole grain, dry bread cubes

Combine all ingredients except pumpkin in a large bowl. Stuffing should be fairly moist so it won't dry out during baking. Wash a pumpkin, cut a lid, scoop out seeds, rinse inside and salt the cavity. Fill pumpkin with your favorite stuffing or one listed above. Dot with butter. Replace lid. Set pumpkin on a rack in a pan with a little water in it and bake at 350° for 2 hours or until done. To test, insert a knife into the pumpkin meat. It will be ready if it is tender. Take to table on a platter. To serve, cut wedges, with stuffing still in pumpkin. The pumpkin will make a very impressive platter.

Variation: Add 1 cup apple slices, nuts, and/or raisins to stuffing mixture. Bake, covered in loaf pan or muffin tins.

THANKSGIVING DAY ROAST

1½ cups cooked, mashed lentils
1½ cups cooked millet
1½ cups cooked rice cereal
OR steamed brown rice
¼ cup rolled oats (or cornmeal)
¼ cup ground sunflower seeds
¼ cup ground almonds
garlic powder to taste
¼ cup ground cashews
¼ cup ground walnuts
1/3 cup melted butter
1 t. ground celery seed
3 t. sage
a few dashes of cayenne
1½ T. dried, minced onions
sea salt/kelp to taste
1 cup cooked soybeans, ground in meat grinder (opt.)

In a large bowl, mix all of the above ingredients together. Soybeans are optional. Add water or more dry ingredients, whatever is necessary to get a stiff mixture. Place in oiled loaf pans. Bake at 350° for 1 hour. Cover with a towel on counter to keep moist until ready to serve. Slice thin and serve with favorite gravy.

Variation: Bake in bundt pan and unmold on platter. Place Cranberry-Orange Relish in center; vegetables around outside. Double recipe if serving more than 6.

NEAT LOAF: Use recipe for Tasty Soyburgers in *Serendipity Suppers.* Be sure to use 2 eggs. Add 1½ t. sage. Mix well and pat into an oiled loaf pan. Top with tomato sauce and bake at 350° for 1 hour and 10 minutes. Let set. Slice and serve.

LENTIL RING MOLD

1½ cups whole grain bread crumbs
2 cups cooked lentils
½ cup milk
OR tomato paste
½ cup finely chopped onion
½ cup finely chopped celery
½ cup grated carrot
1 t. sage
1 t. marjoram or thyme
1 t. oregano
2 T. soy flour OR any flour
2 T. oil OR SunButterBlend
1 t. sea salt/kelp or to taste

Oil a ring mold. Cover bottom and sides with some of the bread crumbs. In a bowl, mix all ingredients together, adding rest of bread crumbs if too soupy. Bake at 350° for 1 hour and 15 minutes. Let stand 5-10 minutes before unmolding onto serving plate. Garnish with carrot curls and fresh parsley sprigs.

PECAN LOAF

1½ cups finely chopped celery
1½ cups whole grain bread crumbs
1½ cups finely chopped pecans
3 T. finely chopped onion
2 cups milk
3 beaten eggs
3 T. finely chopped parsley
2 t. vegetable seasoning
3 T. melted butter
Gravy: 4 T. butter
4 T. pastry flour
2 cups milk
½ cup chopped parsley
½ bay leaf

In a large bowl, mix first 9 ingredients together. Let stand for 20 minutes. Pour into a buttered loaf pan and bake at 375° for 50-55 minutes or until golden brown.

To make gravy: Melt butter in a skillet. Stir in flour and mix well until bubbly. Then add milk, parsley and bay leaf. Stir until thickened; then remove leaf. Serve over Pecan Loaf slices.

HOT MULLED CIDER

1/3 cup honey
1 t. whole cloves
1 t. whole allspice
¼ t. sea salt
dash ground nutmeg
3 inches of cinnamon stick
1 pint water
2 quarts apple cider

Combine spices and water in a large saucepan. Slowly bring to boiling; cover and simmer 20 minutes. Remove spices. Add apple cider and heat, but do not boil. Serve in warmed mugs with a clove-studded orange wedge in each cup.

MINESTRONE WITH PESTO SAUCE

1 cup dried, white, navy beans
water to cover
3 quarts vegetable stock
sea salt to taste
1 small head thinly sliced cabbage
4 carrots
2 medium potatoes
1 pound tomatoes
2 medium onions
¼ cup olive oil or other oil
1 stalk celery
2 small zucchinis
3-5 minced garlic cloves
¼ t. sea salt/kelp
½ cup chopped parsley
1 cup broken, thin spinach noodles or spaghetti
Pesto Sauce: 2 T. softened butter
¼ cup grated Parmesan cheese
½ cup finely chopped parsley
1-4 minced garlic cloves
1 t. crushed basil
½ t. crushed marjoram
¼ cup olive oil
¼ cup chopped pine nuts

The day before, cover beans with cold water. Refrigerate, covered, overnight. Next day, drain. In an 8 quart kettle, add the 3 quarts vegetable stock, sea salt to taste and beans. Bring to a boil; reduce heat and simmer 1 hour, covered. Slice cabbage thin, slice carrots on diagonal, ¼" thick. Cube the potatoes and chop the tomatoes. Add to kettle, cover and cook ½ hour longer. Slice the onion thinly, slice celery on diagonal, ⅛" thick and slice the zucchinis in ¼" thick slices. In a skillet, in hot olive oil, saute the onion slices, stirring, for 5 minutes. Remove from heat. Add celery, zucchini rounds and garlic. Stir in sea salt/kelp and cook with onions, uncovered, for 20 minutes, stirring occasionally. Add to the bean-vegetable mixture with ½ cup parsley and the spaghetti or noodles. Cook slowly, covered, for 30 minutes, stirring occasionally. Serve soup hot, dolloped with Pesto Sauce. In hot weather, serve cold.

Pesto Sauce: Cream butter, cheese, parsley, garlic and herbs in a bowl with a fork. Add oil gradually, beating constantly. Add pine nuts and mix well. Dollop over hot soup.

DIANE'S VERSATILE HARVEST WAFFLES: Separate 4 eggs and beat whites until stiff. In large bowl, beat the yolks with 2 cups cooked, mashed winter squash or yams, 1 t. vanilla and 2 T. oil. Add 1 T. cinnamon to 3 cups Snappy-Quick Mix and quickly stir in wet ingredients. Carefully, fold in egg whites. Add ½ cup sesame, sunflower or pumpkin seeds if you choose. Oil waffle iron with pastry brush. Pour batter in center of iron; waffles are done when steam ceases to escape. Serve with Lemon Syrup.

Variation: Any thick fruit puree can be substituted for the squash or yams and ground nuts can replace seeds for crunch.

LEMON SYRUP: Stir 2 T. butter and 2 T. lemon juice into ¼ cup very hot water. Add ½ cup honey and serve warm over waffles.

SQUASH FLUFF: Separate 4 eggs and beat whites until stiff. Mix in large mixing bowl: 4 egg yolks 1½ cups mashed, cooked danish or butternut squash, ½ cup each honey and Snappy-Quick Mix, 2 T. each SunButterBlend and pumpkin pie spice and dash of sea salt. Carefully, fold in egg whites and spread in large oiled baking dish. Place dish in pan of hot water in a 350° oven for 40-50 minutes or until knife inserted just off center comes out clean. Top with orange yogurt or honey-whipped cream.

CHEESY BANANA PIE

2 eggs
1 cup plain yogurt
1 cup cottage cheese
1 t. vanilla
juice from ½ lemon
¼ cup whole wheat flour
¼ t. salt
3 T. honey
2 bananas, sliced
wheat germ

In a blender, blend eggs, yogurt, cottage cheese, vanilla and lemon juice. Add flour, salt, honey and bananas. Blend again until smooth. Pour filling into an oiled 9" pie plate that has been dusted with wheat germ OR use your favorite pie crust. Bake at 350° for 25-30 minutes. Sprinkle with toasted coconut and serve with sliced peaches or berries.

PETER PUMPKIN EATER BREAD

2/3 cup oil
1 cup honey
1 pound cooked pumpkin
4 eggs
½ to 2/3 cup milk
1 cup whole wheat flour
2/3 cup soy flour
1 1/3 cups flaked bran
2 t. baking soda
½ t. baking powder
2 t. cinnamon
½ t. cloves
½ t. nutmeg
1 t. salt
handful of raisins
2/3 cup chopped nuts

Beat oil and honey. Add pumpkin and mix well. In a separate bowl, beat eggs with milk, then stir into honey-pumpkin mixture. Mix dry ingredients together in a bowl. Stir into liquid mixture and mix. Add raisins and nuts. Pour into 2 well-greased loaf pans (9"x5"x3"). Bake about 1 hour at 350° until a toothpick inserted comes out clean.

Variation: For a lighter texture, separate eggs, whips whites until stiff and fold in just before baking.

MELT-IN-YOUR-MOUTH PUMPKIN PIE

1 envelope unflavored gelatin
¼ cup cold water
3 eggs (separated)
1 cup cooked pumpkin
¾ cup honey
1 T. butter
1 t. cinnamon
½ t. salt
½ t. ginger
¼ t. nutmeg

Soften gelatin in cold water. On top of a double boiler, beat egg yolks; add cooked pumpkin, honey and butter. Stir in cinnamon, salt, ginger and nutmeg. Cook over boiling water until slightly thickened. Stir in gelatin and cook and stir until dissolved and smooth. Cool well. Whip egg whites until stiff and fold into mixture. Spoon into a baked pie shell and chill until firm. Garnish with walnut slices and serve dolloped with Honey-Cinnamon Yogurt or real whipped cream. (See *KIDSTUFF*.)

Keeping The Christmas Spirit

The Christmas season seems to come earlier and earlier each year, and many people become frustrated as they fight traffic and crowds in an attempt to do last minute shopping. When families join in home-oriented activities and gift-making, everyone gets into the Christmas spirit by giving time and energy to each other, rather than frantically driving about to stores, trying to maintain a semblance of calm amidst the confusion.

During a family "Homemade Christmas" you will be recycling used items into attractive and useful gifts, which otherwise might have contributed to non-biodegradable litter; you will be baking with ingredients that you know are natural and nutritious; and the gifts you give will communicate individual creativity, enthusiasm, and celebration from the heart.

Holiday Harmony

The true spirit is love, and love is nurtured by caring, sharing, experiencing and doing things together. This is the kind of busy, noisy, happy atmosphere that transforms holiday frustration into holiday harmony. Following are some positive suggestions for activities and homemade gifts that will get everyone so involved that what might have been hyper- will become constructive-activity.

WHAT YOU CAN DO

1. **Recycle materials around the house and yard into truly beautiful and unusual homemade gifts. Make a party of gift-making one or two nights a week. Everyone can gather at the table bringing the basic materials: pine cones, feathers, yarn, cans, jars, stones, paint, fabric scraps, glue, paper, and wood scraps. There is real enjoyment and satisfaction in making a gift, whether it be a personal gift, a food package or an ornament. Working together can reunite a family. Communication is inevitable as your**

family centers around the kitchen table rather than the television set, and a new closeness develops between family members.

2. **Read stories aloud around the fireplace, wood stove or any favorite, cozy place. Maybe Dad, an older brother or sister, or a grandparent would like to have the opportunity to read. Pop some corn for stringing and eating while listening to stories. Check your library for books for all ages about Christmas. Read the New Testament account of Christ's birth in Luke.** *The Gift of the Magi, Let's Keep Christmas, Petunia's Christmas, The Christmas Mouse,* **and** *How the Grinch Stole Christmas,* **are some enjoyable all-time favorites.** *The Chronicles of Narnia* **by C. S. Lewis are excellent stories for all ages. Start with** *The Lion, The Witch, and The Wardrobe.*
3. **Dig out your dusty musical instruments and play and sing carols together. Younger children can make a kazoo from a comb and wax paper, a drum from an oatmeal box, and a maracca from a can half-filled with dried beans.**
4. **Invite a "foster grandparent" for an evening of stories from his or her past. Our senior citizens and friends have a wealth of memories they are more than willing to share. Many children today know very little of their own "roots," but developing a friendship during the holidays may just result in a kinship all year long.**
5. **Do as much food preparation as you can ahead of time so you're free to spend Christmas Day with your family. Involve everyone in preparing goodies.**
6. **Purchase a live tree from a nursery or live tree farm. Keep outside in a cool place until the week before Christmas and plant before New Year's Day for a special evergreen memory. (Longer indoors may be too much of a shock for the tree.)**
7. **Start the New Year off right. Get together with friends who share your interest in health and have weekly exercise, Bible study and meditation meetings. Alternate homes and continue the relaxed atmosphere with a potluck of crisp, raw salads.**

FOOD RELATED GIFT IDEAS

During the holidays, especially, we attend parties at work, school or friends' homes and are confronted with sugar-sweetened candies, cakes, pastries and beverages. Most of us don't even realize that when refined sugar became readily available to the homemaker, traditional recipes which used honey, real maple syrup, and mashed fruit, had to undergo specific changes to accommodate the texture change of the devitalized white sugar. Now we are changing recipes *back* to the original use of natural sweeteners.

The same care and preparation of natural foods that you give your family's holiday treats can be doubled to share with special friends. All of us are inherently creative; it just takes longer for some to realize their potential, and the holidays are a perfect time to let our imagination run wild. The following gift ideas are positive proof of the variety of festive foods and original containers available without us having to succumb to the over-sweet candies and cookies that permeate pages of holiday magazines and grocery store aisles.

1. FABRIC: Stitch a skirt for a flower pot; then plant a culinary herb; chives are a favorite. Festive prints can be used as drawstring baggies for jars of herb vinegar, herb butter, yogurt facial cleanser, or teas. Personalize an apron and stuff the pockets with some power-packed sandwich recipes and a package of pocket bread. Even the beginner can sew a little gingham drawstring bag to stuff with mint, rosemary, lavender, or a combination of fragrance for a drawer sachet.
2. POTTERY: Make a teapot and a pair of mugs from clay and stuff with a variety of herb teas. Make a honey pot sweet with raw, wild, honey. Fill ceramic shakers with kelp, cayenne, gomazio, or your own special herbs, blended with just a little sea salt. Tuck a package of home-dried soup mixture into a tureen or earthenware casserole.
3. WEAVE, KNIT OR CROCHET: What homemaker wouldn't be thrilled to receive books on whole-istic health (body-mind-spirit), natural foods cooking, exercise, poetry, or self-awareness, nestled snugly into a hand-woven cover, or with a clever needlepoint or embroidered book mark tucked

inside? How about making a set of napkin rings to tuck in with a loaf of homemade whole-grain bread and a jar of honey-butter? A light, airy, woven bag with room for a loofa sponge, some oatmeal soap and aloe vera gel (medicine plant) could hang in a bathroom or easily travel back to college.

4. LETTERING: Sketch some of Nature's most unusual and delectable vegetables, and include wholesome gourmet recipes in caligraphy. Or paint a still-life of fresh fruit that looks good enough to eat. There's so much to be said for the power of suggestion!
5. WOODCRAFT: Build a spice rack to fill with dried herbs and spices, or a mortar and pestle to grind them. A wood chopping block is indispensible for wok cookery, and a wooden cheese board complete with undyed cheese and whole-grain crackers would be a pleasure to give as well as receive. Make a rack for draining jars of sprouts and a cloth cover to "keep them in the dark."

GIFT IDEAS FOR YOUNG CHILDREN TO MAKE

1. Transform plain white shelf paper or tissue paper into colorful wrapping paper. Carve designs in the ends of peeled potatoes; dip into paint, and stamp patterns and designs on the paper.
2. Little plaques or beads can be made with this Play Dough recipe. It's just the thing to keep young hands occupied while older children work with something more difficult. Use your white flour and table salt for this:

Play Dough

2½ cups white flour, ½ cup salt, 1 T. alum
Sift flour and mix ingredients. Add:
2 cups boiling water, 3 T. vegetable oil, a few drops of food coloring
Mix and knead. When cool, store in plastic bags in refrigerator.

3. An infinite number of items, from a cradle to a colander for sprouts, might be made from cans and oatmeal boxes. For a decorative container, you will need a can, white glue, paint, and your old white pastas — wagon wheels, macaroni, noodles, shells, and stars or alphabets. Mix white glue with a little water. Using a paint brush, paint glue over a section of the can. Apply different shapes of macaroni in a mosaic pattern. Let dry before applying to a new section. When totally dry, container may be painted or varnished. The uses are many: pencil can, thread, paper clip, nail, or letter holder. Let your child dream up a use for it based upon the needs and desires of the receiver of the gift.
4. With a little help, young children can make a delicious-smelling Pomander Ball.

Pomander Ball

1 large, firm orange
whole cloves
ground cinnamon
orrisroot

For each ball, select a large, firm orange. Stick whole cloves into the peel until completely covered. (Use prongs of fork or pencil to make holes.) Roll balls in a mixture of equal parts of orrisroot and ground cinnamon. Use about 1½ T. of combined spices per orange. Pat in as much of the spices as will adhere to the orange and wrap in tissue paper. As pomander dries and shrinks, its fragrance develops. Remove from paper, shake off any loose powder and it's ready to use. To hang, attach a piece of ribbon.

5. Recycle packaged instant whipped cream topping by whipping it up as per directions. Divide into bowls, adding a different food coloring to each bowl and mix carefully. Give the child a piece of paper and let him/her fingerpaint. Please supervise to see that none gets eaten. For edible fingerpaint, use real whipped cream, tinted with a little orange juice concentrate, carrot or beet juice, or berry juice.

6. Bath Potpourris: Make a small drawstring bag out of a pretty print. Fill bag with about ¼ cup of dried herbs. The bags are placed directly into the tub of water for a terrific bath. Use peppermint or lavender for a stimulating bath; chamomile or rosemary to aid skin problems; hops to relax; and thyme to aid respiratory problems. SHAKE up some bath salts by placing epsom salts, a few drops of vegetable food coloring and a few drops of scented oil in a jar. These gifts will be appreciated because most of the commercial bath products are largely composed of chemical substances.
7. Make delicious-smelling spice necklaces. Soak whole cloves and allspice in water for two days. Using a strong polyester thread, push needle through center of clove stem and allspice kernel. Experiment with different repeat patterns, than hang finished necklace to dry. Be sure to make long enough to slip over your head.

FOOD CONTAINERS

Save all glass jars that peanut butter, mayonnaise or other foods come in. Glass gallon jars can be obtained from restaurants for a very small price. Use them to store pastas, beans, seeds, and flours. Use smaller ones to fill with food; making pretty labels, tying with a ribbon and giving to neighbors, teachers, ministers, bosses, and friends. For decorative or down-to-earth jar lids for these jars, try this recipe:

Decorative Jar Lids

2 cups white flour, 1 cup table salt, 1 cup water

Knead for five minutes. Press small amounts over jar lids and add decorations made from the dough, like dough flowers, mushrooms, fruit shapes, nuts, or little animals OR impress dough-covering on lid with macaroni, buttons, stamps, or pencil point; then remove objects. Prick a few small holes with a toothpick so that the dough dries inside. Dry naturally for several days or for one to two hours in a very low oven. Stain with shoe polish or varnish; then screw the lids onto your jars. Makes six 2-4" lids.

A sturdy gift box, a basket, a pretty bowl, unusual jars, macrame hangers, stockings, decorative tins with lids, or eye-catching containers of any kind can be filled with limitless combinations of the following: homemade fruitcake, fudge, catsup, chutney, chile sauce, jams, jellies, purees and home-canned goods (all made with natural ingredients, of course). Fill with home-dried vegetables or fruit slices, a dried soup mix, or seeds for sprouting.

Dried fruit, fruit leather, garlic braid, whole grains, beans, seeds and unshelled or shelled nuts, may be placed in these containers. For the truly traditional Christmas gift, arrange a basket of fresh fruit and nuts and deliver it personally with wishes for a happy and healthy Christmas.

If there is righteousness in the heart,
There will be beauty in character.
If there is beauty in character,
There will be harmony in the home.
When there is harmony in the home,
There will be order in the nation.
When there is order in the nation,
There will be order in the world.

Sai Baba

Christmas Menu

Christmas Eve Dinner

Cauliflower-Broccoli Pie* or Mediterranean Melt*

We Love You Truly Tabouleh* on Bed of Greens and Sprouts or Christmas Day Salad

Herb-Buttered Whole Grain Bread*

Steamed Matchstick Carrots

Peppermint Tea* Milk

Diane's Baked Apples Supreme (Later)

Christmas Morning Brunch

High Protein Strata*

Baby Whole Beets with Butter and Lemon Juice

Mock Crab Salad in Avocado Half*

Pineapple Bran Muffins* with Cream Cheese

Hot Lemon Mist Tea Milk

Snack

Kids Parfait* or Cranberry Fruit Gelatin* in Parfait Glasses

Birdseed Banana Bread*

Milk Fruit Flips

Christmas Day Dinner

Mushroom-Asparagus Crepes* or Millet Souffle

Mele Kalikimaka Salad* Cranberry-Orange Relish

Bread Stuffing Baked in Muffin Tins

Wonderful Winter Squash Parsley New Potatoes

Lemon/Garlic Brussels Sprouts

Best Walnut Apple Cake Ever*

Milk Mellow Mint Tea

Evening Snack

Fruitcake with a Variety of Cheeses

Crocked Punch

*Can be prepared ahead of time.

SOME HOLIDAY RECIPES

FRESH CRANBERRY-ORANGE RELISH

2 1-pound packages cranberries
2-3 oranges (use peel if not dyed)
½ cup honey

Put cleaned cranberries and cut-up oranges through a juicer or food grinder. (Reserve most of juice for Spiced Fruit Punch.) Place pulp in bowl, along with a little juice and stir in honey until well-blended. Allow flavors to blend in refrigerator for 2-3 days. Snack idea: Spread rye crisp with cream cheese and top with relish.

SPICED FRUIT PUNCH

½ gallon fresh apple juice
2 cups orange juice
¼ to ½ cup cranberry juice
a stick of cinnamon and/or other whole spices of your choice

Heat all together, but do not boil.

CROCKED PUNCH

1 small can frozen orange juice
3 cans water
1 quart apple cider
5 whole cloves
2 cinnamon sticks
1 t. ground nutmeg
¾ t. ground ginger
orange slices

In a crock pot heat water and spices only on high for 30 minutes to 1 hour. Remove cloves and cinnamon sticks. Add orange juice, apple cider and heat, but do not boil. Garnish with orange slices.

CARAMEL CORN

¼ cup butter
½ cup honey
1 cup roasted peanuts
4 quarts popped corn

Heat butter and honey in a pan until it bubbles for about 2 minutes. Stir constantly; no need to use thermometer — it never fails! Sprinkle peanuts on top of popcorn; then drizzle caramel mixture over all. Toss lightly and serve hot or allow to cool before storing. (If giving as a gift, test for storage time; some popcorn gets tough.)

BUFFET CHEESE ROLL

1 8 ounce package softened cream cheese
2 ounces crumbled Bleu cheese
3 cups grated Cheddar cheese
1 T. minced onion
a dash of cayenne

Combine all ingredients and chill. Then shape into a roll 1½" in diameter. Coat with ¾ cup finely chopped pecans or walnuts. Wrap in wax paper. Refrigerate until firm.

Variation: Roll in alfalfa sprouts or chopped parsley.

SPICY WALNUT RAISIN PIE

1 unbaked whole wheat pie crust
4 eggs
½ cup honey
½ cup maple syrup
2 squirts lemon juice
½ t. cinnamon
½ t. nutmeg
½ t. cloves
¼ t. vanilla
1/3 cup melted butter
1½ cups walnut pieces
½ cup raisins

In a large bowl, mix eggs, honey, syrup, lemon juice, spices, vanilla and butter. Beat well. In 9" unbaked pie shell, arrange walnut pieces and raisins. Pour liquid mixture over nuts and raisins. Bake in a preheated 375° oven for 30 minutes or until set. Delicious warm or cold! Serve with yogurt or whipped cream.

Variation: Use pecans in place of walnuts, OR use 1 cup raisins and omit 1 of the sweeteners (honey or syrup).

VANILLA EXTRACT: Place 2 vanilla beans in 1 quart of inexpensive brandy. Set aside for at least 4 weeks, but preferably 10-12 weeks. Leave beans in and it will continue to improve as you use it. After the bottle is half empty, start a new batch. You may reuse the beans or keep them in the old bottle. If you reuse the bean, you should add another bean.

CRANBERRY FRUIT GELATIN

2 T. unflavored gelatin
½ cup cold water
1 cup boiling water
1-2 T. honey
2½ cups mixed fruit juice — part orange, part cranberry and part apple
2 cups fresh fruit — chopped apple, sliced bananas, sliced oranges

Dissolve gelatin in cold water. Pour boiling water over it, add honey and stir well. Cool. Then add fruit juices and fruit. Spoon into a mold and chill.

Variation: Use pineapple juice in place of cranberry and pineapple chunks in addition to other fruit.

WE LOVE YOUR BODY PEANUT BUTTER CUPS

1½ to 2 cups carob chips
1 cup crunchy peanut butter
2 cups rolled oats
½ cup granola
½ cup finely ground almonds or walnuts

Heat carob chips and peanut butter in a saucepan until smooth and creamy. Remove from heat and stir in oats, granola and nuts. To shape, press into paper muffin cups (about 1/3 full) or 1 oz. paper nut cups. Refrigerate.

Variation: Shape into kisses, freeze, then wrap in foil. Great stocking stuffers.

UNCOOKED FRUITCAKE

1 cup ground raisins
1 cup chopped figs
1 cup chopped, pitted dates
1 cup honey
1 cup chopped, dried fruit (pear, apple, apricot, banana, peach, etc.)
1 cup mashed over-ripe fresh fruit
OR ½ cup frozen juice concentrate
2 cups wholewheat bread crumbs
1 cup ground sunflower seeds
½ cup ground sesame seeds
2 cups broken walnuts

Mix everything together. Pack into oiled pans (1 large or 3 small); ripen, covered, in refrigerator for 2-3 days. Spices may be added according to taste to above mixture.

COOKED FRUITCAKE

½ cup Almond-Cinnamon mixture (See *KIDSTUFF*)
½ cup lightly toasted and chopped sunflower seeds
2 cups whole wheat flour
½ t. salt
1½ cups rolled oats
½ cup flaked bran
1 cup safflower oil
2 t. vanilla
2 beaten eggs
3 cups crushed, unsweetened pineapple with juice
1 cup shredded coconut
1 cup raisins or chopped dates

In a large bowl, combine first 6 ingredients. In a separate bowl, mix oil, vanilla, beaten eggs and then add to dry mixture. Stir in pineapple, coconut and raisins or dates. Divide dough in half and place each in well-oiled 9" cake pans or a 9"x13" pan. Bake at 350° for 40-50 minutes. Cool 15 minutes before turning out. Frost with Honey-Butter Frosting. (See *KIDSTUFF*)

CHRISTMAS DAY SALAD

3 kinds of lettuce — Romaine, iceberg and red leaf
chopped parsley
raw broccoli or spinach
chopped green onions
thin sliced radishes
chopped raw yam
grated carrot
grated red cabbage or red beet
sprouted sun seeds
alfalfa sprouts
mixed sprouts (opt.) about 3 T.

Wash, rinse and pillowcase-dry the lettuces. Tear into pieces in a large salad bowl. Chop broccoli or spinach and add remaining ingredients in amounts desired. Serve with Bleu Cheese Dressing. (See *Labor of Love Lunches*)

MELE KALIKIMAKA (MERRY CHRISTMAS) FRUIT SALAD: Slice a pineapple in half, lengthwise and scoop out pineapple. Cut in small pieces and mix with fresh sliced bananas, chopped apples and orange wedges. Spoon into shells. Top with strawberry yogurt, sprouted sun seeds and granola. Arrange pineapple halves on lettuce leaf-lined platter.

KIDS PARFAIT: In parfait glasses, alternate cottage cheese, home-canned peach slices, and banana slices. Tilt glass when spooning in so you have a diagonal rainbow effect. Top with granola.

TOMATO BROCCOLI-CHEESE CASSEROLE

3-4 stalks broccoli, lightly steamed and chopped
1 cup Easy Pizza Sauce
OR Hearty Spaghetti Sauce
(See *Serendipity Suppers)*
1 handful raw cashews and almonds
Parmesan cheese
butter

Steam broccoli and chop. (Slice stalk before steaming.) Arrange in a buttered casserole dish. Pour sauce over broccoli. Sprinkle nuts and Parmesan cheese over all and dot with butter. Bake, covered, in a 350° oven for 15 minutes, and uncovered, for 10 minutes or until cheese is melted and sauce bubbles.

BEST BROCCOLI SOUP

3 cups chopped, steamed broccoli
2-3 T. sliced green onions
2 T. butter
1½ cups buttermilk or yogurt
1½ cups vegetable stock
sea salt/kelp to taste
dash cayenne
grated Jack cheese

Place all of the ingredients (except cheese) in a blender and blend until smooth and creamy. Heat in a saucepan, but do not boil. Serve in bowls and garnish with cheese and croutons. To take shopping: place soup and some cheese in a thermos and take with you.

Variation: Substitute mushrooms, carrots, zucchini, asparagus or spinach for broccoli. For kids, use milk in place of buttermilk or yogurt. Serve chilled for a summer treat.

BIRDSEED BANANA BREAD

5 T. butter
¼ cup honey
1 large egg
1 T. arrowroot flour
1 heaping T. soy flour
1 T. minute tapioca
2½ t. baking powder
¼ t. salt
½ t. baking soda
½ t. cinnamon
2 scant cups rice-millet flour (equal parts of rice and millet ground into a flour)
3-4 bananas, cut in pieces
¼ cup buttermilk or kefir
10 chopped, pitted dates
½ cup chopped nuts

Cream butter, honey and egg together. Measure dry ingredients in a bowl; then add alternately to the creamed mixture with bananas and buttermilk or kefir. Stir in dates and nuts and spoon mixture into 3-5 (3″x6″) well-oiled loaf pans (filled ½ full). Bake at 350° for 35-45 minutes or until bread is browned and begins to pull away from edges of pans. Remove from pans and cool on rack. Wrap in clear wrap for gifts for teacher, friend or neighbor. Tastes super when spread with Neufchatel cheese (a low-fat cream cheese).

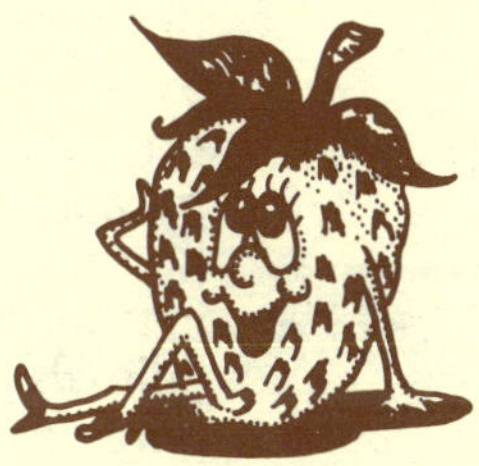

P.S. Stone-Age Food For Space-Age People

You may have noticed the obvious absence of such words as miraculous, mystical, wondrous, etc. from our vocabulary. Although many unique and beneficial results have been achieved through dietary changes, we realized that some of the new foods we were introducing to our families were neither "magical" nor "space-age." They were the respected, time-tested foods of our ancestors which, even today, endure and provide us with sound, sensible nourishment.

We have become increasingly impatient with sophisticated junk food promoters and their effort to debase the entire natural food movement by accusing health advocates of attributing certain foods with "miraculous" qualities. Actually, we have found very few promoters of magic formulas among health-conscious people. Most of them are very much aware of the necessity of consuming many different kinds of whole foods and are reluctant to credit any one food with more than its share of qualities.

Now and then, reference is made to miracles in first-person accounts, where pitifully ill persons (perhaps even considered hopeless by traditional medical diagnoses) started a self-help program of their own. Using one or two particularly wholesome foods and ascribing their rapid improvement to those foods, they may have truly considered the healing of their own weak bodies miraculous.

In essence, however, the foods selected could have simply been high in the very nutrients they had been lacking or not utilizing properly. More than likely, a new attitude was being formed at the same time the new foods were introduced, and an old habit may have been surrendered as well, such as smoking, drinking or inactivity. The "wondrous" results could have been a combination of one or more measures toward better health that frequently accompany the increased awareness of personal responsibility. It wasn't just the food, but the total program, that was accountable for the changes.

We asked our children to observe T.V. and magazine commercials to see if they could find some descriptive words such as marvelous or fabulous, used in reference to processed foods. Sure enough, this terminology is not limited to the ever-accused health food industry, but is a maneuver prolific in junk food commercials as well. Steeped in traditional advertising vernacular, the kids' findings included wonder, wondrous, wonderful, enchanting, dynamic, amazing, adds life, indescribably (delicious), incredible, incredibly, terrific, super, superb, supreme, colossal, fantastic and magical. And that was after only four days of investigation!

A New Lease On Life

We neither condemn nor condone any product just because of the semantics of their packaging and promotion. Let the product stand on its own merits. Each and every *whole* food is a miracle in itself; each and every member of the human race is a miracle in themselves; and the incredible relationship between plants and animals that support life for us all, is the ultimate miracle.

We are certain that if you will incorporate the following time-honored foods into your diet, you will soon relate your own first-person accounts of a new lease on life. Call it a miracle, call it good, common sense, but don't go through life without experiencing it!

Yesterday's Foods That Endure Today

ALFALFA: A plant whose roots reach deep into the earth for nutrients, including trace minerals that we sometimes forget are responsible for keeping the more familiar vitamins in balance. We know alfalfa best for its use as animal feed, but the sprouted alfalfa seeds are gaining steady popularity with the salad and sandwich crowd. Sprouts are live food, rich in enzymes, high in vitamin C and abundant in all the nutrients necessary to grow the new plant. One of Diane's 4-H members continuously raises champion rabbits and contends that alfalfa sprouts are far superior to lettuce in keeping rabbits healthy, so the next time someone makes fun of your kids for eating rabbit-food, remind them that alfalfa sprouts are the original "breakfast of champions."

AGAR-AGAR: A seaweed product used as a thickener in place of gelatin by people who desire to use no animal by-products. One rounded Tablespoon of agar flakes will thicken one cup hot liquid, but don't expect it to set up as firm as gelatin.

ARROWROOT POWDER: A translucent starch used to thicken sauces, gravies and fruits, great for cobbler or pies. Unlike cornstarch, it is not necessary to boil the liquid intended for thickening; therefore, arrowroot is ideal for oriental stir-fry dishes and heat sensitive fruits. One teaspoon arrowroot is equal to one Tablespoon flour; and two teaspoons arrowroot equal one Tablespoon cornstarch. Since it thickens before it boils, be careful not to overcook.

BARLEY: Long known for building strength, barley has been relegated to the bowls of the sickly as a gruel for weak stomachs. If it can build strength into a weak body, then it can add strength to a healthy one. With its high calcium content, ease of digestion and mild flavor, barley blends well with vegetables, adds texture to pancakes and muffins or makes a hearty soup out of clear broth.

BEANS: The seeds that are cradled in the pods of various leguminous plants, and contain every nutrient necessary to begin new life. Beans should be soaked overnight and the first rinse water discarded to eliminate phytic acid, which may inhibit protein assimilation. If they are to be cooked, allow enough time for thorough cooking and season only in the last fifteen minutes to prevent toughness. Begin a crock of bean soup or stew in the morning for a "ready-made" dinner at night; all you'll need to do is prepare a salad and slice some bread. (Be sure all beans and seeds purchased are for human use and not treated for planting.)

BRAN, FLAKED: The outer hull of the whole grain — usually wheat — which is removed in the making of white flour, a practice which has been implicated in diverticular diseases and colitis, two problems rarely diagnosed in people whose diets contain ample cellulose. One-half cup of bran can be added to any loaf or casserole to absorb excess moisture; it has no taste but provides some trace minerals while adding fiber to the diet. Some people seem intolerant to bran but many swear that it "cured" their constipation, among other problems.

BULGUR: A wheat product that is as old as the Bible and is still a dietary staple throughout Asia. Bulgur is to the Middle East what potatoes are to the Mid-West; it stores well on a pantry shelf due to the process of boiling the wheat, drying, then cracking, yet it is almost identical in nutrition to whole wheat. Cook like rice (two cups water to three-fourths cup bulgur) but only for ten to fifteen minutes, and use as a side grain dish, in Tabouleh or pilaf.

BUTTER: An animal fat which has remained controversial because of its high cholesterol content. When the choice is between butter and margarine, we choose the butter and solve the cholesterol problem in another way: exercise more! Margarine is chemicalized and synthesized to the point of being almost as plastic as the container in which it is packaged. We can't help but think that all those people who have been advised to use margarine instead of butter have simply traded a bullet for a bomb. There are some soybean margarines that are chemical free and perhaps they would alternate well with, or mix with fresh sweet, undyed butter. Mix cold-pressed polyunsaturated sunflower oil and butter to make SunButterBlend. (See *Kitchen Keys*).

BUCKWHEAT: An unusual, hearty grain that should not be limited to use as the flour for delicious pancakes, but should be used frequently because of the nutrients it contains. Buckwheat is a good source of rutin, a side-kick of vitamin C normally found in the rind of citrus fruits, and the B complex vitamins so imperative in a vegetarian diet. It is delicious toasted (whole grain) and prepared with sun seeds, tamari, herbs and butter for a main dish; mixed with other cracked grains for a cereal or ground to a flour and made into the traditional buckwheat griddle cakes. Unhulled buckwheat can be soaked, sprouted and grown into lettuce in eight to ten days. (See *Labor of Love Lunches*)

CAROB: The fruit of a Mediterranean evergreen tree, carob is also known as honey locust or St. John's bread, having sustained John the Baptist during his ordeal in the wilderness. Carob fruit is high in natural sugars and strengthening nutrients and was attributed by various early cultures as having provided stamina, resistance and the "staff of life" during famine, pestilence and war. The leathery carob pod, when dried, ground and roasted resembles chocolate in flavor and aroma. Carob, however, is low in fat and does not require the anti-oxidants BHA and BHT — which are usually added to chocolate to preserve its high fat content. Also in contrast to chocolate, carob is rich in protein, vitamins and minerals, but has little sodium and no oxalic acid.

Carob contains the B vitamins needed to assimilate its 50% natural carbohydrate, whereas the sugar added to chocolate (five times its weight) actually robs the liver of stored B vitamins. Carob can be enjoyed by persons who are allergic to or wish to avoid the caffeine and theobromine in chocolate, who are reducing refined sugar intake or who just plain like variety in taste. For you trivia fans, carob seeds provided the goldsmith with a standard of measurement, hence the term "14-carat gold."

DATES: One of Nature's oldest natural sweeteners, dates are the original candy. In almost any recipe, dates blended with a little fruit juice to a thick paste, can be substituted for the sugar if one fifth of the liquid is also reduced. Besides having a distinctive flavor all their own, dates are 70% complex carbohydrate and have a high mineral content. They are, however, concentrated sweets and therefore, should be followed by a thorough brushing of the teeth.

EGGS: Which came first, the chicken or the egg? We aren't going to attempt to answer that one, but both have been around for thousands of years, though perhaps not the way we know them today. At one time the chickens that roamed this earth were free to get ample exercise and to peck and scratch for food. They laid eggs according to a natural dark-daylight schedule and enjoyed the pleasure of a rooster's companionship.

Today's modern egg ranches, however, fit hens into computerized compartments and increase egg production to maximum by means of hormones added to feed and artificial dark-daylight cycles, designed to fool the chickens into laying around the clock. It works, of course, but to what extent the quality of eggs suffer, is a closely guarded secret. There is no doubt about the visual differences, however. Commercial eggs are pale, dull and runny compared to farm fresh "peck 'n' scratch" eggs that are firm, with bright yellow, almost orange yolks that stand high and are nearly spherical in shape. The color of the shell is determined by the variety of the hen, so don't be fooled by commercial producers who market brown eggs using the same methods described for white eggs. On the other hand, you may get white eggs from the farmer that far surpass any brown ones you've ever tasted, so observe the *yolk*, not the color of the shell for quality.

And now for the real controversy: Fertile vs. non-fertile eggs. May we have a drum roll please? Any rooster will tell you, with a twinkle in his eye, that there is something in a fertile egg that just isn't present in a plain one. We don't give as much credit to the rooster as we're sure his ego would like to have, but we herald his addition of lecithin (found in the male hormone) that is needed for the proper absorption of cholesterol, and commend him for his ability to perpetuate his race. Since the protein and vitamins remain stable in either state, we consider the hen's actions (exercise and feeding on insects) to determine the *quality* of the egg. The choice of fertile or non-fertile is up to you.

FRUITS: Almost any fruit can be enjoyed by the majority in its clean, raw, ripe state. One of the characteristics of fruits is that their enzymes don't stop once they reach peak ripeness. Nature has designed them to continue ripening until they decay so that, when naturally dropped from the tree, the seed will sprout and the decayed matter will provide nutrients for the new plant. To preserve ripe fruits, we must either dry, freeze or can them, preferably in that order.

Most fruits can be dried without blanching if they are cut in small enough pieces that will dry quickly. Although a food dehydrator is a wise investment if you plan to do quantity drying, solar energy is the oldest form of food preservation and is quite satisfactory. (See *KIDSTUFF* for more information on drying fruits and making fruit leather.)

For freezing of most fruits, dip cut pieces in orange or pineapple juice, lay on a cookie sheet, being careful not to overlap, freeze quickly, then bag for individual use in smoothies and shakes. Juicy fruits can be frozen in one cup containers so they can be thawed readily for use in recipes. Never sweeten fruits before freezing. Your tastebuds are keener in the summer because of the abundance of very sweet fruits, but will have relaxed by winter and be more psychologically open to the natural sweetness of the fruit (strawberries in the middle of January, anyone?) which will, therefore, need less sweetening.

Canning fruits without sugar takes a little getting used to, but is practical and far better for you than the heavily syruped, commercially canned fruits. Unfortunately, commercially canned fruits without sugar are specialty items and, therefore, cost more than those that contain the sweetener. Try canning without any syrup; if your family insists on some sweetener, make a very light honey syrup, but be careful — some honeys will overpower the delicate taste of the fruit. Be sure to recycle the juice in cooking, smoothies, mixed juices, etc.

GARBANZO BEANS: One of the unusual tasting legumes that requires a little help from herbs and seasonings to be enjoyed by most people. Also called chick-peas, garbanzos take a long time to cook even after soaking overnight, so plan ahead, be patient and use first in a marinated salad, then work your way into the more unusual Eastern-style dishes. Combine with nuts or grains to form a complete protein and mash leftovers into dips and sandwich spreads or use to give body to loaves and patties.

GARLIC: Well-known for its pungent odor and ability to enhance Italian foods, garlic is much neglected for its healthful properties. Long a part of our medicinal heritage, fresh garlic is a digestive stimulant and an intestinal antiseptic as well as a mild laxative. It can be pressed into a poultice and applied to wounds as an infection preventative, but works best from the inside out. Periodically unbelievable powers are attributed to garlic and the local health food stores will be wiped out of garlic pearls — the encapsulated form. These may be okay for the self-conscious person who wishes to avoid the strong smell, but for the person who wants to receive the most benefit for their time and money, fresh pressed garlic is worth the effort AND the odor.

HERBS, SAVORY: The flavors derived from using various herbs are truly sensational in contrast to the mono taste of salt. Although each herb has its own unique flavor, many are adaptable to blending, and with a little experimenting you can turn a nutritious but bland tasting dish into the main attraction destined for many repeat performances. Savory herbs can be nutritious as well due to their trace mineral content. (See *Kitchen Keys* for individual herbs.)

HONEY: If you've ever felt that you were over-worked and underpaid, study the life of a honey bee and count your blessings! Next to the whole fruit, honey is the oldest, most natural sweet known to man. Predigested and containing numerous trace minerals, honey is an EXTRA source of energy and should be kept in that perspective. Every body needs sugar, but in the form of complex carbohydrates which the body will then make into simple sugars. Therefore, reserve the sweet treats to occasional use and then only after the nutritious food has found its way into the body for necessary rebuilding of tissue and resurgence of strength. Beekeepers are special folks, and we've found that when we drive to the country to get raw, unfiltered, unheated honey direct from the source, we have met some of the sweetest people we know!

KEFIR: A fermented milk that tastes somewhat like yogurt and has the effect, when it reaches the intestinal tract, of nurturing friendly bacteria and regulating constipation or diarrhea.

KELP: A seaweed that contains varying amounts of trace minerals, particularly iodine, along with sodium. Vegetarians or people on a salt-free diet need to consider this alternate source of iodine to prevent goiter.

LECITHIN: Derived most commonly from soybeans, this substance is also a component of egg yolks, corn and non-hydrogenated oils. Often added to processed foods as a homogenizer, it is naturally found in every cell in the body, and it helps emulsify cholesterol (keeps the blood flowing through the arteries). Here again we feel that the amount of cholesterol one consumes does not necessarily indicate the build-up levels present in the arteries. Whether naturally occurring in the food or taken as a supplement (available in granules, powder or liquid), lecithin teams up well with vigorous, work-up-a-sweat-type exercise, thus enabling our bodies to stabilize the cholesterol and aid utilization of vitamins A, D, E and calcium.

LENTILS: A round, flat seed, at the top of the leguminous nutrient scale, is often used as a meat substitute because of its protein and B vitamin content. Lentils cook quickly and accompany beans or grains with equal ease. Sprouted lentils are delicious, even if slightly starchy and are an excellent addition to salads or soups. Sprouted or cooked, lentils are one of the most versatile and easy-to-like seeds.

MILK: Certified Raw Milk must meet rigid standards equal to or surpassing those of pasteurized milk. Cows whose milk is destined to be pasteurized may receive chemical-laden feed as well as hormones for increased milk production. The residues from these substances are not necessarily eliminated during the pasteurization process. The high tempera-tures, however, destroy some beneficial bacteria and some nutrients. If you do not have a souce for Certified Raw Milk, consider looking for a farmer with goats and at least alternate raw goat's milk with the pasteurized milk available. Whether you choose pasteurized or raw milk, know the source!

MILK, POWDERED: Non-instant powdered milk is slowly processed at low temperatures to preserve nutrients. It is very fine and can be added in small quantities to almost any recipe without alterations. It is perishable and therefore must be kept in the refrigerator or freezer. Instant powdered milk is processed at high temperatures, is less nutritious and more expensive because it is mostly air, but can be used for fortification if the non-instant variety is unavailable.

MILLET: One of the oldest grains, yet one of the least used today. You may have seen it in a bag of mixed bird seed and wondered what it was. Millet is an alkaline, mild-flavored, pearl-like grain that can be toasted and served alone with herbs and tamari or added to other grains or legumes for complete protein, either as a main dish or cereal or pudding. It can be cracked and added to baked goods for a delightful crunch or ground into a flour and used in place of wheat flour for persons with a wheat allergy. Millet's mild flavor and digestibility make it an ideal candidate for baby's first cereal and provides a change from rice.

MUSHROOMS: Turn many a ho-hum sounding recipe into a gourmet's delight with the addition of these age-old fungi. Purchase in bulk when available fresh and dehydrate for use when the price soars. Look for mushrooms that are firm and sealed on the underside by a thin membrane. Once this seal is broken mushrooms are overripe. These are all right for cooking but for fresh slices for salads, choose the sealed ones. Handle with TLC.

NUTS: Commercial nuts are smothered in oil and salt, cooked at high temperatures, then blamed for being fattening! Granted, nuts are a source of saturated and unsaturated fats, but they also contain protein, vitamins, minerals and when chewed well and eaten raw, are very digestible and filling. Many nuts can be ground into butters, blended with water or other liquids for nut milks or toasted for adding flavor and crunch to cooked main dishes or desserts. Nut meal that results from grinding one-fourth to one-half cup of nuts in the blender can be substituted for eggs in many recipes.

Nuts should be purchased in their unbleached shell, or shelled, from a health store, where they are bulk-packed and refrigerated. If your family relishes the taste of roasted nuts, simply dry roast half and leave half raw, mix together and enjoy the best of two worlds.

PARSLEY: It's a beautiful garnish, but don't leave it on your plate, for parsley can help beautify you, too. Vitamins A and C are both necessary for healthy complexions and the high cholorophyll content counteracts toxins which also helps keep the skin clear, since the skin is the organ that ultimately will have to deal with excess toxins in the system. Use parsley anywhere and everywhere — but as a food as well as a garnish.

RICE, BROWN: For 4000 years rice has been a staple of Oriental diets. Brown rice has the bran and germ intact and therefore is subject to spoilage. To keep nutrients at their peak, keep rice refrigerated. Whether you choose the short grain or the long, you will enjoy the full-bodied flavor of brown rice so much that you will never desire the instant white stuff again. The complete grain is so versatile and so adaptable that everyone from babe to grandparent will be able to find a favorite breakfast, lunch, snack, main course or dessert dish made with brown rice.

SESAME SEEDS: Tiny seeds that are a powerhouse of nutrients. Due to their high calcium content, they are excellent for children when ground into a meal with a little sesame oil added. Called tahini, this butter can be used in place of or in addition to peanut butter. The hulled sesame seeds are lower in nutrients, but more digestible than seeds still in their hull. We enjoy them both ways and find that toasting improves flavor and gives the seeds a crunchiness that encourages chewing, which in turn improves digestion.

SOYBEANS: The only legume that contains all eight essential amino acids, plus B vitamins and a good amount of calcium, granting the soybean a nutrient position alongside meat and dairy products. Ancient civilizations have been very creative with this staple, so if the beans don't turn you on try some of the following varieties of soy products: Soy grits are roasted beans, coarsely cracked and can be cooked and added to loaves and patties. Soy flour can be substituted for a portion of wheat flour in nearly any recipe for added protein. Soy milk powder is an excellent part-time substitute for persons with milk allergies. Soybean curd is described in this chapter under Tofu. Tempeh is fermented soybeans and requires thorough study for preparation.

SPROUTS: If you are looking for a live vegetable that will grow in any climate, rival meat in nutritional value (and tomatoes in vitamin C), matures in three to five days, may be planted any day of the year, requires neither soil nor sunshine, has no waste, is pesticide free, can be eaten raw and stays crisp in a sandwich until lunchtime, look no further, for SPROUTS are your answer! Sprouts are *live food.* They have a high enzyme activity, are easy to digest, are rich in vitamins and minerals and, depending on the individual sprout, contain most or all of the eight essential amino acids. From seed to sprout, the vitamin C content alone can increase over 1000%. All of the life-giving properties of the seed are released and increased in the sprout. (See *Kitchen Keys* for sprouting directions and uses of individual seeds and beans.)

SUNFLOWER SEEDS: Observe a child's fascination when s/he first notices that the sunflower was facing "that way (east) this morning and that way (west) tonight!" The flower actually follows the sun throughout the day, absorbing energy from which we can all benefit when we chew those compact little, oval seeds. While the rest of the world grabs a sugared snack for temporary energy, learn to keep sunflower seeds handy for quick as well as sustained energy. Smokers often try to substitute roasted, salted sunflower seeds for cigarettes, only to gain weight on the seeds — thus giving up and going back to their habit. Try the seeds plain, in the shell, so you have to work to get to the nutmeat, or toast them and mix with some peanuts and raisins for a complete protein, delightfully delicious snack. Grind sun seeds into a meal and extend the nutritional value of loaves and patties or puddings and shakes, or make hi-protein fudges for backpacking trips. Mix meal in gravies, sprinkle on casseroles, or sprout seeds and add to salads and sandwiches, but use abundantly and encourage chewing for maximum digestion. Since the sunflower has few natural enemies, in most cases the oil and seeds will be pesticide free. (See *Better Beginnings: Breakfasts* for sprouting directions.)

TAMARI SAUCE: Soy sauces are quick varieties of this flavorful soybean fermentation. Unfortunately MSG and preservatives are often added to commercial sauces, which really aren't necessary in true tamari that is aged at least eighteen months. You may want to start with light touches of tamari, then work up to such delicacies as tofu slices sauteed in tamari butter, leaving out all salt as tamari is naturally salty. Whatever you do, don't reserve it just for Oriental dishes; it seasons gravies, casseroles, omelets and salad dressings beautifully.

TOFU: A bland-tasting but adaptable source of complete protein that is also known by the awful name of soybean curd, explaining why few people take it off the shelf at their produce counter. It can be sliced, cubed, shredded or blended and used in many places where cheese or cream cheese are better known. It is best combined with other foods, sweet or savory, and provides a delightful change from dairy products, with the added benefit of containing no saturated fat, no cholesterol and no added salt.

YEAST, BREWERS: A rich source of protein and nutrients, this by-product of the brewing industry is used by vegetarians to help meet B complex and protein requirements. It has an admittedly strong taste, but once used to its distinctive flavor, you will find it lends a pleasant tang to salads and hot dishes. Add tiny amounts at first to baked goods, casseroles and fruit juices. One way to introduce brewer's or nutritional yeast to your family is by sprinkling some lightly over fresh, hot, popped corn. (Nutritional yeast has added nutrients.)

YOGURT: This creamy cultured milk product has sustained hearty European peoples for centuries. Its ease of digestibility and assimilation of calcium and B vitamins are attributed to the predigestion activities of the lactobacillus acidophilus bacteria. The tartness may require a little tastebud adjustment but do try to use yogurt in its plain form as the commercial varieties are full of thickeners, colorings, sugar and preservatives. You can make your own for about fifty cents a quart. (See *Better Beginnings: Breakfasts* for recipe.)

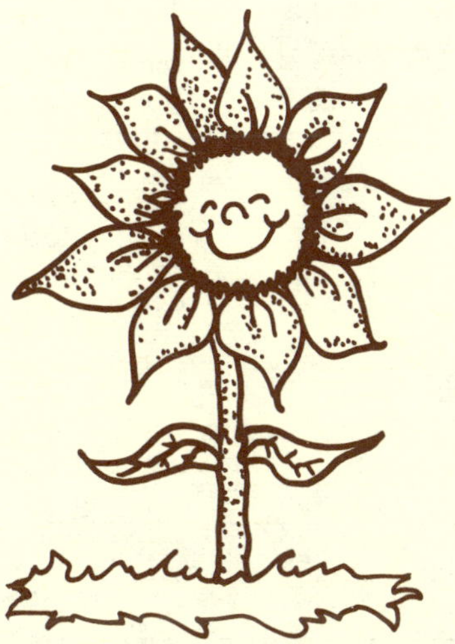

Who's Who?

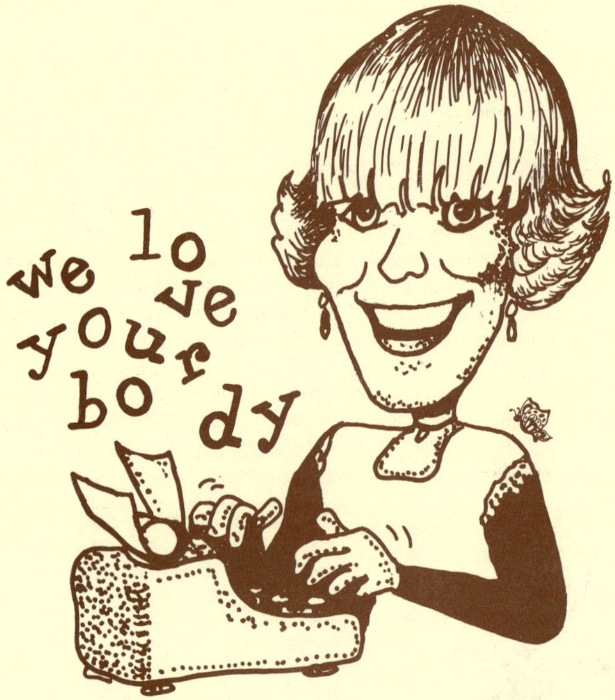

Lani Miller

After 6 years of marriage and two children, Lani returned to the college scene to complete her education and her family — an additional two children. Though her degree was in elementary education she took graduate courses in reading and became a remedial reading teacher. While working with children who had visual perceptual problems, Lani created and published a reading-readiness game (Lil' Smarty) to help teach and reinforce important pre-reading skills.

As her reading and research became more in-depth, so did her observations of the children increase until she began to see first-hand the close relationship of poor diet to learning problems and behavior. What the kids brought to school in their lunch pails seemed to correlate with how long they could sit still. So she and her students mixed nuts and seeds for snacks, grew sprouts, blended hi-protein shakes and made fruit and vegetable salads with the happy results of calmer, more attentive kids and teacher, who became aware, through new eating and learning experiences, of the differences between healthy foods and junk foods. Besides children and cooking, Lani's interests include Hatha yoga, weaving, throwing pots (on a wheel) and bicycling.

Happiness is like a butterfly. The more you chase it the more it will elude you. But if you turn your attention to other things, it comes and softly sits on your shoulder. *L. Richard Lessor*

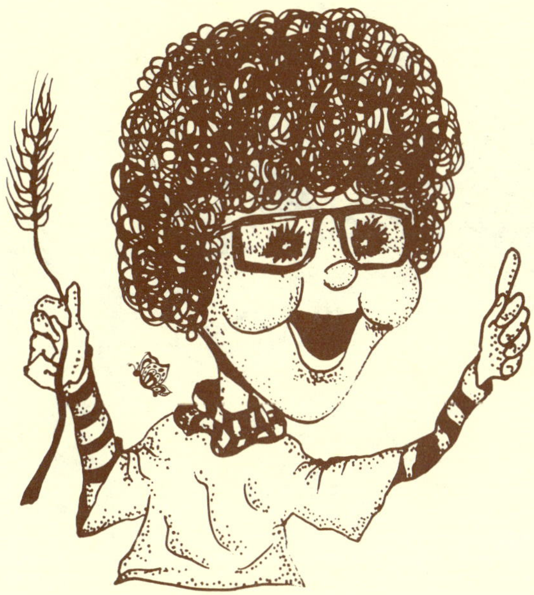

Diane's interest in good health developed out of dietary changes made "cold turkey" as a result of her husband's diabetes. Having always enjoyed cooking, the removal of refined sugars and starches presented a new challenge and opened up, literally, a whole new can of beans. Her enthusiasm for improved health reaches over into her role as a 4-H leader in the areas of cooking, sewing, child development and home improvement.

As a frequent guest on a local television talk show, Diane demonstrates good nutrition and shares recipes and ideas with the viewing audience. She conducts well-being workshops for various community clubs, parent-teacher organizations and classrooms. She enjoys scouting garage sales for interesting furniture finds and spends her quiet hours gardening, writing poetry and transcribing bits of wit and wisdom in italic calligraphy.

Diane Rodgers

In addition to managing and cooking for their "We Love Your Body" restaurant, Lani and Diane have taught nutrition and cooking classes, run a catering service and written a weekly column for the city newspaper. Write in care of this publisher for more information about lectures, workshops and demonstrations.

Joanie's artistic talents are reflected in all facets of her busy life as wife, mother of three sons, and her job as Teacher's Aide at an Elementary School where she is known as "The Artist-In-The-School." She has illustrated several books and the game Lil' Smarty. Her comical drawings have added to her growing reputation as a talented graphic artist.

Gardening and community work through her sorority keep Joanie busy year-round.

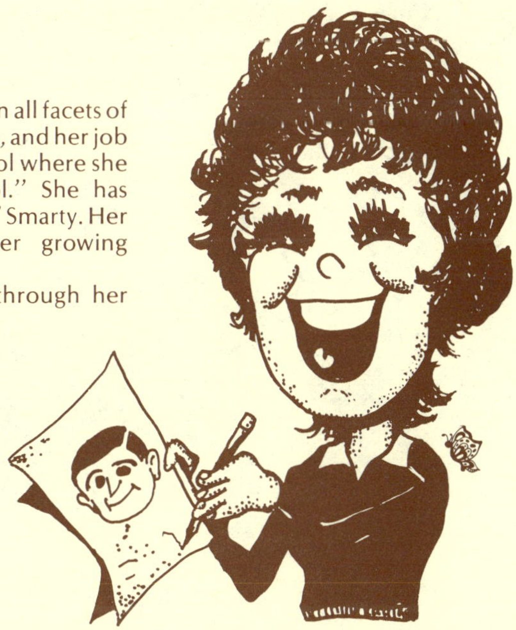

Joanie Oliver

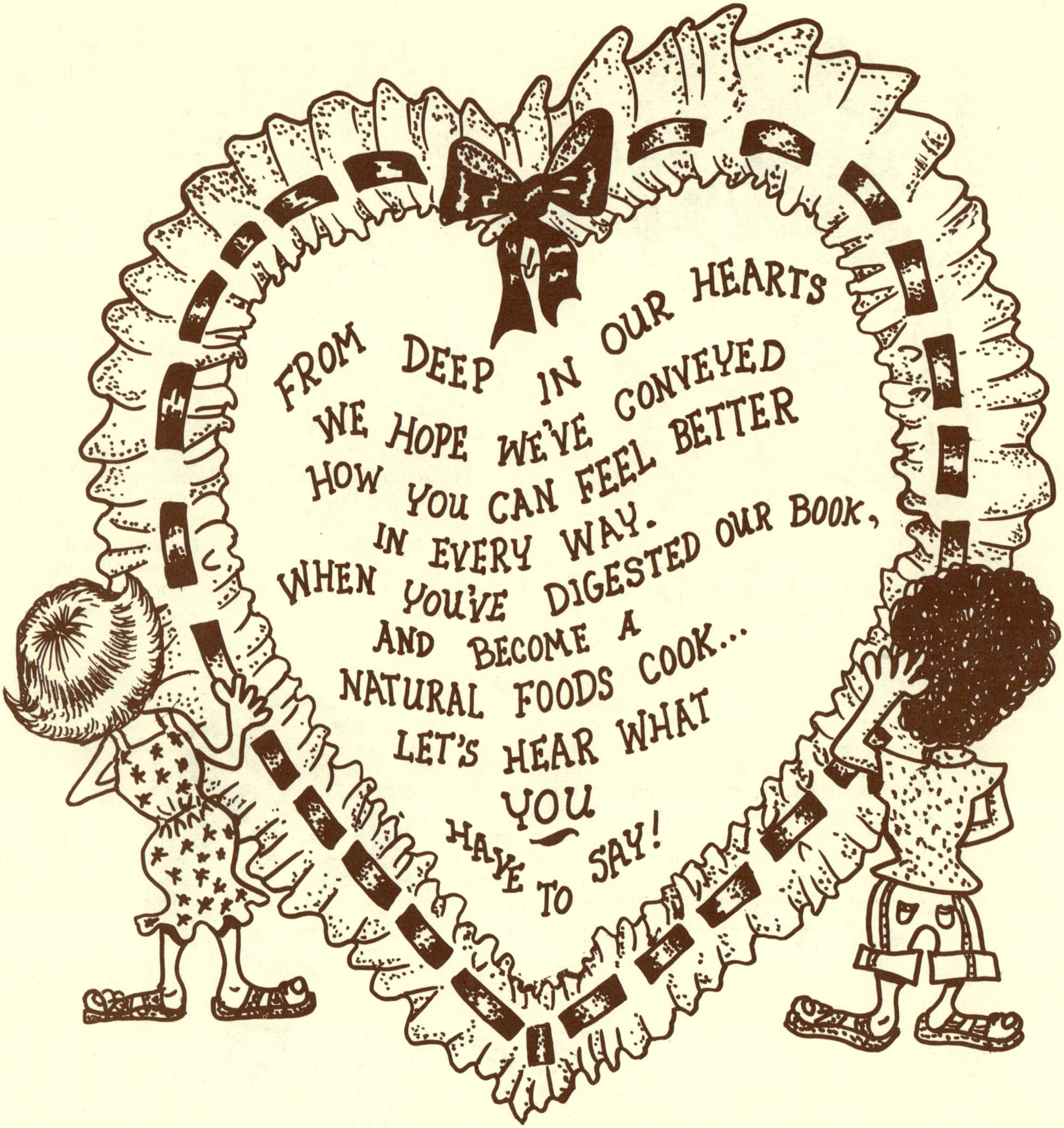

PUBLISHED BY MORSE PRESS, INC.

417 E. Pine

Seattle, Washington 98122

Recipe List

LABOR OF LOVE LUNCHES

SERENDIPITY SUPPERS

AMERICAN POT-LUCK

ORIENTAL OFFERINGS

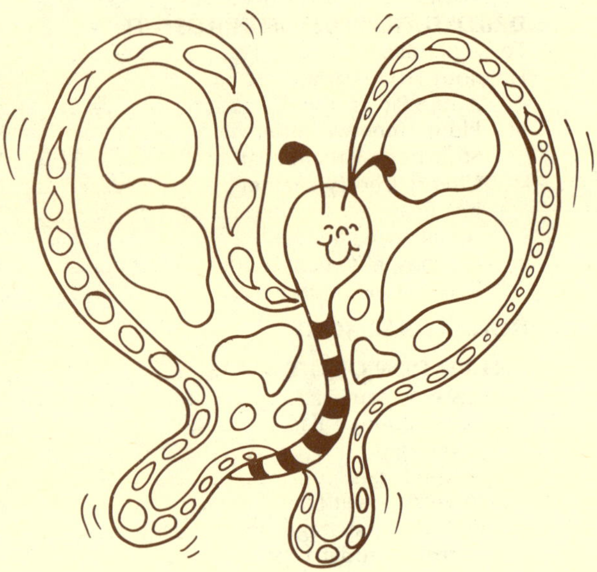

Poem Credits: *"There's a Time," "Fast Food Mania," "Vegetarian ABC's," "Full Circle," "We Love Your Body," "Holiday Harmony,"* 4-line verses in Vegetarian Vitality by Lani

"Kid Stuff" by Lani and Harriet Bergquist

"Do I Work?", "Some Human Rights Issues," "Sunshine for Lil' Sprouts," "Television Schmellivision," "It's a Crime," "Medicine That's Easy to Take," "Self-Renewal" by Diane

Front and Back Heart poems, poem in Count Quality; Not Calories, poem in Better Beginnings: Breakfasts, and *"Phony Phood"* page by Lani and Diane

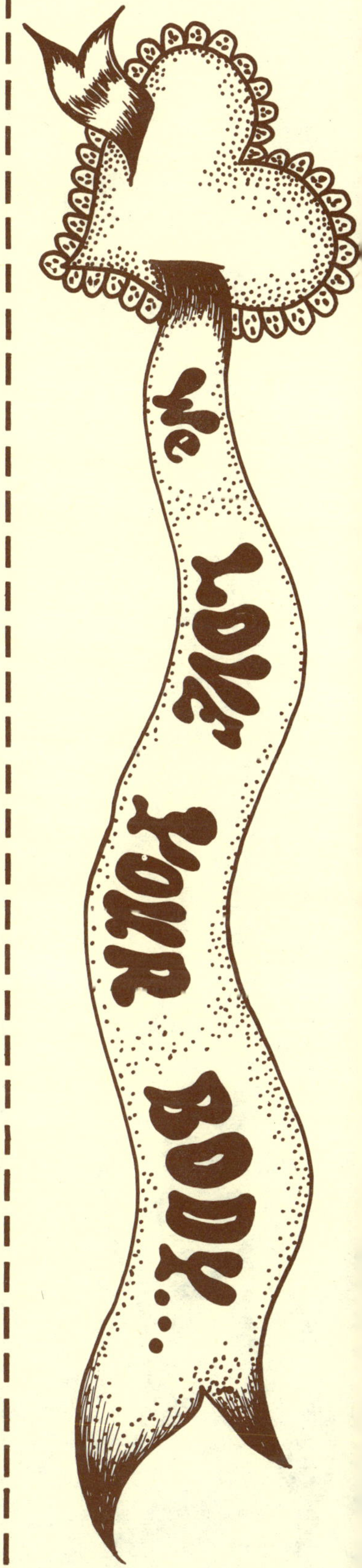

Here's a handy bookmark
for you to use.

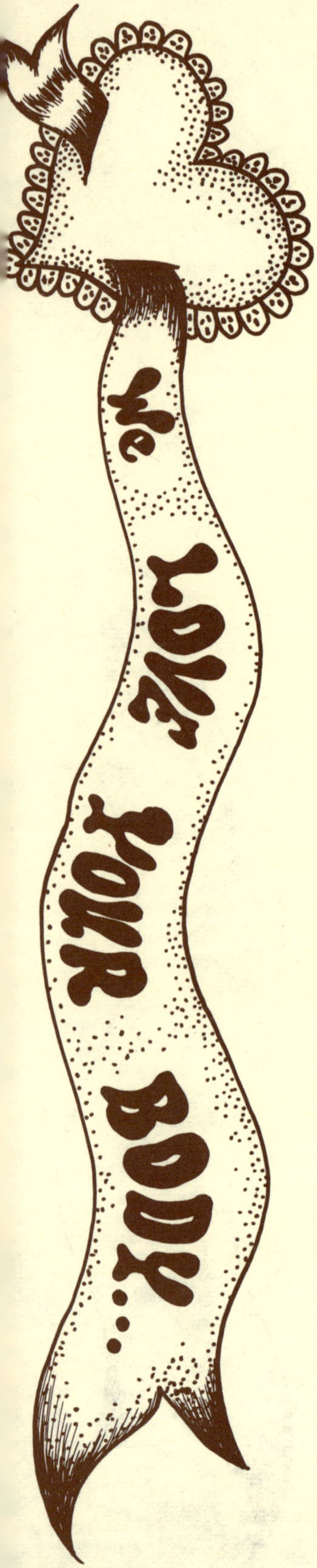

Here's a handy bookmark
for you to use.

Raise the Bar